THE AGING GAME

THE AGING GAME

Frank MacInnis, M.D.

VANTAGE PRESS
New York

Published by Vantage Press, Inc.
516 West 34th Street, New York, New York 10001

Manufactured in the United States of America
ISBN: 0-533-10956-6

Library of Congress Catalog Card No.: 93-94252

0 9 8 7 6 5 4 3 2 1

To Adele
(1912–71)
for twenty-five years
My wife, my lover, companion and friend

And all my children:
Beverley and Frank, Janice and John
Mary and Robert, Ardyth and Jim
And all of theirs

Contents

Acknowledgments

First of all, I must acknowledge with thanks the contributions of the many readers whose letters over the years have graced my newspaper columns, which in turn have made this book possible.

My family, both immediate and extended, have each in their own way, inspired and guided me, particularly through the compiling and editing stage, when often the going was rough and direction uncertain. So I now thank Frank for his sage counsel, Jim for his penetrating wit and sometimes zany advice that I've occasionally used to advantage, John for his rare combination of indomitable optimism and computer expertise that without question hastened the publication date and his twin sister, Mary, whose extensive executive experience in the "Big Apple" has earned her the signal honor of being my (unpaid) New York agent, adviser and publicist.

The typing of the manuscript was no small task and for that I thank my sixteen-year-old granddaughter, Mary (sometimes aided, abetted and gently goaded by her mother, Janice). And here is where I should recognize my lawyer friend and fellow columnist Don McCrimmon, whose popular essays on senior law make up most of the final chapter.

Many others in many different ways have helped me achieve my goal, and here comes to mind seniors' columnist Freda Woodhouse, who read the manuscript in her always critical but constructive way; Dr. Patrick Daley, computer guru, now of Tulsa, who long ago convinced me my project had merit; Hans de Leeuw, whose very personal expertise in Alzheimer caregiving helped in the fine-tuning of numerous columns; and Louise Martin of Edmonton, who also turned a tragic Alzheimer experience into a successful caregiving and counseling career that inspired chapter 5, "Slow Death of the Mind: Alzheimer's Disease."

My special thanks go to many newspapers that over the years have carried my column, "Senior Clinic"; also to Martin Littlefield, vice president; Leonard Zimmerman, director of publications; and Michele Curry, publicity director, all of Vantage Press, for their unfailing courtesy, cooperation and dedication demonstrated in their publication of this book.

Author's Note

The reader should be aware that *The Aging Game* is essentially a collection of questions and answers on medical topics. The questions, submitted by elderly readers of my newspaper column or by their adult children, may consequently overemphasize the importance of certain medical conditions over others, sometimes even to the exclusion of others.

While *The Aging Game* may accurately address a medical condition and offer advice in a general way, it was never intended to be a medical reference textbook and should not be utilized as such. Furthermore, the general advice given may not necessarily apply to you, the reader. For personal medical advice you should consult your doctor.

Introduction

The Aging Game took twelve years to complete. This may seem like an inordinate length of time to write a book short of yet another popular version of the Holy Word!

But many readers will understand. For they will immediately recognize some of the "Dear Dr. MacInnis" questions written by themselves, for which they patiently waited, sometimes for many months, to see in print.

If you haven't yet experienced that rapture of déjà vu, let me explain. This book is an edited compilation of my weekly "Senior Clinic" columns—over six hundred of them, written over twelve years and syndicated to newspapers in Canada and the United States. They address exclusively the medical, surgical, psychiatric, and social issues affecting the elderly and will serve, I hope, as my response to so many of you who wrote asking, "Why don't you make a book of them?" It serves, too, as a tribute to my thousands of readers who, by their contributions, made this book possible.

The selection and compilation of so many columns into book form has been a formidable task. Each chapter deals with a specific subject with only the "best" questions of many very good ones contributed by readers over the years. A small percentage are of the essay type, written by the author and prompted nearly always by correspondents' suggestions and important advances in geriatric medicine. Throughout the book I have tried to maintain a pervading theme of hope without sacrificing realism. And there is no better exponent of hope blended with realism than the senior reader.

Twelve years ago, in my introductory column to "Senior Clinic," I expressed surprise that this weekly feature would be the only one of its kind in the entire newspaper field catering to the elderly person. At that time (1981) the 65 and older population was over 26 million (2.6 million in Canada) and the senior population of our two countries was increasing by 1,800 per day—over 600,000 per year. But here we are, twelve years and 33 million seniors later, and "Senior Clinic" is still the one and only!

Grey power is burgeoning throughout the land. At the turn of the present century, the *average* life expectancy at birth was 47 years. Now, it's 75 years and steadily increasing. And what passed virtually unannounced and unnoticed was that in June 1984 the number of people in the United States 65 and older, for the first time, exceeded its teenage population!

So often I'm asked, ". . . why geriatric medicine?" What is so different between geriatric medical practice and medical practice in general? I share the belief of many that in treating the elderly we should strive to heal when possible, but to care always. If only this maxim was sufficiently taught in our medical and nursing schools, young graduate doctors and nurses would find the care of the elderly more fulfilling and the elderly, in turn, would be much more content.

Opponents of the concept of geriatrics as a medical subspecialty (now recognized in Canada) contend that there are few diseases in the elderly not found in younger folk.

This may be true. But what's different is the older person's *manifestation* of disease. Here we see multiple signs and symptoms from multiple medical conditions—often three or four at any one time. And it's here that we physicians face a dilemma. Should we prescribe for a myriad of signs and symptoms and run the risk of side effects and drug interactions, or should we "tread softly" by recognizing and treating the main problems and "managing" the others? The latter would be the more prudent course, in my view.

Sick old people, more often than not, take their medications haphazardly, if at all. One recent study revealed that 50 percent didn't take their prescribed drugs regularly when left on their own. This could be due to "benign senescent forgetfulness" or to a confusional state from serious mental or physical illness or both. If it's important, then, for an aged ill person to take medicine, it's equally important that he or she is perceived to do so by a trustworthy relative or friend.

Then there's their often abnormal reaction to pain. The old are generally more insensitive to pain than the young. The severe heart attack without pain, the so-called silent coronary, is common in the aged patient and can be perplexing to the unsuspecting practitioner. Acute appendicitis, more often than not, goes undiagnosed until peritonitis sets in, with its much more serious prognosis. Delirium, with its disorganized thinking and marked loss of attention, may be the cry not of a mental condition but the geriatric symptom of an infection such as pneumonia.

Another difference is that medical complaints in the aged are very often stress related. And the stress is often the stress of loss, for old age has been called the "season of loss"—loss of spouse, friends and relatives, security, responsibility, dignity, self-esteem, and, not least, the loss of physical and mental health. Such stress can evoke a multitude of bodily complaints. This may be the voice of depression crying aloud, which, if not recognized and treated, can lead to further mental and physical disability.

The newly arrived resident to a nursing home is a prime candidate for this type of depression. Older people, as a rule, do not accommodate well to situational change, like a sudden transfer from home to institution (often after a recent bereavement). Here the treatment is not anti-depressant pills but copious doses of social interaction between the resident, staff, and family.

Then there's the prevailing misconception that the elderly patient doesn't respond well to medication. This is simply not so as long as the drug is thoughtfully prescribed and, above all, closely supervised.

Finally, there's the pernicious notion that old people's ailments arise mostly "from old age." Again no, for the old can be ill not because they're old but because they're sick!

And when they're well, they're very well indeed. Eighty percent of our senior population are enjoying the good life. They live independently in their own houses or apartments and are an ever-growing economic and political power in our nation. They are the winners in the Game of Life.

The Aging Game embodies my philosophy of geriatric medicine which, over the years, I have endeavoured to uphold both in medical practice and medical journalism. And here it is: To maintain as far as possible and as long as possible the "best years" of our lives. But when, in good time, the game of life is played out, then the laudable practice of "caring" rather than "curing" should prevail.

THE AGING GAME

Chapter 1
Better to Wear Out Than Rust Out

Better to wear out than rust out.
—Richard Cumberland, 18th Century English Cleric.

I wish I could say, "I wrote that," for in seven words it embodies the secret of successful, healthy aging.

Fully 80 percent of our older population are enjoying good physical and mental well-being. Ask them for their secret elixir and the answer may be another old medical maxim—"a sound mind in a sound body"—and many will enjoin you to keep your joints well oiled by daily exercise and that old mind razor sharp by constant honing with creative thinking and not passive "boob toobing."

Still they're realists, knowing full well that the ravages of time will eventually wear them out. But like a venerable Rolls Royce, their aging can be gracious, even elegant. Rusting never!

I recently received a letter from one of these "medical elite." He's a pretty active fellow with lots of things to do but limited time. He's got to rev up that motor to stave off rusting, or "carbonizing," as he puts it. Here's how he handles things.

Before the Carbon Hits

Dear Dr. MacInnis:

It's an expression I've read about and have experienced the physical syndrome over the years.

I'm a lone country lad, with much maintenance work to do on my shack and grounds, and often this old syndrome comes to the fore.

1

I awaken at the normal morning hour and feel spright and nimble. In fact, I could almost jump fences with both feet in a bag! After cereal and citrus intake, I proceed to the mailbox to retrieve whatever—including the daily paper.

Perusing the news, I get hooked on the crossword puzzle. Then I get drowsy and start "hammering fence posts." That Dagwood couch appears most inviting. Why not?

That's it. I've succumbed to the temptation and will pay dearly for it. My day's work plan and projects are ditched. The clock ticks on. My body is in a comfortable state of lethargy. The snuggling sensation of that old couch is indescribable!

The phone rings. Let it ring. I can't leap and bound. Too dangerous. A knock on the unlocked door. A neighbour walks in. He caught me napping, the old frinker. "Shame on you," says he. So what? And he ambles out muttering other sassy remarks.

By around 3:00 P.M. I've shaken it off and miserably arise from my couch and supporting the most intense inner guilt. Why didn't I stay up in the first place?

Now at this time of year, there's only three or four hours of daylight left to tackle the projects. So I get real busy, feeling real good. I'm just getting into the heat of battle, moving stones, chopping wood, winterizing the shack, you name it. I always get it done.

Could it be that our mammal co-inhabitants, the like of groundhogs (marmots) and bears, along with others, who fall into a lethargic state to hibernate, take as long as six months to dispose of their carbon residue?

The Dagwood of the comic strip is pictured as a young fellow. Does this carbonizing syndrome affect all ages?

Your valued comments on these matters are highly anticipated.

Hopefully yours,
Mr. L.M. (80) Ontario

Answer

You said it all, Mr. M., and eloquently.

I guess that old carbon starts to hit at the moment of birth, ever so lightly and it piles up as you get along in life.

But somehow, I feel the rust of time will treat you gently. Decarbonize, yes, but never like the marmot who takes six months. We want people like you up and at 'em 365 days a year.

Age 250 Years!

Dear Dr. MacInnis:

We are three so-called seniors who make this lodge our home. Our combined age is 250 years! It looks bad in print so let me break it down. Our oldest member is 90, next to him is an 85-year-old, and I am a mere youngster of 75 and am serving as our corresponding secretary. We all are enjoying good health and indulge in all of the social activities here, including a fling with the ladies who always enjoy our company. Maybe it's because we still have our "marbles" and hope to continue wowing them with our remarkable feats of memory, particularly memories of the past which stand out much better than recent happenings. Question number one: How does aging affect memory? In other words, are we aging normally?

Our second question has to do with defining our aging status. Granted, we are all getting up there. We are sometimes called "seniors," "elderly," "aging," "older people," "young old," "old old," and so forth. So how would you designate my pal of 90, my 85-year-old companion, and not forgetting myself at 75? In other words, are we all just classified as "young old," "old old," or just plain "elderly?" I'm sure most of your readers would like to know where they stand in the age line-up.

Mr. T.P. (75) and friends

Answer

Your vitality and sheer joy of living flies in the face of the mournful aging stereotypes we are so tired of hearing about. Unfortunately, most of them tend to become self-fulfilling prophesies. We age and expect physical and mental deterioration will follow. We nurture it and the inevitable happens: we not only grow old, we act old. So yours is a refreshing departure from the "norm."

Some years ago, a theory was advanced that human beings are endowed with two kinds of intelligence. One was called "fluid intelligence" and had to do with the processing, storing, and memory retention of *new* information. The second kind of intelligence was termed "crystallized intelligence," which concerns *old* information, i.e., the accumulated knowledge of our past experiences.

According to recent research in gerontology (study of aging), the aging process appears to have no effect on the recall of "crystallized" information while it does to some extent the recollection of recently acquired information (memory for recent events). Research scientists are quick to point out, however, that older people are still able to process, store, and recall new intelligence but only require more time and motivation to achieve it.

So to answer your first question, "Are we aging normally as far as memory is concerned?" the answer is yes; and I needn't add that you have the necessary motivation to enhance those "recent memory" problems you mention.

I answered your second question for a correspondent several years ago, and I believe it's worth repeating. I know it made many readers feel quite young again!

The new redefinition of various age groupings is based on the technical life span (TLS), the greatest age yet attained by a human being. This was achieved by a Japanese man who died recently at the authentic age of 120 years. Here are the new definitions based on a TLS of 120 years (from *Clinics in Geriatric Medicine* Vol. 3, No. 2, May 1987).

AGED: ninety years and older, who have survived at least three-quarters of TLS

ELDERLY: eighty through 89, who have survived at least two-thirds of TLS

AGING: seventy-two through 79, who have survived at least three-fifths of TLS

MIDDLE-AGED: sixty through 71, who have survived at least one-half of TLS

So there you are. At 75 you are "aging" and successfully too! Your 85-year-old buddy is "elderly," only to be outdone by his 90-year-old companion, who earns the title of "aged" (and probably resents it!).

"Seventy-Five-Plus," a Poem

Dear Dr. MacInnis:
   Someone showed me your column on "Benign Senescent Forgetfulness." There's lots of nostalgia in it for an oldster.
   A few years ago I consented to be interviewed in connection with a Law Society history of the profession. I guess the meeting lasted too long and the memory efforts were too much, because I finally went blank, which scared the female lawyer interviewer more than it did me!
   However, upon recovery, I sat down and expressed myself thus:

Seventy-Five Plus

When your minds fills with confusion, and you say it's no illusion
That your memory isn't what is was before,
It's such luscious compensation when you get that new sensation
That you're sure that once again you know the score.

It is worse than being frustrating when you're simply ruminating
About things that happened not so long ago,
And some fellow about fifty, with an air he thinks is nifty,
Says, "I wasn't even born. Hoho, Hoho."

But with age some independence seems to gather in abundance
Once you've sort of put your mind in proper frame;
When you should attend a meeting or express a formal greeting,
You can always say, "I'm sorry," without shame.

If the simple fact of living is the source of some misgiving,
Make your mind up just to live from day to day,
And by gosh, before you know it ('Cause I'm sure that you won't
blow it),
You'll be seeing everything the brighter way.

Growing old, I can assure you, must not ever quite allure you
Into thinking you're as good as once before.
Have a drink and say, "I'm grateful for this life which is so fateful,
So at my age I'll accept a bogey score."

Yes it's fun philosophizing
For the new group who are rising,
But I think that if I'm wise I'll say no more!

Note: For best results read it aloud and get into the swing of the meter.

As I've said before, growing old is a great adventure and a greater blessing.

I took up Norwegian folk painting at 70, but having been forced out of it by serious toxic and allergenic problems, I began wood carving at 80.

I would be glad to show you my original style and "Silken Primitives."

Sincerely,
Eric H. Silk (Queen's Counsel), Streetsville, Ontario

Answer

If you forget and you remember you've forgotten, that's normal; it'll come back to you in time, it's benign senescent forgetfulness (BSF), a comforting diagnosis on which Mr. Silk, now 82, rhapsodises so well in delightful rhyme.

And many more good years ahead, sir!

Greying Baby Boomers

Dear Dr. MacInnis:

I'm one of your so-called baby boomers and read your column regularly because it won't be so very long before people like me will be called "geriatric." I believe the image of the "old" person is changing for the better and would like to think that we "boomers" will add even more lustre, productiveness, and longevity to our "golden years" come next century. Do you agree?

Mr. F.M. (44), Westport, Connecticut

Answer

You'll be a "young" oldster of 65 in 2014, twenty-one years down the road. Yes, I agree the time-worn "geriatric" stereotype of being "toothless, sexless, and worthless" is slowly changing for the better. By the turn of the century, "middle life" could mean 60 or more. But we still tend to emphasize the negative aspects of aging and thus perpetuate a myriad of myths.

Even now, fully 80 percent of our elderly are enjoying healthy, successful aging, living independently in their own houses or apartments.

I have written several columns on the extraordinary resilience of the aged in major surgery. Just two decades ago these people would be excused treatment because they were considered "too old."

Remember what I said before: "The old can be ill, not because they are old, but because they are sick." No question about it; "grey power" is an ever-growing social, political, and economic force that you "baby boomers" will some day greatly enrich.

It's the "Right Stuff" and They've Got It

Brilliantly written letters from the very old (85-90) have graced my columns on many occasions. I hope more of them will continue to write, for it gives "young old" people like ourselves something to hope and strive for. We like to think we too are made of that "right stuff."

But are my 85- to 90-year-old correspondents representative of that exceptionally old group or merely exceptional stand-outs—geriatric aristocrats as it were?

I'll try to answer this question by summarizing a very interesting and informative report titled, "A Community Survey of Mental and Physical Infirmity in Nonagenarians" (90 year olds). This survey was conducted in an English community and was published in *Age/Aging,* Vol. 18: 411–414, 1989. The principal investigator was Dr. D. W. O'Connor.

During a twelve-month period, 132 people with a mean age of 92.5 years were visited, interviewed and examined.

Quoting from the report:

Only three persons were older than 100 years and 108 were women. Of the ninety who lived in the community (not in nursing homes) fifty-two continued to live alone. Overall, 33 percent were cognitively (mentally) impaired of which 14 percent were mildly demented, 11 percent were moderately demented and 8 percent were severely demented. More than half of the non-demented persons were able to cook, do light housekeeping and dress, and 20 percent did their own shopping. In contrast, demented individuals were more seriously disabled and required greater assistance with even the most basic activities.

So much for mental function. How did they fare physically?

"There were no significant hearing impairments in 55 percent of respondents," reported the survey, "and no visual impairments in 73 percent." Multiple impairments including "mental, physical and sensory abnormalities," the report concluded, "were common and most people had difficulties in at least one area."

Using the "half full or half empty" water glass analogy, I conclude that 67 percent were not cognitively impaired, over half of the non-demented could do housework and cook, and 20 percent did their own shopping; surprisingly, 55 percent could hear okay and 73 percent could see well.

All in all, a very creditable showing and really something for us youngsters to strive for!

Again, in Praise of Older People (Nonagenarians)

Traditional belief has it that when old people, particularly the very old, develop muscle weakness, it's downhill all the way and no amount of structured exercise can turn back the clock. Right? Wrong!

Just recently, I came across an astounding report published in *JAMA* (the *Journal of the American Medical Association*), where the "feasibility and physiological consequences of high-resistance strength training for frail elderly persons were determined in ten institutionalized volunteers (mean age 90 years)."

The results (in brief) were as follows: The conclusion was that "a high intensity weight training program can induce dramatic increases in muscle strength in frail men and women up to 96 years of age. The rise in lower extremity [leg] strength ranged from 61 percent to 374 percent over baseline. The volunteers had increases of 3 to 4 fold on the average in as little as 8 weeks" (Fiatarone and Colleagues, Tufts University; Harvard Medical School; Hebrew Rehabilitation Center for Aged, Boston, *JAMA* 263[1990]:3029–34).

All we know is that it can happen, and that's what matters. Think of the effect of regained muscular strength in the reduction of falls and fractures—not to speak of enhanced well-being.

"I Never Feel That I'm Old"

In a recent column on the "geriatric elite," I asked the question, "What makes nonagenarians (90-year-olds) tick?" Two "medical aristocrats" from Rochester, New York, were the first to answer, and I believe that their letters, both beautifully handwritten, let us in on the secret for a long, useful, and happy life.

Dear Dr. MacInnis:

I was so pleased with your article today. I wrote you three years ago how I felt about growing old. I still feel the same way.

I will be 96 in January. I am still in my own home, alone. I take care of myself and home. I have a nice yard, with vegetables and flowers. I work in my yard every morning until I feel tired.

I have so much to thank God for—a good daughter and so many real, good friends. They take me shopping twice a week.

Three years ago, some people at the hospital thought I should go into a proprietary home, but the doctor told me that I should go back to my own home because I had the mind and body of a 60-year-old-woman!

I am in excellent health. My hearing is perfect, my eyes are bothering me, and I can't take the long walks I used to. My friend takes me to my senior club and all their parties.

I don't think I can complain about anything.

Ethelyn L. Maloney, Rochester, New York

Answer

Yes, I remember you well. I've saved your letter of three years ago and am sure many readers would like to know more about you—so here are some excerpts from that letter: "I've been a widow since 1953 and have lived in my home (an eight-room house) for sixty-five years [now 68]. I do all the yard work except snow removal and grass cutting. I cook nourishing meals and have a good appetite. I enjoy a cool glass of beer, wine, or a cocktail when the fancy strikes me.

"I never feel that I'm old. I don't have many friends near my age but my younger ones seem to think I'm special!

". . . . my memory so far is perfect, I can remember when I started school and the names of all my teachers . . ."

Another delightful letter arrived the same day:

Hi, Doc:

How's this for the "right stuff"?

I am 90 years old, never had a headache or flu, never catch a cold or take medication. I bowled in three leagues until my late

10

seventies when I tripped on a raised pavement and dislocated my shoulder.

I still drive my car and need no glasses for driving. I had two accidents; a man backed into my car; another man made a U-turn (a no-no) and crashed into my rear end!

I've been married fifty-three years and I'm ten years older than my good husband. I have no wrinkles and am proud of my brown hair—thanks to a good hairdresser!

Hang in there, Doc.

Mrs. Virginia Overhaus, Rochester, New York

Answer

Yes, I agree. You were certainly endowed with the "right stuff," for which you must thank your ancestors!

At present I'm immersed in compiling and editing the best of my columns written over the years for publication in book form. The subtitle will be "Better to Wear Out Than to Rust Out" and come to think about it, who better can it apply to than you and Mrs. Maloney?

And I'll sure try to hang in there!

Can I Make a Hundred, Doc?

Dear Dr. MacInnis:

I am a 65-year-old man in good health. What are my chances of living to 100, or is that asking too much?

A.L., Toronto, Ontario

Answer

Longevity experts tell us that the average life expectancy of a 65-year-old Canadian or American person is now 16.9 years. Take note, this is the average. You as an individual may live a shorter or longer life. A healthy woman of your age, as an individual, could expect to live several years longer.

Living to 100, however, is another matter. Statistics Canada reports that our 1991 census showed there were about 3,700 people (80 percent of them women) who have beaten tremendous odds to achieve the status of a centenarian. And in 1992 another 1,200 will make the honor roll.

So what makes centenarians tick? Gerontologists are trying to find out, and what they already know is that our elderly elite are endowed (genetically?) with a superimmune system that protects them from the ravages of mortality. In addition, they seem to exhibit that firmer will and a more positive attitude toward life's problems than lesser mortals.

Life expectancy has increased tremendously over time. In the Bronze Age (3000 B.C.) the average life expectancy is said to have been 18 years. During the early Roman Empire it was about 25 years. By the year 1900, it had increased to an average of 47 years. Our present (1992) average life expectancy at birth is a whopping 76 years. Put another way, the average life expectancy over the past 90 years has increased by the same amount (29 years) as it did in the previous 5,000!

For the information of my American readers, your centenarians, as in Canada, will soon be the fastest-growing age group of the population.

For example, there are now (1992) 36,000 in the U.S. By the year 2020 it's estimated that there will be 266,000 centenarians in your country.

Now, Mr. L, I know this doesn't answer your question. But if you're endowed with the "right stuff" (thanks to your ancestors), you just might make it to that elusive Senior Hall of Fame!

A Real Extended Family

Dear Dr. MacInnis:

I am a great-grandmother of 71 years and in good health. I would, however, be more contented and happy in my old age if it were not for my mother, just short of 90, who insists on treating me like a child, always demanding obedience and sulking for hours if I don't toe the line.

Our relationship, which is strained, would be vastly improved if Mother would agree to move out to an apartment. She too is in excellent health and can look after herself quite well. She insists on running our home and our lives as well. She treats my husband (76) like a little boy, and I believe he's actually scared of her. We have partly solved the problem by going on extended trips all over the country visiting with our grandchildren, some of whom have children of their own.

I honestly believe Mother is glad to see us go so she can have the house to herself with the cat and dog. The neighbors tell us she is then a very gracious host.

Mrs. A.L., Ottawa, Ontario

Answer

Your letter is truly a sign of the times! Never before in our social history could a letter like yours have been written, for never before have there been so many grandparents, great-grandparents, and, yes, great-great-grandparents around as today. A baby born at the beginning of this present century could expect to live on the average about 47 years. But that baby's great-great-grandchild born in 1993 can look forward to an average life expectancy of about 78 years.

It's clear why in the "good old days" so few adults lived long enough to be grandparents, let alone great-great ones like your mom. Nowadays our 85-year-olds are the fastest growing segment of the general population.

So in these times of domestic turmoil, with so many children in peril, thank heaven for the extended family.

Writing on this subject recently, Colleen Johnson, a medical anthropologist at the University of California (San Francisco) said, "Grandparents are increasingly necessary as a stabilizing force in the American family."

As you describe her, your mom is hardly a "stabilizing force" in your family. But despite her shortcomings, this can be said of her—she's dependable in an arrangement that is mutually satisfying. You enjoy your grandchildren and she evidently enjoys your absence.

Aspects of Longevity

As a writer on geriatric subjects, I'm often asked questions on longevity, i.e., the duration of human life. Invariably, readers get the terms "life expectancy" and life span" mixed up and, unfortunately, some think the two are one and the same thing. Nothing could be further from the truth.

Let's first deal with "life expectancy." If I were writing this column around 1900, I could report with confidence that the average life expectancy of a baby born in 1900 would be about 47 years. If you (the reader) are now around 70, this average life expectancy (47) is what your parents could expect at birth. Of course in reality, your parents (as individuals) may have lived longer than 47 years or one or both of them may have lived less. Remember we are speaking of average life expectancy.

But I'm writing this column ninety-three years after the turn of the century and can tell you with even greater scientific confidence that your grandchild born this year will enjoy a whopping average life expectancy of over seventy-five years. Longevity specialists tell us that this spectacular increase in life expectancy from 47 to 75 in about ninety years is mainly due to the great advances in preventive medicine and other public health measures that have practically eradicated the rampantly infectious and often deadly diseases of infancy and childhood. Contrary to popular belief, the well known dramatic breakthroughs in modern clinical medicine and surgery have played only a relatively minor role in this increased life expectancy.

What can we reasonably expect over the next century? Many eminent researchers are capping average life expectancy at around 85 years, contending that the human chassis and its organs will have by that time reached their limit of endurance and can take no more. They say that to reach this average 85-year milestone, all heart disease, cancer, stroke, and diabetes would have to be eliminated—a tall order it would seem. But there are optimists in the research field who believe that a baby born this year (1993) will have a life expectancy of 100 years! So there you have it , to which I will add my sage and "scientifically secure" opinion that "only time will tell."

The term "life span" varies with the species and is genetically determined. Thus, a human being can ideally (not succumbing to disease, accidents, and ravages of environment) attain a mean maximum life span of 110 years, a Galapagos turtle 175, an elephant 75, a cat 25, and a mouse 3.5 years. And just as there are exceptions to average age expectancy, there are individual stand-outs from the maximum life span, such as the Japanese gentleman who died a few years ago, having lived a medically authenticated 120 years, the longest ever for a human. This man was undoubtedly endowed with the "right stuff" and gerontologists still don't know what it is but are beginning to get interested in what makes our nearly five thousand Canadian centenarians tick.

So we can see that although life expectancy has, over the years, increased, the human life span has remained practically unchanged in recorded history. But there is, none the less, a linkage between the two. Our increase in life expectancy reflects our ambition to attain as far as possible this mean maximum life span. How far can we go from here? Prof. Leonard Hayflick, who has contributed so much to the biology of aging, has said in effect that even if we could live out our lives free from disease and accidents and fear of premature death, we must still face the reality that normal wear and tear of the human organism dictates death at around 100. It is the feeling of Hayflick and others that more research time and funds should now be expended on efforts to increase the human life span, which if in time successful "no fixed endpoint can be ruled out" (Hayflick, *Perspectives in Biogerontology*).

"Who's the 'Champeen'?"

Dear Dr.MacInnis:
We enjoyed your column on longevity. Now that the Japanese gentleman who lived to be 120 years is gone, who is the reigning champion?

M. L. Toronto, Ontario

Answer

Identified by the *Guinness Book of Records* three years ago when 116 years as the world's oldest living person "whose age can be authentically documented," Jeanne Calment of Arles, France, celebrated her 119th birthday on February 21, 1994.

On the advice of her spoilsport gerontologist, she had to quit her daily cigarette and glass of port for "health reasons," but it's reported that she cheated on her recent birthday.

Although bothered with failing sight and hearing, her memory for past events remains remarkably sharp, such as remembering Vincent van Gogh buying canvases at her father's art shop in Arles. "He was ugly as a louse." Mademoiselle Calment recalls.

Life Span Can Be Doubled—at Least in Fruit Flies

Dear Dr. MacInnis:

In a column you wrote some time ago on longevity you stated that the life span of a species has remained constant since recorded history. But you also said (quoting Leonard Hayflick) that more research time and funds should be expended on efforts to increase the human life span. Is there any research currently in progress with that end in view?

Mr. T.Y., New York

Answer

Yes, it was Hayflick who said, in effect, that if science could lengthen the life span, "no fixed endpoint can be ruled out."

There is some interesting research going on at the present time and although it is confined to laboratory fruit flies, worms, and mice, it may have human implications.

In his book, *Evolutionary Biology of Aging* (N.Y.: Oxford University Press, 1991), bioscientist Michael Rose of the University of California states that "aging can now be regarded as a problem that is well on its way toward a scientific solution."

In his experiments on fruit flies, for example, Rose has shown that aging can be postponed so that life span can be doubled "or the pattern of deterioration with aging can be vastly slower," he said.

Such experiments involve manipulating so-called aging genes in an effort to slow the aging process.

Body Parts

Dear Dr. MacInnis:

Perhaps you could write an article for us old geezers on what parts of the body keep growing for life. I know the finger- and toe-nails keep growing as does the hair on our head. How about the rest of our body hair? Someone told me the ears keep growing. What parts of your body grow and then stop? And when? How about your teeth, tongue, nose, spine, and fingers?

And when does the Creator tell our brain, "Stop, that's enough"?

If there isn't enough material for a column, perhaps you could reply to me. I'm enclosing fifty cents. Thank you.

J.G.B., Macedon, New York

Answer

Your questions are a gerontologist's delight! You've given me enough material for several columns.

First, about nails and head hair: You're right about the nails; they just keep growing along. But head hair loss varies, being determined by a multitude of factors—sex, genetics and race. Male pattern baldness is inherited from the mother. Body hair elsewhere? Two researchers in 1959 surveyed the underarm hair in 169 males and in 189 females past age 60 and found that in one-sixth of males and in one-half of females nearly all the hair was lost. And the eyes? Vision deteriorates with age. It is said that if we lived to be 130 years we'd all die blind!

You ask about ears. They just look bigger because of a generalized loss of subcutaneous (under skin) fat causing a shrinkage of the face and a sharpness of facial contour. For the same reason, all bony prominences become exaggerated in old age. (Observe your nose past and present.) In general, aging causes a decline in lean body mass where, it has been aptly said, "the engine shrinks within the chassis." The spine shrinks too, especially in elderly women with osteoporosis, who may lose three or more inches in height. And the aged brain? It shrinks 6 to 7 percent from the bloom of normal adulthood. Somewhere beyond that range our Creator becomes the Attending Physician.

Real Women Don't Wear Slacks

Dear Dr. MacInnis:

Remember us? We are the three ladies in our early 60s living in a high rise and having a ball! You may recall we asked you how many more years were in the cards for us and you guesstimated "at least 17," which pleased us no end. Now we have another question on this subject and hope you don't think we're completely bonkers— so here goes again.

A noted authority on women's fashions, Marilyn Brooks of Toronto, is reported to have said that "high fashion isn't just for size-nine women under 30— it's for seniors too." Bless her.

Ms. Brooks further says that if a woman has shapely legs in her youth, she'll have them forever. All three of us are well endowed in that department, so we are wondering whether or not a slit skirt might look too brazen. We again will be guided by your excellent judgment in all matters of concern to mature readers. And no slacks, please. We're completely convinced that real women of mature age shouldn't wear slacks. They simply don't look nice in them as slim young folk do.

Three Swingin' Grannies, Vancouver, B.C.

Answer

Yes, I remember you well, also the three jolly bachelors (in their 80s) who wrote to me for your address and phone number!

Many thanks for the newspaper clipping featuring high-fashion items. I'm sure readers will be pleased to know that Ms.

Brooks heartily endorses slit skirts—at any age—if the legs are right.

And a useful tip to you out there whose weight is settling on the midriff and hips. If you can't slim down, hide it by wearing your blouse outside your skirt and not tucking it in.

So Real Women Don't Wear Slacks! (Rebuttal)

Dear Dr. MacInnis:

So real (older) women don't wear slacks. You've got to be kidding!

Well, I may not be a real woman. But I am, always have been, and, I pray, always will be a real lady. No slit skirts for me, thank you. I wear slacks exclusively.

And I'll tell you why. Because I look good in them and I feel modest and comfortable in them. I have no fanny, so they are not immodest, and, anyway, I wear all my clothes loose, just as you advised. I have a large stomach and my legs are too thin for the rest of me, plus I have varicose veins. Get the picture?

So I may not be what you call a real woman (I've had my day) but I am a real lady—no smoking, no swearing, no dirty stories, no fooling around, and no torrid fantasies.

So put that in your pipe and smoke it!

Mrs. A.B. (81)

P.S: When skirts go down all the way to the floor, then I'll be that "real woman" of yours.

Answer

Good heavens, the lady's right. Why did I get myself in this mess? I promise you all, from now on, I'm sticking to "doctoring." But just in case someone may have missed the point in that column, let me repeat the old stereotyped view of aging: Aging dictates (1) that you should act as old as your age; (2) that you should be totally disengaged from the frivolous, wanton world of youth; (3) that you should continually recount the past and bore people; and (4) that you should be properly inflexible in thought, word, and deed, and, of course, be totally nonsexual.

I hope, gentle readers, you are not unconsciously promoting this image of agism. If so, take heed and correct your ways before it's too late.

And thanks for your letter, Mrs. B. You're a Real Woman—slacks or no slacks!

Has the Fountain of Youth Been Tapped?

Dear Dr. MacInnis:

There's lots of excited people around the Seniors' Lodge these days. Last night a group of the boys and gals (ages 60 to 90) saw on TV the realization of our wildest dreams. "Scientists have tapped the Fountain of Youth," so said the announcer, and he had the bodies right on the TV screen to prove it. There was one old guy pretty close to 90 who took this injection three times a week for just six months and he didn't look a day over 70! It made a 70 year old look like his middle aged son. At age 60 and a former amateur boxing champion, I should be able to regain the crown I lost forty years ago!.

A group of us, all candidates for the elixir of youth, decided to write to you for an unbiased opinion, even if you are now taking it yourself. We would like to know the name of the drug and especially how much it costs. As for myself, if I can't afford it now, I can be patient and wait for a year or two for the price to come down, but there are a couple of old boys (around 90) who tell me it's important they sign on right away, for obvious reasons.

Mr. M.F., Toronto, Ontario

Answer

Human growth hormone (HGH), that's what all the excitement is about. When I first heard a brief news account about it on the radio, I harkened back forty, fifty, even sixty years ago—right back to the monkey-gland injection craze in the roarin' twenties when ecstatic oldsters were pictured swinging from chandeliers and flying trapezes. You must recall the zany ads for Kruschen Salts, depicting an octogenarian deftly clearing a ten-foot clothesline! And within recent memory is the infamous novocaine-injection "clinic" in Romania that allegedly bestowed immortal youth on its thousands of well-heeled clients, which included high-ranking politicians, churchmen, erstwhile princes of European dynasties, and fading stars of stage and screen.

But there's nothing quackish about HGH. It has been around a long time. We have long known that this hormone, secreted by the pituitary gland situates at the base of our brain, stimulates the growth of bones and organs in children. But more important, we've been aware that a deficient secretion of the hormone causes stunted growth sometimes leading to dwarfism. We also know that an overproduction of the hormone in a fully grown adult may lead to excessive size and structure (acromegaly). Oversecretion in a growing person might lead to a condition known as gigantism. Scientists have long surmised that HGH promoted healthy tissues in older people, which led to the hypothesis that HGH might reverse some signs of aging. As we get older our body composition changes. For example, lean body mass consisting of bone, muscles, and organs account for 80 percent in a healthy young adult but after 30, lean body mass is very gradually replaced by fat at the rate of 5 percent per decade until, at the age of 65–79 the percentage of fat to lean is roughly 50-50.

Researchers at the Medical College of Wisconsin and the Veterans Affairs Medical Center in Milwaukee gave twelve men between 61 and 81 synthetic HGH by injection three times a week over a six-month period. All twenty-four men (twelve controls and twelve receiving HGH) ate identical diets and continued their same lifestyle.

Result: All the HGH men maintained their original body weight but with 4 percent less body fat and 9 percent more lean body mass than the twelve controls. Human growth hormone levels rose to that of men under 40. The participants felt and looked younger. The researchers reported that in their opinion the treatment reversed in some respects as much as one to two decades of aging.

But they emphasize that these results are preliminary involving a very small group. *The long-term effects are still unknown.*

And to answer your all-important question— the cost? Currently, a year's supply of the hormone is reputed to set you back about $12,000 should you ever be able to buy it!

Update: Human Growth Hormone (HGH) has been produced synthetically since 1985, making it available in ample supply for its proven value in treating stunted growth in children. However, early optimistic reports, such as the one cited above (1990) and a few others, have not been satisfactorily duplicated in more recent studies. While current researchers agree that HGH can enhance growth in under-height children and in the old for healing of fractures, bone building in osteoporosis and rapid convalescence after surgery, they don't believe it will ever reverse the aging process and indeed, over the longer term, they feel it might produce serious side effects.

My advice: At 60 you can afford to wait another 10 years, when the long-term effects of HGH will be better known. As for your three pals (including myself), we'll just have to await the verdict of natural mortality and hope for the best!

Chapter 2
Thoughts on Retirement

Within the framework of each life exist unrealized possibilities and long ignored talents that may be developed and pursued. These hidden potentials can be used to create new challenges and interests. They can make life more satisfying and can enrich the individual personality.

—*Guide to Health and Well-Being after Fifty*,
American Medical Association

Dear Dr. MacInnis:

I recall a column that you wrote a long time ago on the subject of retirement, where you told the story about a retired and depressed old man who had all but given up, when a family tragedy shouldered him with a responsibility and purpose that gave him a new lease on life. Little did I realize that my own recent retirement (compulsory and unplanned) would be just as disastrous. And thanks to that story, I sought and found a purpose for life again. I'm sure many of your readers would benefit from it as I did.

Thank you.

Mr. L.T. (66)

Answer

I say so often that one should retire not from something but into something. So many people retire from something into nothing. This is often the case when retirement is forced—like yours. And life quickly disposes of this person, for the less expected of the brain, the quicker it withers, condemning its owner to a passive and eventually useless existence.

The retired person who awakens in the morning with nothing to do and realizes (correctly) that nobody cares whether or not he or she gets up or stays in bed is well on the way to a depression—a depression that never responds to pills. One must regain a sense of self-worth by assuming responsibility for someone or something.

Retired persons must feel that they are part of the world around them and that their world, however small, must need them. The story I've told so often is from a stage play I saw many years ago titled *On Borrowed Time,* whose theme was the sad plight of the aged in a world that didn't seem to need them anymore. A depressed grandfather, well along in years, convinces himself that life had nothing more to offer.

One night Death edges into his room and addresses him: "Grandfather, it looks like your time has come." "Yes," answeres the old man, "I'm tired and I'm ready. But just give me a few hours to write some letters. Come back at nine in the morning."

That night the old man's son and his wife are killed in an auto accident, leaving an eight-year-old boy with no one to look after him but a tired old grandfather.

Promptly at nine the next morning Death again enters the room, whereupon the old man springs out of bed and, whacking the spectre with his cane, exclaims, "Death be on your way—I'm not going, I've got something to live for." And Death skulks away to bide its time.

The play's message is powerful and one well known to caregivers treating the old, the lonely, and the depressed. The grandfather would never have responded to pills or potions alone. He was "cured," literally overnight, when prescribed a mantle of responsibility and a sense of self-worth. As many of my colleagues can attest, such "miracles" are commonplace.

In my early years of medical practice among the elderly, I soon became aware of, and was puzzled by, two distinct personality types: the perpetually young at heart, who seldom saw or needed a doctor, and the opposite, the frequent clinic visitor needing ongoing support for a myriad of maladies, real or imagined— the latter often more devastating than the purely physical illness.

I think I have the answer now. One had "retired" *into* something or had never really retired at all. The other had duly retired from a busy life into nothing but a sterile existence that rendered life literally "a pain in the neck" and the so-called imagined ills were often the cries of mental depression.

What's on the Other Side of the Hill?

Dear Dr. MacInnis:

There seems to be a large number of people who are disappointed with retirement. When we were very young we displayed unlimited curiosity. We had to investigate everything to find out why and how things ticked. It seems that the workaday world takes all this out of us. We no longer have the urge to climb the hill to see what's on the other side. We have no interest in something "because it's not in my department." Or, "I'll leave that to the experts for I know I can't do it." Or, "That's a woman's job." Such negative feelings are endless.

If we older people could only stir up that curiosity we exhibited sixty years ago and get it going again, we'd be much happier.

I am a retired mechanic. I once knew another mechanic who discovered, much to his surprise (even shock!), that he could make the prettiest cushion covers you ever saw. He was a darned good mechanic; I worked with him. There's no way of seeing what talents are hidden under that shock of white hair or, in my case, a bald head.

If you're turned on by pretty paintings of landscapes or flowers but you're "sure" you've no artistic talents, maybe you should give it a try anyway.

To start with, don't go to the hobby shop and buy three or four hundred dollars' worth of equipment. Get the little tin box the kids use at school. If it turns out not to be your "cup of tea," you've only lost a few dollars and you can then try something else.

This "starting from scratch" can be applied to 90 percent of all known hobbies and amusements. A model train system is a good example. We are floored with that five thousand-dollar lay-out, not realizing that it could take thirty years to reach that stage (and we haven't all that time left!). A friend of mine started off with one engine and a few pieces of track. His grown-up kids got a kick watching the system grow and almost took possession! And forget about living long enough to "finish a job." Start it and enjoy it while you can.

Mr. G.W.C., Ontario

Answer

Take heed what Mr. C. says about *not* "finishing a job"; for it's the unfinished business in work and recreation that makes life worthwhile. You with the cluttered desk, unanswered letters, unread books, and places and friends to visit; you can always look forward to tomorrow and the next day and the next. You may never quite get there, but you travel hopefully along the way.

And therein may rest the secret of "eternal youth."

The Myth of the "Empty Nest"

Dear Dr. MacInnis:

My husband, a physician, has recently retired, which coincided with the last of our four children leaving the "parental roof." We now find ourselves victims of the "Empty Nest Syndrome." We've heard a lot about it producing symptoms of depression, but in our case it was a mixture of sadness and gladness tinged with a sense of relief from worry now that our goals and responsibilities toward our children have been fulfilled. They are all doing well and in a way they are now more our best friends than our children—if you know what we mean.

Is our attitude normal for "empty nesters"?

Mrs. A.M., Edmonton, Alberta

Answer

It would seem that the so-called Empty Nest Syndrome clinically characterized by anxiety, depression, and a sense of loss was "concocted" by professionals treating empty nest parents who in reality were undergoing a mid-life change brought on by retirement, job change, or the menopause. In a recent San Francisco study, 160 women were asked how they reacted to the empty nest. Only one experienced the above-noted symptoms. And in a Colorado State University questionnaire, the majority of parents stated that the experience was "beneficial," gave them a "new sense of freedom", "increased marital expression," and, like yourselves, they got to know their children as "best friends."

According to sociologists, the best way to ensure a symptomless "empty nest" is to prepare well ahead for a change of lifestyle and stick to your plan.

So you see, your attitude is quite normal. Enjoy your retirement.

Retired Doctor Announces Remarkable Research Breakthrough

Dear Dr. MacInnis:

I am a retired doctor whose greatest accomplishment to date is having survived with my prostate reasonably intact. But this is not the subject of my letter. On your advice, I retired not from something but into something and that something is trying to analyze signs and portents in the lifestyles of my friends and neighbours. So I'm relaying an important observation that will become apparent (immediately after my preamble) and I would appreciate your valued comment. It has to do with certain signs or trappings that might indicate who rules the household roost, the husband or wife. For instance, if a farmer's barn and other outbuildings outshine the house, he and he alone wears the pants and vice versa.

Now that you got the idea, I'd like to let your readers in on my own very personal observation—personal, because it can only be observed in the privacy of your host's toilet. It's the toilet seat that won't stay up by itself and needs to be held upright by the male guest who is simultaneously trying to keep things on the straight and narrow—an exercise doomed to disaster. I recall with horror one that would only rise halfway, choked by a shroud of thick sheepskin!

Result of Study: In all ten (as depicted above), the lady of the house was dominant. The men ranged from indifferent to servile with a few I would class as henpecked.

Respectfully submitted,

Dr. C.H.S., Westerose, Alberta

Answer

A remarkable study in deductive reasoning, Doctor. Move over Sherlock Holmes!

Factually, the inner workings of our modern toilet have little changed since its invention in the eighteenth century by the redoubtable Sir Thomas Crapper.

I'm sure Sir Thomas would be even more frustrated than you, had he encountered such a cumbersome snafu in his wonderful flushing machine.

Especially, if Lady Crapper wore the pants!

How Old Is "Old Old"?

Dear Dr. MacInnis:

We're having an argument here at the Seniors' Retirement Lodge about the term "old." We hear expressions like "young old" and "old old." Where is the dividing line? Is it just pretty well how one acts *his or her age?*

Dr. MacInnis, are you "old old," or if not, then when do you expect to be? And when will you retire?

Miss K.M., Edmonton, Alberta

Answer

Good gracious *no*. How can you say such a thing!

I'll consider myself "old old" when I have geriatric children to worry about. Then I'll be too busy to retire.

28

Fun with Figures

Dear Dr. MacInnis:

Several years ago in a column on retirement, you said that France's greatest contribution to gerontology (science of aging) was in producing Maurice Chevalier. What did he do to merit such a distinction?

Mrs. M. M.W., Brookville, New York

Answer

It's not what he did; it's what he said (older retirees take note).

Quote France's supersex symbol (male), "The difference between 30 and 70 is 40 years of experience!"

Now that's really retiring *into* something!

We Chose Spain

The one and only place in the world we chose for future retirement was Spain. This was in the late sixties. After braving the bitter January cold of north central Spain (which I could have done without), our journey ended in the lovely little town of Marbella on the sunny Costa Del Sol where a comfortable, well appointed seaside villa (summer cottage to us) could be purchased on excellent terms for as low as $15,000! In those days, retirement planning involved renting out the villa to tourists for months, sometimes years, until the day of the "great move" when we would join our expatriate friends from Canada, the United States, and Europe already luxuriating as new and happy "citizens." But as fate decreed, our "Castle in Spain" was not to be.

What I've just said will serve to introduce a review of a delightful travel book on Spain, tailor-made for both leisurely tourists who can spend weeks or months or, better still, a full retirement there. It's definitely *not* for those who want to "do" Spain in a fortnight!

Choose Spain, a comprehensive new guide to enjoying Spain and Portugal combines the experience of a long-time American resident of Spain, Bettie Magee, and travel writer, John Howels. Loaded with details on costs, legal requirements, local customs, and language, *Choose Spain* is designed to make even the short-term visitor feel like a resident.

The authors offer practical advice on affordable short-term apartment rentals that can provide vacationers and prospective retirees with a base for exploring Spain and Portugal's cities and countryside. A chapter on camping and RV (recreation vehicle) travel should prove invaluable to those who want to try the European approach.

The best news is that these newly democratic countries are still among the least expensive in Europe.

(Choose Spain, Gateway Books, 31 Grand View Avenue, San Francisco, CA 94114, 252 pages, illustrated, maps, $22.95 in U.S. funds. Available in many book stores. Add $1.75 for mail orders direct from the publisher.)

Chapter 3
Other Grey Matters: A Discussion of Patient-Doctor Communication

A common complaint of elderly correspondents is that their doctor is always in a hurry and doesn't listen to them. Here is a letter that illustrates my point.

Dear Dr. MacInnis:

I have hesitated to write this letter for fear my doctor will read it in the paper and recognize himself. But on second thought, maybe it will be all for his good.

My criticism is that he never gives me time to converse with him. During the short visit, which is never more than ten minutes, he very rarely sits down. He paces the floor, monopolizes the conversation, never gives me a chance for complaints, and before I know it, he's scribbling a prescription on the fly and buzzes for his next patient.

I don't want to leave the impression that I am the so-called difficult patient who drives doctors up the wall. Mostly, I just want a simple explanation of what a drug is for and what are some of its side effects, for example. When he does get around to explaining something, it requires a medical dictionary to translate it into familiar English. He seems to be preoccupied, but at times can be funny. So to sum up, I never, after leaving his office, feel better than when I stepped in. On a scale of one to ten he rates five.

My question. Should I chuck this young man (he's in his mid-thirties, I would think) in favor of a more understanding doctor who takes the time to sit down and listen, even if it's only for ten minutes?

Mrs. X. (age 69)

PS: I'm not a neurotic and only visit the clinic every two to three months.

Answer

My short answer is yes, "chuck him," as you say. It would seem that your very occasional visit is a waste of your time and, most likely, of his. I suggest that you make some enquiries from your friends, and I believe you'll find that the majority are well satisfied with their doctors. In this way you may discover Dr. Right!

******

Mrs. X's complaint is a familiar one that my reader mail will verify. Some elderly patients tell me that doctors don't take the time to explain what's wrong and that they always seem to be in a hurry. But when the doctor takes time to sit and talk with them they are satisfied.

This was the consensus of a study recently published in the journal, *Evaluation of the Health Professions,* where it concludes that "patients are more satisfied with physicians who are courteous and express personal warmth during interviews." They also found that patients expressed "high levels of satisfaction when physicians volunteered information regarding their condition, expressed emotional support and trust in the patient, and used plain language similar to the patient's during the interview."

It is reassuring to read from the study that poor communication between patient and doctor is now being recognized, and something is being done about it. According to the report, many medical schools are now providing programs to students and physicians on doctor-patient communication. Although this study deals specifically with younger patients, the important conclusions apply even more so to the elderly, who are not always capable of expressing their complaints and other concerns and who, in some cases (particularly in the very old), forget to ask the doctor pertinent questions.

As I have said on many occasions, the elderly patient who has memory problems should, if at all possible, be accompanied by a younger family member to the doctor's office. And it's important that this family member remain with the patient during the whole interview. In my experience, most elderly patients appreciate this.

Are Doctors Nutritionists?

Dear Dr. MacInnis:
Every time I go to the doctor and ask him advice on nutrition he seems to shy away from the subject as if he didn't care to discuss it. I tried another doctor with the same results. Why do they have this attitude towards nutritional counselling? I'll be blunt. Could it be that they don't know anything about nutrition and really don't care?

Mrs. N.Y.

Answer

I too will be blunt. Doctors receive little or no training in nutrition in medical schools. Consequently, this important aspect of medicinal practice is denied to both them and their patients. It is impossible for them to give counsel when they have little or no knowledge of nutrition.

A few doctors, embarrassingly aware of their shortcomings, have taught themselves by reading, attending seminars on nutrition, and promoting it in their practice. Personally, I spent many years practicing medicine, blissfully unaware that nutrition counselling was a part of it!

According to a study conducted by the University of Minnesota, most physicians considered it appropriate to counsel their patients on dietary and nutritional matters but actually, few did.

The objectives of the study were to determine (1) whether M.D.'s considered nutritional counselling appropriate for patients who did not specifically request it, (2) the proportion of patients given such counselling, (3) physicians' reasons for not providing it. Their answers appeared in the study published in the medical Journal *Preventive Medicine,* Vol. 13 (March 1984): 219–25.

Sixty-two percent agreed that dietary counselling was appropriate. Twenty percent disagreed and 18 percent were undecided. The most common reason given for lack of counselling was the absence in some of the heart patients (who made up the study group) of risk factors such as high cholesterol, hypertension, and obesity. The majority also reported giving counselling to fewer than 40 percent of their patients.

Another reason was "a perceived disinterest in or noncompliance with dietary recommendations by the patients." The report stated that in its opinion the major barrier was the doctors' belief that only a small proportion of patients would benefit.

The report concluded: "To play a role in reducing the (cardiovascular disease) burden, physicians must be taught the rationale of the community approach to disease prevention. They must also be taught that patients are seeking nutrition information and will change their behaviour in response to an intervention."

Doctors: Old *versus* Young

Dear Dr. MacInnis:

I hope this doesn't offend you, but I just got fed up going to old doctors (like you). All they do is sit and talk and trying to get them to do tests is like pulling a hen's tooth—in short, impossible.

My present doctor is a young fellow who right away ordered lots of tests—twelve to be exact. No fuss, no bother, no idle talk. "Come back in a week," he said, "and we'll see what the printout says."

"You're just fine," he congratulated me. "Your tests are all good." Now this made me feel real nice, and I left that young doctor's office a very satisfied customer.

After getting home I recalled that the old man had told me the same thing. But somehow it didn't get through to me. He just didn't back up his words with written proof. That's where the difference is. Don't you agree?

Mrs. B.M. Westport, Connecticut

Answer

My main reason for printing this long letter (abbreviated) is because it places in excellent context a recent study by researchers of the Harvard Medical School who investigated the differences between U.S. and British doctors in ordering diagnostic tests for hypertension (high blood pressure). The results were published in the October 5, 1984, issue of the *Journal of the American Medical Association.*

They found that U.S. doctors ordered 41 times more electrocardiograms, 6.8 times more chest X-rays, and 2 times more upper intestinal X-rays than their British colleagues.

A co-author of the report, Dr. Arnold Epstein, believes that the great (and unexpected) differences "are due to our greater dependence on technology in all our life's pursuits—including medical diagnosis."

Another co-author, Dr. Robert Hartley, said in a related interview that he had a strong suspicion that the U.S. doctors' tendency to order more tests "is not limited to hypertension patients."

Dr. Hartley was asked if more and more tests mean better care. His answer: "I don't see that we're buying any better health." Apart from such international variance in ordering habits there is a vast difference amongst American and Canadian doctors in their diagnostic approach to illness.

Could it be that a younger generation of doctors are also utilizing more and more technology and losing the "Art of Medicine" in the process?

Or put another way, could we "old" doctors be still mindful of the seemingly endless clinical bedside teaching in our student and intern years, and where a technical test was ordered solely to assist, confirm or negate a strong diagnostic impression?

You have believed, Mrs. M., because you have seen. "Blessed are those who believe and have not seen" (John 19.29).

The Waiting Game

Dear Dr. MacInnis:

Why do patients always have to wait and wait in a doctor's office—sometimes as long as an hour or more. In all my years going to doctors, not once have I been met at the door by a smiling nurse/secretary who says, "Ah, Mrs. M., you're right on the dot and here's your doctor." I suppose if that really happened, I'd faint dead away and would truly need a doctor!

Seriously though, I can't help surmising that doctors in training must take special courses from old veterans, maybe like yourself, who can, from long years of experience, teach them the fine art of mismanagement of their personal and professional morning chores so that it virtually guarantees getting to the office late for the first appointment, which compounds itself into an hour or more past midday when unfortunates like myself arrive.

Admit it, Dr. MacInnis, professionals from other disciplines would never dream of inflicting long and tedious waiting games on their paying clients.

And when I finally gain admission to the holy of holies, my doctor is usually so tense that he hasn't had time to sit down but keeps pacing while enjoining me to "take it easy and relax"! What do you think of the idea of a professional like myself submitting a bill to the doctor for my time lost in waiting?

Mrs. A.M. (42), Olds, Alberta

Answer

I have long espoused the art of medicine, Mrs. M., but not the nefarious "art" you accuse me of so glibly. But I'm not offended. Rather, I'm kind of relieved to have you as a correspondent and not as a patient. But perhaps you're getting to me and I should restrain myself.

Now, with this off my chest, I agree with you that inordinately long waits in doctors' waiting rooms have been the norm since Hippocrates set up general practice in Cos. And the wonder of it is that patients have seldom complained. It was just something they expected—just a minor sacrifice on the altar of great expectations, be they joy or grief.

Happily, I perceive a trend for the better. Doctors are becoming more sensitive to the great inconveniences they sometimes unconsciously inflict on their patients. These are the doctors whose practices will grow and prosper with satisfied "customers." Those who gauge their success by quantity of patients rather than quality of care will, in time, discover their once crowded waiting rooms strangely silent and deserted. Their patients will have simply opted for a more personal touch—elsewhere.

Charging the doctor for your waiting and wasted time is a novel approach, Mrs. M. Whether you realize it or not, you're practicing extra billing in reverse, where the doctor pays up instead of the patient. So there's no harm trying.

Few waiting patients rant, rankle, and rage like you, Mrs. M. Indeed, some lonely retired folk frequent clinic waiting rooms solely for the social adventure. They enjoy robust health and attribute their good fortune to the exceptional, high quality care from their doctors and nurses. What fine psychotherapy, especially for first-time, timid, nervous patients who are dreading their "ordeal" ahead.

"?%##%?*"

Dear Dr. MacInnis:

Why is it impossible to make out a doctor's writing, like "?%##%?" on a drug prescription? I believe they don't want the patient to read it. How can the pharmacist make it out? Or does he know the secret code?*

Miss M.N.M., R.N., Ottawa, Ontario

Answer

It's a God-given gift to pharmacists on graduation. But every now and then it fails. Like the time a bewildered pharmacist confronted the physician with a totally illegible prescription. Sputtered the good doctor, "When I wrote that, God and I both knew what it was. Now, God only knows!"

Some Doctors Think They're God

Dear Dr. MacInnis:

What do you think of doctors who think they're God? I am 55 years old and now in good health. Two years ago two doctors told me that I had chronic disease of the pancreas. One gave me six months to live; the other was more generous—he gave me ten months. Well, both were wrong. I only had yellow jaundice from my liver. It's now all gone and I feel fine and already I have outlived one of them who sentenced me to death!

R.J.W., Glen Head, New York

Answer

As you give few details I hesitate to pronounce judgment on your medical advisors, who both obviously saw you in the same light. It is true that some doctors try to play God, but it can be a dangerous game beset with pitfalls that you mention. Of course, it can happen the other way around as illustrated by the following story: A world-famous doctor of Medicine died and went to heaven. He was immediately welcomed by Saint Peter, who escorted him around to see the celestial sights. On his heavenly rounds, the famous doctor's eyes fell on a distinguished-looking, grey-bearded gentleman, gowned and masked, stethoscope in hand, intently listening to an angel's chest. And there was a long retinue of angels waiting for examination. A busy day at the office it would seem.

The famous physician could no longer contain himself and exclaimed, "Saint Peter, how come you have doctors in heaven where there are no sick people? To which Saint Peter replied, "Of course, we don't need doctors here. But, shush, lower your voice please. That's not a doctor. That's God. He often likes to play doctor!"

In the Doctor-God Game, Here's How They Rate

I recently received a literary contribution from a physician friend who, along with being distinguished in his profession, is a very funny man and well armoured for "the slings and arrows" so often directed at his specialty—psychiatry.

This classification of medical specialties is based on the well-known attributes of our late-lamented Superman, where you can see the specialty of psychiatry falls short, but thanks to my friend's generosity, geriatric medicine gets full marks. I thank him for this outpouring of adulation, but the reader should remember that this is only a fun game with any specialty attaining top honors if the perpetrator so wishes.

And one more thing. My friend, who is known for his occasional modesty, does not claim authorship. He would like to know the creator and I would too. So would the author please step forward for well-deserved recognition!

The PATHOLOGIST, being the perennial custodian of Truth (and lots of money), comes first on Superman's rating list. Well, almost. For he leaps tall buildings in a single bound. Is more powerful than a locomotive. Is faster than a speeding bullet. Walks on water. Gives policy to God.

A close second is the INTERNIST (specialist in internal medicine), who leaps tall buildings in a single bound. Is more powerful than a switch engine. Is just as fast as a speeding bullet. Walks on water. And gives policy to God—only when requested.

Next comes the SURGEON, who leaps short buildings with a running start and favorable wind. Is almost as powerful as a small trolley. Talks to God when permission is granted—but not often.

The DERMATOLOGIST and RADIOLOGIST can barely clear a Quonset hut and lose tugs of war with a locomotive. Can fire a speeding bullet. Swim well, and are occasionally addressed by God.

The GYNECOLOGIST makes high marks on walls trying to leap over tall buildings. Is run over by locomotives. Can sometimes handle a gun without inflicting self-injury. Talks to animals.

The PSYCHIATRIST runs directly into closed doors. Can recognize a locomotive two times in three. Is not issued ammunition. Floats on water with a life jacket. Talks to the water.

The MALE MEDICAL STUDENT (new special category) falls over doorsteps trying to enter buildings. Exclaims "Look at choo-choo." Wets himself with a water pistol. Plays in mud puddles and mumbles to himself.

The GERIATRICIAN, replete with paranoid delusions from advancing senility, lifts tall buildings and walks under them. Kicks locomotives off the tracks. Catches speeding bullets in teeth and then eats them. Freezes water at a single glance. In Truth, IS GOD!

You Have a Right to Ask (Your Doctor)

When my medical colleagues taunt me (gently) about my geriatric column, their commonest question is, "Do readers really write in those questions or do you just make them up?" And my pat answer goes something like this: "No, I'm not that creative, but I can tell you one thing, if most of my elderly readers, on visiting their doctor, asked him or her the same questions they later mail on to me, I would soon be out of business for lack of correspondents!"

In many cases, it is quite apparent that the patient, on arriving home with prescription clutched in hand, has very little or no idea what it's all about and when goaded by the spouse as to *why*, invariably replies, "I forgot to ask," or "I didn't want to bother the doctor," or "the doctor said something about it but I didn't understand and I didn't want to ask again." This is the scenario of the all-too-common unsatisfactory medical consultation.

Patients generally, but particularly elderly patients, are often intimidated by doctors and hospitals, and as in the "White Coat Syndrome," where normal blood pressure shoots up at the sight of a doctor, the elderly patient, with best of intentions for a "good visit" often "blows it" and arrives home empty-handed of information.

I have often thought of writing a manual for seniors advising them how to approach the doctor in his den and get the most out of an office call, but Zelda Freedman has beaten me to it and eloquently at that! Ms. Freedman was at one time the medical librarian at the Elizabeth Bruyere Health Centre, a long-term/palliative-care teaching facility affiliated with the University of Ottawa. It was here she became acutely aware of the frustrations experienced by the elderly on visiting their doctors in office and hospital, which made it clear to Ms. Freedman that there was a serious gap in communication between the elderly and their physicians.

This experience extending over eight years gave birth to an admirable little booklet of fifty-four pages entitled, *Pleased to See You—You Have a Right to Ask: A Guide to Visiting Your Doctor.*

"This book," the author points out, "will assist you to improve communication with your doctor so that as equal partners you will make informed, educated decisions about those things that affect your health. You will learn how to ask, not to be afraid to ask, and to ask the right question at the best time. Communicating is not as difficult as it seems."

Pleased to See You . . . is well laid out and exceedingly easy to read. The author deals specifically with questions the elderly patient might wish to ask about: aches and pains, bladder and bowel control, health care costs (for U.S. patients), hearing, heart/blood pressure/stroke medication, memory, osteoporosis/fractures/falls, sleep tests, X rays, surgery, and vision. (There's ample space on each page for the patient's own questions and notes.)

And there are many more penetrating but realistic questions to ask about, e.g., emotional health, loss/grief, and one I particularly liked—"Things I've Been Afraid to Ask." Example: "I would like a second opinion, doctor. Would you be offended by this?"

I wish I had more space to further extol the merits of this little book dedicated to the author's parents: "To My Father Who Was Afraid to Ask and My Mother Who Didn't Know How to Ask." The dedication tells the story better than any review of mine! Needless to say, I heartily endorse this handbook to help the older patient get the most from "seeing the doctor."

41

(Pleased to See You—You Have a Right to Ask costs $5.96 in Canada (plus 7% GST) and $5.35 U.S. in the United States. On all orders please add postage and handling charge of $1.50 per single book and $0.50 for each additional book. Order from Canadian Public Health Association, Suite 400, 1565 Carling Avenue, Ottawa, Ontario. K1Z 8R1.)

Chapter 4
Benign Senescent Forgetfulness

I could have titled this short chapter "Age-related Memory Impairment" but I opted for a more elegant and far more comforting diagnosis—"Benign Senescent Forgetfulness" (BSF). Comforting, because it assures us that all those pesky mid- to later-life memory problems are, at worst, just bothersome and with patience and perseverance may be improved. More importantly, though, it reassures us that it will likely remain "within limits" and not evolve into a more serious situation where the lifestyle of the patient and family are affected.

Some memory experts believe that this age-related memory trouble is due to the reduced speed of the aging eye, ear, and brain in processing information. How often have you had something "on the tip of your tongue" and couldn't retrieve it until later when you least expected it and then when you probably didn't need it?

The letters, the essay, and the poem in this chapter deal with benign senescent forgetfulness with the possible exception of one letter, where the memory problem is on the fringe of normalcy. Here, only time will resolve the outcome and I often wonder if my worst fears have indeed come true.

If You *Remember* You've Forgotten, That's Okay, It's BSF

Dear Dr. MacInnis:

I am 82 years of age and greatly alarmed as my memory is gradually failing. It was recommended to me to take improved

43

lecithin, choline, and garlic capsules. Would you recommend tak-
ing all three or something else? Or should it be taken in modera-
tion? Thank you,

Mrs. E.R.

Answer

Among the commonest memory problems besetting older
people are forgetting names, faces, phone numbers, where the
car is parked, and "where in the world are the keys?" But just
give us time and we will recall. We learn to adapt to our failings
by writing down phone numbers and addresses for easy reference, by taking our bearings when we park the car, and by
always leaving the car keys in the same pocket—always. Some
I know have developed elaborate memory aids.

We have a delightful diagnosis for such lapses in memory.
It's called "benign senescent forgetfulness." Here forgetfulness
is termed "benign" (not serious) because like you (my correspondent), we *remember* we've forgotten and can then take steps to
improve our lot.

I've written numerous columns on memory problems in the
elderly and have always reminded the reader that the old saying, "If you don't use it, you lose it," applies to more than sex!
You can hone the mind razor-sharp by creative, intellectual activities such as solving crossword puzzles and other word games;
one of the best card games being cribbage. Reading is excellent
mental exercise, which is enhanced by writing notes on what
you read and discussing it with your friends (in moderation!). I
stress the more active creative activities over passive pastimes
like chronic "boob-toobing."

Although everyone is not fortunate in discovering stimulating company, it's often possible, especially in retirement lodges.
I have found excellent study groups operating in senior citizen
homes, one of which "graduated" a member to a university arts
degree. Another lodge encourages oil painting.

Now back again to "failing memory." We can all live with
benign senescent forgetfulness because we can learn to adapt.
But when a patient's memory gets progressively worse despite

all efforts to overcome memory loss and his lifestyle (and that of his family) is seriously disrupted, then we must consider brain impairment, and here medical help should be sought. (Before a clinical diagnosis of a dementia like Alzheimer's disease may be made, other causes of loss of memory and awareness must be ruled out, for some of them may be reversible and treatable.)

I believe that you (the writer) are bothered with BSF because you *know* you have a memory problem and are seeking help. I would therefore advise you to follow, as best you can, the creative mental exercises and socializing activities suggested earlier in this column.

There are simply no scientifically controlled studies indicating that lecithin and choline are beneficial in improving memory. Glowing reports are mainly the word-of-mouth variety. When it was discovered several years ago that the nerve transmitting messenger, acetylcholine, was deficient in Alzheimer's disease, it was thought that by feeding choline and/or lecithin (building blocks of acetylcholine) to the Alzheimer's patients, their memory might improve. But despite negative results, both choline and lecithin are still widely touted by certain practitioners and advertised in so-called health magazines—some of dubious reputation. My opinion? They're a waste of money.

As for garlic, far be it from me to decry the medicinal virtues vested in that noble bulb. So, brethren, I say unto you, take it for thy health's sake. For who knows what secret source of memory lurks in the heart of a single clove!

Demented People Don't Write Poems

Dear Dr. MacInnis:

Several years ago you published a delightfully humorous poem by an unknown author bemoaning her awful lapses of memory. Would you kindly print it again. I liked it so well I put it away for safekeeping, but now I can't remember where. I'm sure many of your readers would appreciate it if they are as forgetful as I am.

Mrs. T.P.

Answer

As I've said so often, if you forget and don't remember you've forgotten, that's not good. But if you remember you've forgotten and it comes back to you sooner or later, then it's that old "benign senescent forgetfulness" again. And we can live with that.

Now what did I start out to do? Oh, yes, the poem.

Our unknown author titled it "Senile Dementia," a misnomer because demented people don't write like this.

Just a line to say I'm living
And I'm not among the dead
Though I'm getting more forgetful
And am mixed up in the head.

For sometimes I can't remember
When I stand below the stair
If I must go up for something
Or if I just came down from there.

And before the fridge so often
My poor mind is filled with doubt
Have I just put the food away
Or come to take some out.

And there are times when it is dark
With the curlers on my head
I don't know if I'm retiring
Or I've just got out of bed.

So if it's now my turn to write you
There's no need of gettin' sore
I think I may have written
And don't want to be a bore.

So remember, I do love you
And wish that you were near
But now it's nearly mail time
So I'll say "good-bye, my dear."

Here I stand beside the mailbox
With my face so very red
Instead of mailing out your letter
I've just opened it instead!

I Can't Remember What He Just Said

Dear Dr. MacInnis:

Could you please answer a few questions about memory changes in old people? I am 75 years of age and find that I am becoming very forgetful. For instance, I can read several pages in a book and will not remember a word of it. I try to listen to a public speaker and often my mind gets so sidetracked with my own private thoughts that I catch very little of what's said. But I find if I can shut out distracting sounds from radio or TV, I can concentrate on what I am reading and that helps me to remember. Are my memory problems all due to aging? Are they inevitable? Please comment.

Mr. A.Y.

Answer

I'm no expert on memory matters, but psychologist Dr. Alan S. Brown is and I'll be reviewing his memory book in the next column. Here's a "sneak preview" of chapter one, where Dr. Brown deals with memory changes unaffected by age. Dr. Brown tells us that there are some memory functions that don't deteriorate with age. First is the brief sensory memory of something you hear (auditory sensory memory), e.g., when you're asked the time. Here you hold the question long enough to answer, after which the mind loses hold of it and it's gone. Visual sensory memory is used when you quickly act on something you see in print like a road sign. Here again, you record it only for a moment, follow the directive, and then forget about it. This is raw, unprocessed memory that is not always stored because there's often no need to retain it.

The second type of memory that aging doesn't change is called short-term memory. You look up a number in the phone book, repeat it to yourself several times, and then dial it hoping you won't "lose" it in the process. Short-term memory lasts about thirty seconds and is said to be the workshop of memory because it's where new information may be stored and "solidified" for later use. If you really want to remember that phone number you will keep memorizing it for storage in your long-term memory compartment for later recall.

Long-term memory is what we use in the recall of current (day to day) personal happenings as well as knowledge we have learned in the past of the world around us. "Aging apparently does not diminish our ability to access our long-term store of information," says Dr. Brown.

What aging may impair is the smooth transition of information through the three aforementioned stages—sensory, short-term, and long-term memory. For instance, if no great effort is made to deposit sensory memory into short-term memory or short-term into long-term memory, recall may be elusive or lost for good.

I hope Dr. Brown answers to some extent your last question on memory and aging. Next column I'll address your concerns about "mind meandering" and the inability to concentrate and I'll review Dr. Brown's "memory book."

I Can't Remember a Word of It

In his letter, Mr. A.Y., age 75, seems worried about his memory failing him. "I can read several pages in a book but can't remember a word of it," he writes. It's the same when he tries to listen to a speech. "My mind gets so sidetracked with my private thoughts that I catch very little of what's said," he continues.

Mind meandering is common in the elderly. As we age it becomes increasingly difficult to ignore distractions. But Mr. Y. comes up with a remedy. Before sitting down to read he "shuts out" distracting sounds of radio and TV or any other noise that competes for his reading attention. He then finds that he can concentrate on what he's reading and that helps him to remember.

Mr. Y. is telling us that by blotting out this constant barrage of noise (auditory sensory bombardment) he can facilitate the reception of visual sensory imagery (from the book) and store it in his memory for later recall.

And why does Mr. Y. always forget what the speaker said? Most likely he concentrates more on how the speaker looked (his dress, physical features, gestures, etc.) than on what he was saying. In other words, visual sensory memory (how the speaker appeared) competed with auditory sensory memory (what the speaker said) and won. It was just too powerful for the aging mind to mask out.

What should Mr. Y. do to turn the competition around where audio wins over video? He can "turn off" the visual distraction by gazing elsewhere or by simply closing his eyes and concentrating on what he hears. This is not easy at first but with patience and perseverance Mr. Y. should succeed.

Elderly people beset with annoying memory problems have devised ingenious schemes to store and retain new information. What I've briefly reported here is how some have succeeded in hearing and reading better.

Have you retained pretty well what I've just written? If not, you had better turn off that TV or whatever's competing for attention!

I promised to review what in my opinion is a good memory book. It's titled *How to Increase Your Memory Power* (Note: currently out of print. Check your library.), by alan S. Brown, Ph.D., Associate Professor of Psychology at Southern Methodist University, Dallas, Texas, who specializes in memory problems. He has written several books on the subject of memory but this, his latest, deals specifically with memory processes in the years after 50 and is the response of the author to the inquiries of a "continual stream of mature adults who posed the following question to me: 'How can you help me improve my memory?'" (From author's Introduction; excerpt reprinted by permission).

The book has 178 pages of easy reading and has 13 chapters. The first chapter describes how memory works (referred to in my previous column) and what age-related changes are considered normal. (This is calculated to put your mind at ease!)

Chapter 2 describes how memory may be affected by physical problems arising from acute chronic illnesses and nutritional disorders, and there's a very helpful listing of prescription drugs that frequently cause confusion or memory problems especially in the elderly. Psychological disorders impairing memory are discussed in chapter 3.

Chapters 4, 5, and 6 deal with general principles of memory and how to effectively "store" incoming information for later recall.

Chapter 7 provides useful techniques on how to remember names and chapter 8 tells us how to retain information from conversations and reading (referred to earlier in this column). Chapter 9 deals with "remembering what needs to be done" and chapter 10 is about "keeping track of what you did."

What to do when your memory "gets stuck" is discussed in chapters 11 and 12 and the final chapter, 13, wraps everything up by presenting suggestions on "how to change your memory habits."

The Aging Brain

Dear Dr. MacInnis:

Could you please give some information on aging of the nervous system? Do all parts of the brain shrink at the same rate?

Mr. A.G. (age 60), Winnipeg, Manitoba

Answer

Before I answer your questions, let me give you a few facts about the greatest of all computer systems—the human brain. It's hard to imagine, but the mature adult human brain has over one hundred billion nerve cells or neurons. Each of these neurons is equipped with a thousand projections or filaments connected to adjacent neurons. This marvellous and intricate circuitry makes possible our thought processes, our consciousness, memory and everything that makes us a distinct personality different from everyone else. And any process that disturbs these neuronal interconnections, be it degenerative disease or aging, affects how the brain functions, however insidiously at first.

Loss of brain cells (neurons) begins at 30 years of age at the rate of thousands per day with no replacement. By the time we reach 80, our brain will have lost about 7 percent of its weight in the prime of our life. Not all areas of the brain shrink at the same rate. The grey matter of our cerebral cortex that mediates all of our highest intellectual functions shrinks the fastest in old age, losing about 50 percent of its neurons.

This may help to explain our often bothersome memory problems as we approach middle life (and often earlier!) forgetting names, faces, telephone numbers, and the like, shrugging it off as "benign senescent forgetfulness," which it nearly always is. But who of us has not given a thought to the morbid memory changes and destruction of self in Alzheimer's disease.

Morbid Forgetfulness: When BSF May Cross the Line

Dear Dr. MacInnis:

Your recent column on the early memory changes in Alzheimer's Disease dismisses that common aging syndrome, benign senescent forgetfulness (BSF), as of little account. Certainly this is true when compared with the dreadful memory loss in Alzheimer's disease. But I ask you can nothing be done to help someone for whom the "benign" problem becomes a daily misery? The fact that one is aware of memory difficulties, or even that the answer does eventually come (sometimes after minutes or a half hour or days later) doesn't help the total blankness and mental confusion that robs you of self-confidence. And even more—it makes you start avoiding some people and situations and begin "playing for time."

Such evasions and "playing for time" become so commonplace that you begin to feel like half of yourself, always waiting for your brain to "kick in" and give the appropriate verbal response.

Would you please discuss.

(No initials)

(Normally, I never publish "nameless" letters. But this one is the rare exception because it expresses so well the plight of a presumably elderly person with severe memory impairment who is acutely aware of his/her deficiency.

51

I regret that the writer will have waited for four to six months to read my answer in his/her paper when it could have taken only a few weeks to receive a personal reply by mail—something I always do as a courtesy in the case of a letter deemed suitable for publication.)

Answer

Benign senescent forgetfulness (BSF) has always been a comforting diagnosis for those of us beset with the memory problems beginning in early old age and considered part of the normal aging process. Some examples are difficulty remembering names—"I know your face but I can't for the life of me recall your name and it's just on the tip of my tongue"; or "I forget where I've placed things"; or "Where did I park the car?" or "Now that I've found it in the parking lot, I can't find my keys!" Another senior writes, "I always go over the grocery list (my wife writes) before I leave home, just in case I might misplace it. Well, one day I did, and do you know, when I got to the store, I couldn't remember a single item and had to phone home for another list!"

Most of us have in time adapted well to memory frustrations with some developing clever memory "enhancers" for remembering names, such as tagging a facial "feature" with such an outrageous designation that it always comes to mind and provides the clue for the real name.

A BSF reader admonishes, "Never walk away from the parking lot before establishing a 'land-sight' for your car. It always works." To which I might add, always put your car keys in the *same* pocket and you'll always find them on the first try.

Admittedly, the above examples of BSF in our daily activities are minor nuisances. "But when memory problems," I recently wrote, "begin to affect the person's lifestyle and perhaps that of his/her family, then we may be looking at a more serious disorder."

It is apparent that our correspondent's lifestyle is being affected by serious memory deficits even though they are still "remembered" and agonized over.

I would therefore strongly advise that this person seek professional help from a clinical psychologist or psychiatrist.

(This is a fitting column to end chapter 4, for the "morbid forgetfulness" so strikingly depicted in this reader's letter, even though "remembered," may portend an evolving dementia of the Alzheimer's type, featured in the next chapter.)

Chapter 5
Slow Death of the Mind: Alzheimer's Disease

Alois Alzheimer was born in Bavaria, Germany, in 1864, graduated in medicine in 1888 and practiced for fourteen years in a psychiatric clinic in Frankfurt. Later he joined the great psychiatrist Emil Kraepelin and the then world famous brain pathologist Franz Nissl and published research papers on epilepsy and mental illness. In 1907 he presented to his medical colleagues at the Kraepelin Research Institute the autopsy findings on his patient, a 51-year-old woman who died from dementia and exhibited peculiar brain tissue "plaques" and "tangles" in a disease that will forever be associated with his name. He died in 1915 at the age of 51.

******

In the Introduction, I noted that people over 65 as a group are growing faster than any segment of the population, with our 85's and older leading the pack. No wonder, then, that age-related disorders like Alzheimer's disease, known at the turn of the century as "senility" and relatively uncommon, now affect at least 40 percent of patients over 80 and more than half the nation's chronic nursing beds are occupied by its victims. But this is only the "tip of the iceberg," as you'll learn in one of the more arresting statements in this chapter.

Public health authorities call Alzheimer's disease the "scourge of the century" and assert that we are now facing an ongoing epidemic of historic proportion.

On a personal note, most of the comment and essays you read here have been written from the perspective of the clinical director of a large hospital department admitting annually over a hundred elderly patients with far advanced dementia of the Alzheimer's type. We always encouraged families to bring along personal mementos of their loved ones to make their residence, as far as possible, "a bit of home." Family photographs adorned the walls, recording tales of better days. There, the patient was the "center-person" so much alive, so happy and secure. This stark contrast between past and present impressed upon us, more than any "case" presentation, the great human tragedy unfolding before our eyes and I believe made us better caregivers.

What is the meaning of "dementia"—a word you'll run across frequently in this chapter? It's from the Latin *de* meaning "out of" and *mens* meaning "mind"—literally "out of one's mind," where the mind disintegrates slowly but relentlessly, leaving the victim devoid of cognition or awareness that leads in time to complete destruction of personality and self.

Over the past two decades a prodigious amount of research has been expended on finding the cause of Alzheimer's disease, with each year getting closer to the still elusive prize. I have attempted to keep the reader updated on scientific progress over the past three years, sometimes at the expense of being repetitious, but Alzheimer's research is an evolving process and an exciting one as we near the home stretch.

Here, then, is the "Alzheimer's Story" as chronicled in my newspaper column over the years.

******

Alzheimer's Disease: The Beginnings

Dear Dr. MacInnis:

My mother, age 73, has just been diagnosed as having "senile dementia, Alzheimer type." What is the difference between this condition and "Alzheimer's disease"? Also what are the chances of her two sons and two daughters coming down with it?

Mrs. J.K.

Answer

Dr. Alois Alzheimer's celebrated patient was a 51-year-old woman, who (in 1907), after several years of progressive mental deterioration, died in a state of advanced dementia. The post mortem revealed marked atrophy (shrinkage) of the brain along with peculiar microscopic findings such as plaque formation and "tangling" of neurons (nerve fibers). Dr. Alzheimer's picturesque description of his patient's brain is unequalled and since 1907 (the year of discovery) it has served as the ultimate diagnostic criterion of the disease. Hence the designation "Alzheimer's Disease."

From 1907 to the mid-1960s, the term "Alzheimer's disease" was restricted to an age range of approximately 40 to 65 and was, at least in later years, most commonly known as pre-senile dementia, because it occurred before the senium (old age). Pre-senile, or classical Alzheimer's dementia was (and still is) relatively uncommon.

On the other hand, we were well aware of a very common kind of mental deterioration found in old age. This was called "senile dementia," which we unquestionably attributed to hardening of the arteries of the brain. It just never occurred to us that senile dementia and pre-senile dementia might be the same condition occurring at different times of life.

Then came the seventies when British researchers (studying blood circulation in the brain) demonstrated that only a very small proportion (about 15 percent) of their demented elderly patients had any degree of "hardening," or narrowing of brain arteries. Furthermore, the majority at autopsy demonstrated the same plaques and nerve tangling described by Alzheimer many years before in pre-senile dementia. Could pre-senile and senile dementia then, be the same clinical condition? Subsequent American studies seemed to confirm this view (which serves to answer your question).

And so was coined in mid-1970 (mainly in U.S. and Canada) the term "senile dementia, Alzheimer type" (SDAT), denoting Alzheimer's dementia occurring at 65 or older. Later, for convenience, both the early and late varieties were lumped together as Alzheimer's disease. Such "lumped terminology" widened the overall age spectrum tremendously from 40 to 80 plus years.

This change in terminology, coupled with the current phenomenon of extended aging and its associated incidence of brain degeneration, answers the oft-repeated question, "Why are we hearing so much nowadays about Alzheimer's disease?"

Every year we admit to our service a hundred or more cases of advanced dementia (mainly Alzheimer's disease). And the number one concern of relatives is the same as yours, "How will we children fare?"

If your mother has no brothers or sisters affected, she is a "sporadic" case of SDAT. As her child, your chance of getting Alzheimer's disease is not much higher than for one without an affected parent. (But read in an upcoming column what recent genetic research on this subject suggests.)

The majority of our admissions are fortunately of this sporadic late kind of SDAT. But early Alzheimer's disease (under 65) seems to be on the increase with its greater sibling involvement and a higher than normal risk for Down's syndrome and certain malignancies of the blood and lymph glands.

And, finally, there's the devastating "familial" type running through many generations. Once considered quite rare, it too is seen nowadays more frequently (estimated to constitute about 10 percent of the Alzheimer's population). But this perceived increase may be due to our now better methods of diagnosis and a higher index of suspicion when taking the family history.

Addendum 1993: The "familial" type of Alzheimer's disease is the kind most often investigated in Alzheimer's research, as witness Duke University's lead scientist, neurologist Allen Roses, reportedly "scouring the globe" to find Alzheimer's families where two or more siblings developed the disease in later life. This long and painstaking research led to Roses' recent finding that a formerly known cholesterol-carrying protein called ApoE, important in the genesis of heart disease, also transports amyloid to the brain where, in time, the accumulated deposits may destroy certain areas of the brain subserving, e.g., memory, often the earliest function to be impaired in Alzheimer's disease. This "shared gene" finding has tremendous implications not only for the early detection of heart disease but for the early diagnosis of Alzheimer's disease as well and a more scientific rationale for its treatment.

We're Trying to Cope

Dear Dr. MacInnis:

We could see our 65-year-old mother going steadily downhill in her mind for about five years. Now she's totally confused, not able to dress herself properly or go to the toilet or eat by herself. She wanders aimlessly around the house most of the night and sleeps in fits and starts during the day. She doesn't recognize any of us. Just recently a doctor told us. "It's Alzheimer's disease," he said.

Thank God Dad's health is holding up. He not only nurses Mom but has to do all the housework, too.

We, the children (two of us), have our own families but we try to relieve Dad two or three times a week to give him a break for a few hours, otherwise he wouldn't be able to leave the house.

I often wonder how many families are trying to cope with this tragedy.

Mrs. A.N., California

Answer

There's an estimated four million cases of Alzheimer's disease in the United States and about 400,000 in Canada. The age range is roughly 40 to 90 plus, with the majority of cases occurring after 60.

Let me briefly describe the clinical picture of Alzheimer's disease. It begins in a slow, insidious way, most frequently with progressive memory loss. Over a period of years there is increased confusion, a marked narrowing of interests, and impaired judgment and insight in all aspects of intellectual function. In time, the patient reverts to infancy, requiring spoon feeding and diapering.

The cause is still unknown, but theories abound—the better known being (1) genetic, (2) infective (of so-called slow virus

59

origin), (3) immunological (where the patient's own immune system damages and ultimately destroys brain cells), (4) environmental (where extraneous substances like aluminum accumulate in the brain, (5) biochemical (where biochemical deficiencies adversely affect nerve messaging transmission in the brain), and (6) brain trauma, acute and chronic (a good example of the latter being "dementia pugilistica" or "punch drunk" syndrome frequently seen in older professional boxers from constant brain battering). Currently, the genetic theory is receiving the most attention.

I am frequently asked, "How do you diagnose Alzheimer's disease?" In the early stage, diagnosis is practically impossible. Here, such symptoms as memory loss and occasional confusion are not discernable to the observer although the patient may sense something wrong. Often a year or two may pass before it becomes obvious to the spouse, a family member, or a friend that "there's something wrong with Dad."

So what's happening to Dad, now age 60, who only three years ago held down a responsible executive position and was very much in control? It was his secretary who first noticed the change. He lost his drive, he couldn't concentrate or make decisions, and pondered needlessly over trifling matters. His interests narrowed. Once a meticulous dresser, he would often arrive at his office unshaven and carelessly dressed.

He stayed on the job for almost a year—thanks to a superefficient, understanding, and diplomatic secretary, who, sensing the "boss's" plight, carried his load without letting him be aware that he wasn't in charge any more!

At home, the change in year three was not so obvious as in the office, as his general intellectual capabilities were not so severely tested. What the family did note as year three progressed was that he lost interest in everything. He stopped reading the paper and watching TV. He would follow his wife around like a child, getting in her way and becoming irritated, even hostile and threatening, if reprimanded. He still went to the office.

It was about the end of year five that mental impairment began to accelerate with rapid deterioration of memory, orientation (ability to locate himself in time and place), and personality.

He dressed more slovenly, mismatched socks or more often put two socks on one foot—that sort of thing. He would insist on going down to the office, would often get lost on the way and would have to be brought back home.

By the end of year six his confusion worsened. He became practically unable to look after himself. He could still eat by himself after a fashion, and, as is usually the case at this stage, his appetite and physical condition remained robust. He looked well.

But soon after this he lost control of his bowels and bladder. At night he would pace the floor and would sometimes wander out and get lost. Special locks had to be put on all outside doors.

He is now in the state, Mrs. N., your mother is in and is looked after by a spouse, this time the wife. You ask if there's any hope at all in Alzheimer's disease. There is still no cure or treatment for it and the duration of life is from five to ten years after the disease has peaked. The younger the patient is at onset, the shorter the life expectancy, as a rule.

The majority of Alzheimer's patients are still at home looked after by a dedicated but understandingly harried spouse like your father working the "thirty six-hour day." If there's a supportive family (like yours), that's a bonus.

An Alzheimer's Society or support group is of inestimable help in a situation like this. A typical Alzheimer's support group consists of spouses, families, and concerned friends of Alzheimer's patients. The object of such a group is the provision of mutual support of its members. They learn everything they can about the disease, from providing social interaction with the patient as long as possible to preparing themselves to cope with the relentless downhill course that never fails.

So you see, the main function of this laudable society is one of group therapy, this time not for the afflicted but for those who suffer more—the spouses and families. There's one in nearly every city everywhere.

Your help is as close as your nearest Alzheimer's Society and the number is in your telephone book.

Come Fly with Us

An Alzheimer's Support Group Call to Action

Next autumn, when you see geese flying south in a V formation, you might be interested in the scientific explanation of why they fly that way.

As each bird flaps its wings, it creates an uplift for the bird immediately following. By flying in V formation, the flock can fly at least 71 percent farther than a bird flying on its own. People who share a common direction and sense of community can reach their destination quickly and easily because they share one another's energy.

A goose that falls out of formation suddenly experiences the drag and resistance of trying to go it alone. The goose quickly gets back into the group. If we have as much sense as that goose, we'll stay in formation and travel with others headed in the same direction.

When the lead goose tires, it rotates back in the wing and another goose flies point. It pays to take turns doing difficult jobs.

The geese at the back of the formation honk to encourage those up front to keep up their speed.

When a goose gets sick or is wounded by a gunshot and falls out of formation, two geese fall out with him and follow him down to help and protect him. They stay with him until he is able to fly or until he is dead. Then they launch out on their own to join another formation so they can catch up to their group. If we had the sense of the geese, we too would stand by another like they do. (From Alberta "Perspective," *Alzheimer's Newsletter,* Vol. 3, no. 4 [1992].)

The Doctor Suspects Alzheimer's Disease

Dear Dr. MacInnis:

My father, age 73 and a widower, is still active in politics. Over the past two years, I've noticed that although he's able to engage in light superficial conversation, he becomes confused, particularly when he speaks in public. He tends to wander in thought and sometimes doesn't bring a sentence to its logical conclusion—or just stops in "midair" as it were, forgetting what he was saying.

Is this just due to age, or could it be something more serious? I've watched this happening for about a year now and had hoped that it was just a temporary thing. But it's definitely getting worse and I'm beginning to think it's becoming noticeable in public.

When I mention it to him, he either denies it or has some sort of improbable explanation for it. He has given up reading and doesn't watch TV any more—not even the news that was once so important to him.

I got him to a physician on the pretence of an annual physical examination. The doctor suspects Alzheimer's disease. From what I've told you, can you give an opinion?

Mrs. E.L., Utah

Answer

I regret to say, I'm suspicious, too, based on your lucid description. Just about all of us past middle age experience mild memory problems, like forgetting names, faces, phone numbers, car parking, and the like. But don't let it bother you too much. By this chapter you're aware of these "normal" memory lapses because I mentioned them time after time; it's our old friend and bugbear, benign senescent forgetfulness (BSF).

But when such forgetfulness worsens and begins to interfere with one's way of life, something may indeed be wrong. Recent memory is often the first thing to go awry. And a good rule of thumb is this: If you forget, and you remember you've forgotten, that's normal. But if you forget, and it's plain that you don't remember you've forgotten, then you may be in trouble.

Often it's the spouse or a family member or a close friend, particularly one who has been absent for a while, who first sees the early change, and the change may be subtle, indeed. It would seem that the fine edge of his/her intellect is now dulled. A wife remembers it well: "At times he seemed like another person, but it was hard to put your finger on it, for just when I'd be sure I had a stranger in the house, he was back to his old self again." But such lucid spells are fleeting, and one thing we can be sure of—cognition (mental awareness) goes slowly, insidiously and relentlessly downhill.

People in public life and subject to public scrutiny, like your father, often show the first signs of brain deterioration on the speaker's rostrum, particularly when they attempt to speak without memory aids or "off the cuff." Here, mental lapses and errors in syntax may be painfully evident.

What I have briefly described are some of the early signs of senile dementia Alzheimer type (SDAT), a brain disease that afflicts from 5 to 10 percent of people around the age of 65 and to a lesser degree in the 40 to 60 age group, when it is known as pre-senile dementia.

Over the years I've written numerous columns on various aspects of Alzheimer's disease based on my day to day experiences with many patients in an advanced state of the illness. From their old hospital records and also from further interrogation of relatives, it was often possible to later discover some very *early* symptoms not considered significant by the doctor or relatives when the patient's initial history was taken.

Alzheimer's Disease: Is It Reversible?

Dear Dr. MacInnis:

The doctors diagnosed my husband, age 75, as having a dementia, specifically Alzheimer's disease. This was later confirmed in the hospital by a specialist. I am one of those people who never gives up, so when I was told by both that there was no chance for his getting better, it overwhelmed me, so I am writing to you as you have written a lot about dementias, including Alzheimer's disease. Is there, in your opinion, any chance of this being a "reversible" condition?

Mrs. T.A., Rochester, New York

Answer

I regret to tell you, Mrs. A., that Alzheimer's disease is not a reversible condition. Its progress is slowly but surely downward, and I believe you will have to accustom yourself, however difficult, with this gloomy outlook for the future. There are other chronic dementias, the best known being due to circulatory disease (brain or heart) called "multiinfarct" dementia, characterized by the development over time of multiple brain lesions causing "little strokes." While the progress of multi-infarct dementia may be erratic, with spells of relative stability and seemingly signs of improvement, the long term outlook is the same as Alzheimer's.

There was a time, only a few years ago, that great emphasis was placed on the "reversibility" of many dementias, and elaborate tests such as electrocardiagrams (ECGs), electroencephalograms (EEGs), and computerized tomography (CT) scans, etc., were recommended to "flush out" the so-called reversible dementias, and many doctors and clinics faithfully followed these recommendations. In our own department of two hundred beds we found in a period of over two years, that most of the dementias, regardless of cause, showed no evidence of reversibility on our screening program. So we first modified and later discarded screening as being nonproductive in the light of good clinical observation.

It is now generally conceded that reversible dementias are much fewer than originally thought. Dr. A. Mark Clarfield,* one time head of geriatric medicine at McGill University Medical School in Montreal, critically reviewed thirty-two studies investigating the causes of dementia. It was found that 13.2 percent were *potentially* reversible but in eleven of these studies where the patients were followed up, "only 8 percent had partial reversal and 3 percent showed complete reversal." But even in some of these apparently "reversible" cases, additional follow-up showed symptoms of further decline in cognition (mental awareness).

---

*Now director of academic affairs, Sarah Herzog Hospital, Jerusalem, Israel.

So the widely touted screening program to detect potentially reversible dementias is now considered in most cases to be unnecessary and was the principal subject at the annual meeting of the American Geriatric Society in 1989.

A suggested routine workup for reversible dementias is now much toned down. The emphasis is on a good clinical history and physical examination along with simply performed tests like thyroid, B_{12}, folate, SMA_{12}, and sometimes specialized (imaging) tests in particular cases.

In our department of psychogeriatrics we admit yearly over a hundred cases of dementia of which 75 percent are Alzheimer's disease. For over two years we routinely performed B_{12} tests in the hope of discovering a reversible dementia that could be successfully treated with vitamin B_{12}. Since our quest proved fruitless we discontinued this screening program.

As before mentioned, a thorough history repeated periodically and coupled with a careful physical examination with good follow-up can provide a diagnosis of Alzheimer's disease 75 percent of the time, in our experience. Dementias in the remaining 25 percent can usually be diagnostically resolved over time.

Alzheimer's Disease: A Strongly Inherited Genetic Disorder

The most important evidence ever that Alzheimer's disease is a strongly inherited genetic disorder was published in the May 1987 issue of *Archives of General Psychiatry*.

The study, conducted by researchers at the Mount Sinai School of Medicine in New York City, and the Bronx Veterans Administrative Medical Center, also in New York, establishes Alzheimer's to be among the most prevalent of genetic diseases.

The scientists found that the risk for developing Alzheimer's disease is four to five times greater in first-degree relatives (parents, children, brothers, and sisters) of Alzheimer's patients than for people without immediate relatives with the disease.

The data strongly suggests the presence of a "relatively common dominant, autosomal [non-sex linked] gene for late Alzheimer's disease, *the expression of which is delayed until old age, but is largely complete by 90 years of age when the risk among first degree relatives approximates 50 percent."* Put another way, the study suggests that by age 90, half of the first-degree relatives of people with late-onset Alzheimer's disease would themselves be stricken with the disease.

"The major reason," they explained, "why many Alzheimer's patients have not had close relatives with the disease may be that those relatives who had inherited the genetic predisposition died of other causes before developing the disease."

Although there has been evidence that *early-onset* (before 60) Alzheimer's disease suggests that autosomal-dominant inheritance carries a 50 percent risk for first degree relatives (familial Alzheimer's), this is the first study to suggest a similar risk for relatives of late-onset Alzheimer's patients, the common so called sporadic type that we thought, up to recently, just "popped out of the blue." Now it would seem that both kinds, the familial (incidence 10 percent) and our common sporadic variety, share the same genetic background.

One of the most frequently asked questions by relatives is, "Why is there so much Alzheimer's disease around now?" Everybody seems to know someone with it or has a relative with it. The main reason is the tremendous increase in our life expectancy at birth, from 47 years around the turn of the century to over 75 years in the 1990s. Our "aging" (70 to 80 year olds) are now living on to become our "aged" (80 plus) with our 85 year olds the fastest growing segment of our population! And all this sets the stage for that time programmed (late) Alzheimer's gene to emerge as a full-blown disease.

Aspects of Alzheimer's Disease: Three Letters

Dear Dr. MacInnis:
You write a lot about Alzheimer's disease. My husband has just been diagnosed as having it. As he is still very much aware of what's going on, I am wondering if he should be told and what do you think would be his reaction?
Mrs. L.K., Toronto, Ontario

Answer

Another way of putting your question is to ask whether or not Alzheimer's patients are aware of their condition, and the answer would depend on what stage of the disease the patient is in. You state that he's still aware of things but you do not elaborate. I therefore can only answer in a very general way. In the early stage of the disease when cognition (intellectual awareness) is fairly well preserved, the patient may be very well aware of his memory problems and may have thought of Alzheimer's even before the family did! (There are studies verifying this very point.)

I believe that in such circumstances, the patient should be told. Whether it would apply in your husband's case is something that would have to be decided between you and his doctor.

Dear Dr. MacInnis:

What is the best treatment for Alzheimer's disease? My wife, age 65, is in the early stage and, although she suffers a serious memory disorder, can look after herself and enjoys company.

Mr. L.Y., Rochester, New York

Answer

There is no specific treatment for Alzheimer's disease but there are medications that are effective in controlling behaviour problems like anxiousness and agitation, and psychiatric symptoms, such as delusions, depression, and hallucinations that are sometimes present in the later stages. Your wife does not appear to have such secondary symptoms so your main challenge is to maintain her quality of life at her present level for as long as possible.

To achieve this goal, it is important to maintain her physical health by periodic medical examinations with particular attention to her nutrition and special senses, such as vision and hearing. You say your wife enjoys company. This is a positive sign that should be cultivated further by lots of recreational and social activities.

Dear Dr. MacInnis:

My husband, age 72, came down with Alzheimer's disease four years ago and has now become very suspicious and paranoid. For instance, he accuses me of infidelity and other members of the family and several neighbours of conspiring to steal some of his possessions. He can become quite angry about this. Should I ask my doctor to send him to a psychiatrist for a consultation. Is there treatment for this?

Mrs. M.M.

Answer

As mentioned above to another reader, psychiatric symptoms such as hallucinations and paranoid delusions can occur in some cases of Alzheimer's disease, especially in the more advanced stage. Why it occurs in some cases and not in others, we don't know. An attractive hypothesis is that a person who has a tendency to be suspicious and mildly paranoid in "normal" life can usually get by without problems as the paranoid tendencies are normally repressed. In Alzheimer's disease these repressed tendencies are "let loose" and a full-fledged paranoid state can develop.

Your husband should see a psychiatrist in consultation, as there is medication available that might help.

1990 Update on Incidence of Alzheimer's Disease

Studies done in the mid-1970s estimated that there were approximately 2,500,000 older people with Alzheimer's disease in the United States and about 300,000 in Canada. These were the figures we've used until recently. Now a group of scientists supported by the National Institute on Aging (NIA) have conducted an in-depth study of Alzheimer's disease in one community suggesting that these figures represent the tip of the iceberg.

In the November 10, 1989, issue of the *Journal of the American Medical Association*, Denis Evans, M.D., and colleagues at

Brigham and Women's Hospital in Boston, Massachusets, report their findings of the prevalence of dementia in the community of East Boston. Overall, the investigators found that 10.3 percent of people over 65 had what they termed "probable" Alzheimer's disease. This figure is as high as previous estimates for Alzheimer's disease *in addition to all other causes of dementia in the elderly.*

In 1982, Dr. Evans and his co-workers began their study of older people living in East Boston, a well-defined, stable working class community. Since that time, more than 2,800 residents over age 65 have participated in a study that included a questionnaire concerning medical and social problems, a brief memory test, and, for 467 individuals, an extensive medical evaluation to rule out the presence of conditions other than Alzheimer's disease.

In addition to their overall findings, the researchers found the prevalence of Alzheimer's disease to be 18.7 percent in the 75 to 84 age group and a striking 47.2 percent over age 85—a figure nearly twice previous estimates.

According to Dr. Zaven Khachaturian, NIA associate director for Neuroscience and Neuropsychology of Aging, these data call into question the estimates for Alzheimer's cases in the U.S. "Given Dr. Evans' data coupled with Census Bureau estimates for the numbers of people 85 and older, the actual number of Alzheimer's cases in the U.S. might be close to four million," says Dr. Khachaturian (400,000 in Canada).

What does this mean for the future? "Since the numbers of people over age 85 are the fastest growing segment of the population, there could be as many as fourteen million Americans with Alzheimer's disease by the middle of the twenty-first century," said Dr. Khachaturian. (About half the current population of Canada!) "Also, the lifestyle will result in an even greater proportion of people living in extreme old age than the census data predict, meaning even higher numbers of Alzheimer's patients in the next century."

The East Boston study is unique in several respects. First of all, the investigators focused on people living in their own homes or with family, where some four-fifths of all dementia patients are thought to live. They also examined large numbers of older people, including people who had little or no obvious memory problems. "As a result, these estimates might lay the groundwork for developing the most accurate picture of Alzheimer's disease in the population to date," stated Dr. Khachaturian.

According to Richard Gehring, chairman of the Alzheimer Association (U.S.), "This study confirms the growing magnitude of Alzheimer's disease as a major public health problem and emphasizes that both public and private sectors of our society must place a higher priority on research into finding a cure and treatment."

This work was supported by research funds from the National Institute on Aging, a component of the National Institute of Health. (My special thanks to the National Institute on Aging *"News Notes."*)

Outlook in Alzheimer's Disease

Dear Dr. MacInnis:

My husband, age 70, has recently been diagnosed as having a "mild case of Alzheimer's disease," with symptoms of poor memory and difficulty finding words to express himself, also trouble with names. He sometimes gets lost driving in unfamiliar territory. Some of his co-workers tell me they see a decline in his work performance at the office (he is a male secretary). As he doesn't seem to have got worse over the past year, should I expect him to go gradually downhill as the doctors predicted?

Mrs. K.L., Los Angeles, California

Answer

I would be extremely hard pressed to make a *definite* diagnosis of Alzheimer's disease at such an early stage simply because there are age-related conditions that can mimic some of his symptoms.

According to the classification I use, your husband would rate about a 3 on a scale of 1 to 7, and I would classify him as having *possible* Alzheimer's disease and would wait and see how things progress.

Should you expect him to proceed downhill from here? It's a hard question to answer, particularly since his symptoms have remained static for the past year. I can report that Dr. Reisberg, whose Global Deterioration Scale is widely used in diagnosis, noted that about 85 percent of patients in grade 3 (where I classify your husband) experience no serious deterioration in cognition (awareness) and general mental function after three to four years (from Michael A. Jenike, *Geriatric Psychiatry and Psychopharmacology,* [Year Book Publishers, 1989]).

Early Alzheimer's Patients May Benefit from Memory Training

Dear Dr. MacInnis:

I have a question about Alzheimer's disease. My husband, age 72, has been diagnosed as having what the neurologist called "early" Alzheimer's. For the past two years or so his memory has been getting worse but he has no other serious symptoms.

My question: Is there any value in trying to improve his recall by mental stimulation? Can it be done at home?

Mrs. B.C., California

Answer

Contrary to general medical opinion there is evidence that early Alzheimer's patients can, in many cases, benefit from memory training.

In the July/August 1991 issue of the *American Journal of Alzheimer's Care and Related Disorders & Research,* there is an excellent article on this subject written by Sharon M. Arkin, M.Ed., a certified clinical mental health counsellor of Fort Wayne, Indiana. The article is unusual in that Ms. Arkin's mother (with "probable Alzheimer's") contributed substantially to the author's optimistic observations and predictions.

The purpose of the article was "to encourage caregivers and treatment providers of early Alzheimer's patients to try various memory stimulation strategies since, the article will show, some patients do benefit cognitively, emotionally, and psychologically from the cooperative effort" (from abstract of article).

Space restrictions do not permit me to adequately review this in-depth study of the current literature. So my advice to you, Mrs. C., is to get a copy of the article from your local Alzheimer society.

If the journal named above is not available locally than I would strongly recommend that they and every other Alzheimer society and support group write to the *American Journal of Alzheimer's Care and Related Diseases & Research,* Circulation Department, 470 Boston Post Road, Weston, Massachusetts 02193 for information on individual and institutional subscription rates for this outstanding journal.

Behaviour Problems in Alzheimer's Disease

Dear Dr. MacInnis:

My mother, age 60, has Alzheimer's disease and we are still caring for her at home. She has serious behaviour problems such as spells of shouting and wandering, sometimes out of the house at night. One doctor prescribed chlorpromazine (brand name Largactil), but this made her so sleepy during the daytime that she suffered many falls. Another put her on haloperidol (brand name Haldol) which subdued the yelling but had no effect on her wandering.

We are getting pretty well to the "end of our tether" and would appreciate your opinion on the use of these drugs or any others that in your long experience with Alzheimer's disease might be of help.

Mrs. M.H., Owen Sound, Ontario

Answer

You seem to be living the caregiver's "thirty-six-hour day" with Alzheimer's disease in its late stage. Apart from fecal incontinence there's probably no more exasperating strain on the family than those shouting periods throughout the night. This is often the final straw, wherein the family reluctantly decides on a nursing home.

In my opinion, chlorpromazine has little or no place in the management of behaviour problems, such as wandering and shouting that occur sometimes in Alzheimer's disease. The dose required for control of shouting would be so high that the well-known side effects (dry mouth, constipation, and urinary hold-up) would be overwhelming and totally impractical. The same would apply to wandering, which so often occurs at night. (You have found that out for yourself.) I have found that chlorpromazine in extremely small dosage, e.g., 10 milligrams at bedtime to be a good "sleeping pill" for the elderly. In that dosage the side effects are minimal as well as dependency. Unfortunately, what applies to the normal older patient is not usually effective in advanced Alzheimer's disease but could be tried for sleep in the early stage.

One of the better drugs for behaviour problems in the demented elderly (and younger folk) is haloperidol. The trouble with haloperidol is that it is prescribed as a catchall for everything, making it the most widely prescribed neuroleptic drug in medical practice. But it is not a good *sedative* and should never be used as such. So when not much sedation is necessary and control of shouting and/or aggressive behaviour is the goal, then haloperidol can be a very useful drug. For instance, 2 milligrams of haloperidol is equivalent to 100 milligrams of chlorpromazine as a neuroleptic and while it may control aberrant behaviour (in that relatively small dose) the patient usually remains alert. In the aged, I would recommend as little as 0.5 milligram of haloperidol three times daily (to minimize any possible side effects).

There's another neuroleptic I would like to mention that has all the good qualities of haloperidol but fewer side effects. It's called loxapine (brand name Loxapac). It is a good drug for patients of all ages suffering from aggressive and disordered behaviour, hallucinations, delusions, and paranoid thinking. Like haloperidol, it is classed as a "high potency" neuroleptic but as aforementioned, produces milder extrapyramidal side effects (such as muscle stiffness and rigidity as seen in Parkinson's disease).

I have no magic potion for night wandering in Alzheimer's disease. What we have tried with moderate success was keeping the patients awake during daytime hours (sometimes a formidable task) so as to make them tired and more amenable to sleep at night. Here's where a tranquilizer like chlorpromazine in 10-milligram bedtime dose might be helpful as adjunct therapy.

The Aluminum Link?

Dear Dr. MacInnis:

I have been reading a lot about Alzheimer's disease lately and there seems to be the feeling that ingesting aluminum may be the cause (or one of the causes) of this dreadful condition. I know you have written on Alzheimer's many times, but I can't recall that you ever mentioned anything about aluminum being involved. What is your opinion?

Also, does Alzheimer's disease run in families?

Mrs. M.Y., Ontario

Answer

You're right. I've written many columns on Alzheimer's disease—much more than on any other topic. That's because I head a large hospital department that admits about a hundred Alzheimer's patients every year. Another reason is that the disease is age related, with the highest incidence in the 75-plus age group. But younger people succumb, too. The youngest patient with Alzheimer's disease admitted to our service was 42 years old. This is by no means a record, for there are many authentic diagnoses of Alzheimer's patients in their 30's.

Does Alzheimer's disease run in families? Yes, indeed. Anyone who sees large numbers of demented patients soon becomes aware of this. I can recall admitting four brothers in the course of about five years—all of whom came down with Alzheimer's around the age of 60. Another two brothers who were diagnosed in their mid-50s exhibited strikingly similar abnormal patterns of behaviour. It's apparent that the earlier the onset, the more rapid the mental decline with global dementia pretty well complete after three to four years. This is in contrast to a much longer decline period (average ten years) in the more common late onset variety. The genetic background of the so-called younger familial Alzheimer's disease is now well established. This I have alluded to in many previous columns.

The "aluminum connection" is a favourite topic calculated to drive a Tupperware saleslady into conniption fits! Anytime I give a lecture on Alzheimer's I can expect to be asked, "Do we throw away our aluminum pots and pans and anti-acids and underarm deodorants?" (both contain aluminum salts), and I'm never disappointed. My short answer to the question is, "No, nothing as drastic as that." I used to give the pat answer, "The presence of abnormal deposits of aluminum in the brains of Alzheimer's patients is not the *cause* but probably an *effect* of Alzheimer's disease." But the latest research published in 1993 in the British scientific journal, *Nature,* casts doubt on this so-called link between Alzheimer's disease and the presence of aluminum in the brain.

The Oxford University scientists headed by Dr. Frank Watts concluded that earlier findings of aluminum in the brain tissue of Alzheimer's patients most likely resulted from contamination by the stains used to test for the metal.

The researchers used a highly sensitive technique known as high voltage nuclear microscopy to examine post-mortem brain tissue from five Alzheimer's patients. Although some traces of aluminum were detected, similar levels were found in tissue from patients without Alzheimer's disease.

Said Dr. Watts, "We now believe that previous evidence that aluminum is involved in causing Alzheimer's disease should be reviewed to take into account probable contamination of tissue by aluminum compounds present in most reagents."

Is There a Lab Test for Alzheimer's Disease?

Dear Dr. MacInnis:

My mother developed Alzheimer's disease at the early age of 55 and died seven years later. I have read that early onset Alzheimer's in a parent places adult children at risk. My questions: (1) Is there an accurate early test that can discover the presence of Alzheimer's disease before any of the usual symptoms occur? (2) If there is no such test currently available, what are the chances of its development in the near future? I am 40 years old and healthy.

Mrs. A.B., Ottawa, Ontario

Answer

Alzheimer's disease is popularly ingrained in the public mind as an "old person's" malady. While the prevalence increases with age (averaging over 40 percent in the 80 to 85 age group) it is not at all uncommon in early middle life. Indeed, Dr. Alzheimer first reported the condition in 1907 in a 51-year-old woman.

You're right. Early onset Alzheimer's disease (the so called pre-senile dementia) occurring before the senium (old age) definitely runs in families and often happens relatively early. Far more common, of course, is the better known senile dementia Alzheimer's type that occurs in later years. This, too, places relatives at risk for Alzheimer's, but they will more than likely succumb to another disease before reaching the "Alzheimer's age."

You ask if there is a reliable (sure-fire) test available to detect Alzheimer's disease in people at risk like yourself. Unfortunately, my short answer now will have to be no. But there's hope, if not right around the corner, I hope maybe a block or so away!

There are several tests nearing their final stage of development, but to answer your question I will mention those that may probably turn out to be the most practical and definitive ones. One is called the "Ala-50" test being developed by Dr.

Peter Davies and co-workers at the Albert Einstein College of Medicine, Bronx, New York.

Basically, Ala-50 is an antibody that detects a protein that is virtually present only in the brains of Alzheimer's patients. In other words, it reacts very strongly with the brain tissue of those patients but hardly at all with that from normal persons. There is good scientific evidence that this abnormal protein occurs very early in the course of Alzheimer's disease. Another somewhat similar test has been developed by Abbott Laboratories, where Alzheimer's disease associated proteins (ADAP) specific to Alzheimer's disease can be detected.

Of great practical and clinical significance is that most of the Alzheimer's disease patients being tested have Ala-50 and ADAP in their spinal fluid, inciting hope that someday soon we'll have a simple spinal fluid test to detect the presence of Alzheimer's disease before the onset of even early symptoms for which, I hope, we'll have preventive treatment.

Are There Good Drugs for Alzheimer's Disease?

Dear Dr. MacInnis:

My wife has had Alzheimer's disease for five years now. Every once in a while a new drug for treating Alzheimer's is announced in the press with great fanfare but as time goes on we hear less and less about it until it fades away with the rest of them. Over the years specialists who saw my wife always had information on some "new drug" that always was "coming out soon" and, again, that was the end of it. I do recall a drug called "THA", for short, which was highly touted in prestigious medical publications as the be-all and end-all of treatment that went into disfavour for many reasons, not the least being that it proved to be very toxic on the kidneys and, as I understand it, was put on the back burner by the FDA, which has so often been accused of being too strict in releasing drugs to the public. This time I think it did the right thing.

The reason for my long diatribe is that after five years, my wife has still not received any treatment, even on an experimental basis, for her Alzheimer's symptoms. I saw in the paper recently where another new drug called linopirine was undergoing trials in this country to determine its usefulness in improving memory. I presume this drug, if anyways effective, would only be so in early Alzheimer's where memory loss is usually the first problem.

I wonder if you could briefly bring me up to date on the question of these so-called Alzheimer's drugs? Over the years I've read a lot about them (for obvious reasons) but it would seem I am more confused (and pessimistic) than ever.

Mr. R.Y., California

Answer

You're not alone in your confusion. Thousands of Alzheimer's spouses, relatives, and friends (and frequently Alzheimer's support groups) are well aware of your predicament. I know of several support groups that are constantly warning their members to be very wary about those so-called "breakthroughs," but that is not to say they would be adverse to participating in any drug research if given the opportunity.

Although not as specific as you, Mr. Y., many readers ask if there is a drug that cures Alzheimer's disease, or if there is a good drug on the market that helps.

My usual answer is that there is, as yet, no cure for Alzheimer's, although we often use drugs to manage its sometimes bothersome behaviour problems, such as noisiness and striking out, and prescribe psychiatric drugs for depression and delusions that are often part of the picture.

You speak of THA (tetrahydroaminoacridine). The THA story is a long and sorry one that does no credit to its original researchers. The FDA had been agonizing over this drug for five years and in March, 1991, their advisory committee, after reviewing the finding of long clinical trials, was "unable to make a recommendation" presumably because of its well-known toxicity in the face of arguable memory enhancement. In December, 1991, the FDA announced that it would make THA available (now known as tacrine HCL and marketed as Cognex by Warner-Lambert) under one of its treatment programs to eventually

3,000 more patients (on higher dosage than in the large clinical study, where the FDA's lower dosage was disputed by the families of the participants). Now the Alzheimer's families will be able to evaluate the drug publicly. So, if nothing else, this demonstrates democracy in action—even in research!

Most of the forefront drugs currently in Alzheimer's research are those that have demonstrated the ability to enhance memory by turning up the volume of certain brain chemicals like acetylcholine, dopamine, and serotonin. Examples of such drugs are tacrine (Cognex) and linopirine, the latter nearing the end of its clinical trials and reporting "interesting" results. And then there's a hormone called pregnenolone produced in the body, which was discovered in the forties and was used to treat arthritis; this hormone has recently been found to have the ability to help neurons (brain nerves) to form new connections and enhance their chemical and electrical activities, thus apparently improving memory, learning, and even general health. Another hormone, called "nerve growth factor" (deficient in Alzheimer's disease), is undergoing trials in Sweden with initial "remarkable" results.

My Husband Is Getting Short-Tempered

Dear Dr. MacInnis:

I have a question. My husband has Alzheimer's disease. He is able to get around by holding on to chairs and walls. In the last couple of weeks he's been real short-tempered. He gets provoked easily and then starts to throw things around. He picks on the great-grandchildren, and I'm afraid they won't come over to see us anymore.

Is there anything we could give him to calm down his nerves? We now belong to the Access Program that has become available in our county and that has given me some help. I get a sitter to come and stay with him so I can get out. I sure hope help comes soon for all people with Alzheimer's disease.

Mrs. J.B., Williamson, New York

Answer

This short plaintive note speaks eloquently, not for the victim of Alzheimer's disease but for the one who suffers more, this time the harried spouse through whose window you can catch a glimpse of her "thirty-six-hour day."

Mrs. B, one of the common problems of Alzheimer's disease is the temper flare-up often associated with noisy and destructive behaviour. Usually the episode soon blows over, only to repeat itself time and time again. It's no wonder you ask for "something to calm his nerves." My long experience with Alzheimer's disease has convinced me that although there is no cure for it, a great deal can be done to alleviate some of its well-known symptoms. The medication I have found most useful for the behaviour symptoms of Alzheimer's disease, such as angry outbursts and striking out, is haloperidol. You do not state your husband's age but if he is up in years, say 75 or 80, I would suggest a small dose of 0.5 to 1 milligram by mouth two or three times a day. This drug will calm him without oversedating him, which is important, as I gather from your letter that he is quite frail.

I am glad you are getting some help from the Access Program. If your husband does not have a personal doctor, I suggest that you ask Access to recommend one who is conversant with Alzheimer's disease.

Finally, I suggest that you contact your nearest Alzheimer's society or support group for more help I feel you so desperately need.

Delirium in an Aged Patient

Dear Dr. MacInnis:

My mother, age 80, is a patient in a chronic care hospital. One evening during visiting hours, I noticed that she had become very restless and apprehensive and appeared confused. The nurse was called and found her temperature to be 102, which she said was very high for a person Mother's age. The doctor diagnosed

her condition "delirium" as a result of the fever. The cause of the
fever was pneumonia. She only partly recovered and is now a
chronic invalid. My question: What is delirium and is it common?

Mrs. N.H., Sun City, California

Answer

It's too bad the time honored term "acute confusional state"
has given way to "delirium," which in my opinion is not nearly
as descriptive.

Delirium has been described as a sudden change in cognition or mental awareness in a patient, especially an elderly one,
and is one of the earliest and most sensitive signs of a serious
impending or actual acute illness. You describe some of the
symptoms accurately and infection is only one of several causes.

In "A Prospective Study of Delirium in Hospitalized Elderly
Patients" (*Journal of the American Medical Association* 263
[1990] 1097–1101): researchers at the University of Pittsburgh,
studied delirium in 229 people. Here are the commonest causes
in this population: (1) fluid and electrolyte imbalance, (2) infection, (3) drug toxicity, and (4) metabolic disturbances (from such
causes as low or high blood sugar and uremia). Patients with
advanced dementia, such as Alzheimer's disease, are particularly susceptible to delirium, which amounts to an acute confusional state superimposed on a dementia (chronic confusional
state).

I recall many times being called at night by a concerned
nurse reporting that "there's something wrong with Mrs. X."
We all knew that there was indeed something wrong with Mrs.
X. She had Alzheimer's disease! But what the nurse was telling
me, in effect, was that Mrs. X. had departed from the "normal"
Alzheimer's course and was exhibiting signs of delirium. That's
what was "wrong" with Mrs. X.

Delirium is often followed by progressive mental decline, as
illustrated in your mother's case. In severe cases the mortality
is high—not from delirium, but from the illness causing it.

Alzheimer's Research Update (1993)

Beta-amyloid protein continued to play a leading role in Alzheimer's research in 1993. Readers will recall that large deposits of this sticky, gluelike protein have been consistently found in the brains of Alzheimer's patients and indeed is the main ingredient of the well-known brain "plaques" that, along with nerve "tangles," still serve as the hallmark of diagnosis since first described by Dr. Alzheimer in 1907. Although we have long known that these protein deposits destroy brain cells subserving memory and awareness, the mystery has always been how did it accumulate there and why is it more prevalent there in some people than others? Another question comes to mind. Where did it come from in the first place? Much has been written on this subject, which I've reported numerous times in these columns. Briefly, let me say that most Alzheimer's scientists have felt that the source of beta-amyloid is from the abnormal breakdown of a so called precursor protein and a great deal of research has been currently devoted to understanding this precursor breakdown and preventing it with a drug that might do away with beta-amyloid and possibly Alzheimer's disease.

But in June of 1993 this precursor amyloid research was put on the back burner, at least temporarily, by the startling discovery of Dr. Allen Roses, leading Alzheimer's researcher at Duke University Medical Center in Durham, North Carolina. Dr. Roses, a brilliant scientist with maverick tendencies, who has often been at odds with mainstream Alzheimer's research, announced that his laboratory had located the approximate site of a suspect gene in families with *late-onset* Alzheimer's. They discovered that this particular gene was located in the same region as a gene or genes already known for the production of a protein called Apo E, whose sole job, it was always thought, was to shuttle cholesterol in and out of cells and tissues. But Roses' research revealed that it also transports amyloid to the brain where in time it can accumulate, clogging brain arteries and causing brain-cell destruction.

The extent that amyloid is transported to the brain depends on the number of genes directing the production of Apo E. Researchers have found that the genes involved in Apo E production come in three varieties, E_2, E_3, and E_4. Everyone has two of the genes—one from each parent. For example, the Roses' group and others have found that persons with two E_4 genes are eight times more at risk for developing Alzheimer's disease than people with a pair of E_3 genes. It should be pointed out that not all people with two E_4 genes come down with Alzheimer's disease nor do all Alzheimer's patients necessarily have an E_4 gene. However, the genetic correlation is striking enough to spark a rush of activity in this new area of research, for it could very well lead to the development of a good diagnostic test* enabling doctors to identify at least some patients who are virtually certain to come down with Alzheimer's disease in their later years. And more than that—having two copies of the E_4 gene was also linked to people developing the disease at an *early* age, the so-called presenile dementia. In a recent (August 1993) interview, Dr. Roses declared, "It looks like virtually all will develop it [Alzheimer's] by the age of 80 if they have two copies" (of the E_4 gene).

Dr. Roses and his Duke University researchers did gene testing on 234 members of 42 families where at least one family

---

*According to Dr. Judes Poirier, Associate Director, McGill (University) Centre for Studies in Aging, "No reliable test exists today [1994] which can determine if an individual will develop Alzheimer's Disease." Dr. Poirier is a co-discoverer of a genetic test that demonstrates possible relationship between the presence of the Apo E_4 gene and sporadic Alzheimer's disease. Scientists are now working to develop a more reliable predictive test for Alzheimer's disease.

To date (August 1994) Alzheimer research seems to indicate that if a person is carrying the E_4 gene from *both* parents, he/she runs a very high chance of developing Alzheimer's disease between ages sixty and sixty-five. If the individual is just carrying *one* E_4 gene from a parent, his/her chance of developing Alzheimer's disease is apparently delayed for about ten years, i.e. after age seventy. But as Dr. Poirier points out, the absence of the E_4 gene does not rule out Alzheimer's disease appearing in late life. In fact up to 20 percent of people with *no* E_4 gene will still develop Alzheimer's disease. Research continues. (My thanks to Dr. Poirier and Alzheimer's Canada for this information.)

member had late-onset Alzheimer's disease. The disease was diagnosed in 95 members and 139 were unaffected.

Dr. Zaven Khachaturian, a director of Alzheimer's research at the National Institute of Aging, said that this new genetic development "has caused a great deal of excitement among Alzheimer's researchers because it links the disease with a specific gene factor. We may be able to screen for this [Alzheimer's] and be able to make judgments about whether a person's likelihood of getting the disease is high or low or early or late," Dr. Khachaturian said.

Suggested Reference Literature for Caregivers on Alzheimer's and Related Diseases.

Donna Cohen, and Carl Eisdorfer, *The Loss of Self: A Family Resource for the Care of AD & Related Disorders* (New York: NAL Penguin, 1986.)

Lori Kocia, and Myrna Schiff, *Alzheimer: A Canadian Family Resource Guide* (Scarborough, Ontario: Mc-Graw Hill Ryerson, 1989).

Miriam K. Ironstone (ed.), *Understanding Alzheimer's Disease* (New York: Scribner's and Chicago: A.D. & Related Disorders Assn.).

Nancy L. Mace, and Peter V. Rabins, *The 36-Hour Day: A Family Guide to Caring for Persons with Alzheimer's Disease and Related Dementing Illnesses* (Baltimore: The Johns Hopkins University Press, 1991).

On General Caregiving

Howard Gruetzner, M.Ed. *Alzheimer's—a Caregiver's Guide and Source Book* (New York: John Wiley, 1992).

Chapter 6
Depression in the Elderly

Major depression is uncommon in otherwise healthy seniors living in the community—about one half that found in younger age groups. But in institutions the prevalence is much higher, ranging from 12 to 45 percent in two recent studies. What particularly besets the aged is a milder, more chronic depressive state, often the extension of loneliness suffered from a myriad of losses. Here the aging patient reflects on a happier past while resenting the present and dreading the future. In the United States, where the elderly (over 65) comprise about 12 percent of the population, they account for 25 percent of all suicides, with the rate for elderly white men four times the national average and twice that of elderly women.

I have included in this chapter two ancillary columns, one on the grief of bereavement, the other on suicide pacts, both of which evoked an unusual number of reader responses.

Depression Questionnaire

Dear Dr. MacInnis:

I recall that some years ago you printed a questionnaire on mental depression. If the answer was yes to most of them, the chances you were severely depressed and required treatment. I was one of those who answered yes to all of them. I received anti-depression treatment from my doctor and in a month felt fine and chucked the pills for good over a year ago.

I believe many readers would benefit from that questionnaire again as well as an article on depression in later life. Many thanks.

Mrs. M.E. (65)

Answer

Do you wake up early and can't get back to sleep?
Do you feel "real down" in the morning as well as fatigued?
Do you fear the future?
Are you preoccupied with past "sins"?
Have you become irritable?

These questions are just for a start. If your answer is yes to the majority of them, then take a good look in the mirror.

Is that face you see haggard and wan?
Has it forgotten how to smile?
Are you losing weight because you don't care about eating anymore?
Do you feel sometimes that life is not worth living like this?
Do you find it hard or impossible to laugh?
Are you secretly hostile to those who do laugh and joke and are having a good time?
Are you worried about your waning sex life?
Do you have trouble making everyday simple decisions?

The above are some of the manifestations of depressive illness common to all ages. A note of caution: Don't "diagnose" yourself on the basis of just a few isolated *yes* responses. You must answer *yes* to at least five or more of the thirteen questions. Then seek medical help.

Depression is far commoner in the elderly than in any other age group. And in many cases it expresses itself differently because it's most commonly associated with loss—loss of spouse, close friends, and relatives; loss of self-worth, and dignity, and personal possessions; and not the least, loss of good health. And add to this retirement (with loss of livelihood), particularly when retirement was compulsory and unplanned.

Depression in the elderly is characterized more by apathy than by the intense sadness often seen in younger folks. It has been described as "failure to thrive" in an emotional sense.

Fatigue is a common symptom of depression at any age. However, in the older person it may be attributed to "just old age," and the patient goes without treatment and further down-hill. So if an old person looks unhappy, it's often attributed to getting old.

Remember that the fatigue of depression is *worse* in the morning, while the fatigue of physical illness is *improved* in the morning (after a restorative sleep). Depressional fatigue is often accompanied by a sickly feeling in the pit of the stomach that makes the sight of food unattractive.

It might be unwise to make a diagnosis of depression in the face of bereavement and its attendant grief. In uncomplicated grief, the intense symptoms gradually abate and disappear in a matter a months. But occasionally it goes on and on to a state of "chronic grief" that, unfortunately, in some cases responds poorly to medication.

Alcoholism, nowadays a common affliction of the elderly, sometimes signals a depression, particularly if unexplained heavy drinking begins in later life.

Depression: Is It Different in Old People?

Depression in the elderly differs in some respects from that seen in younger age groups. Before discussing the older patient, let me enumerate some of the main manifestations of depression regardless of age. There are two main classification of symptoms: (1) *Vegetative or biological symptoms*—Examples: Loss of appetite and weight, difficulty in concentrating, pervading sadness, no joy in anything, loss of sexual interest, early morning awakening, constipation, severe agitation or the opposite, mental sluggishness; (2) *Psychological (in the head) symptoms*—Examples: Psychomotor (mind and body) slowness, feelings of guilt, low self-esteem, and suicide preoccupation.

If 50 percent or more of these problems are present, the patient should seek medical attention because we may be dealing with a *major depression*.

As I have often mentioned, elderly depressed patients frequently confront the doctor with bodily complaints, such as bowel troubles, headaches, low back pains, sexual or genital problems—just about anything but what they really came in for. The discerning doctor, when approached in this way by an elderly patient, immediately thinks of depression and gradually zeros in by asking pointed questions: Has the patient ever had problems with sleeping, appetite, sadness—indeed, anything listed above? And on receiving a positive response, lets the second shoe drop: Does the patient think he or she is sad and lonely? Does he or she feel that life is worth living? In most cases the depressed elderly patient is relieved to be given the opportunity to discuss his or her innermost thoughts and leaves happy in the thought that the doctor has made a diagnosis and something good will come out of it.

How common is depression in the elderly? Very common, indeed. European studies report a prevalence rate of 2 to 10 percent, and in one Swedish investigation gave an estimate of a lifetime risk of 8.5 percent for men and 17.7 percent for women up to the age of 80. In other studies, women showed higher rates for depression than men in all age groups below 65, after which the incidence in men tends to approach that in women and, in some cases, surpass it. The incidence of depression in chronic hospitals and other old age institutions is very much higher than that found in the community.

In this column our elderly patient is suffering from what is known as a major depression (referred to previously). This being so, I will have no problem advising antidepressant drug treatment. The reason? I have only two drugs to choose from, both relatively free of bothersome side effects such as dry mouth, blurring of vision, slowing of urinary flow, constipation, and fast heart beat. These side effects are exceedingly common in the elderly and, as I remarked previously, they handle them poorly. My first choice is fluoxetine (brand name Prozac). It has few of the bothersome side effects listed above and the daily dosage for an elderly patient is usually no more than one capsule (20 milligrams). In my experience, 10 milligrams (a half-capsule) diluted in fruit juice is usually sufficient and results in practically no side effects, such as nausea, headache, insomnia, and anxiety (reported at higher dosage). In most cases of major depression fluoxetine may begin working in two weeks. (I always prescribe it in the morning to minimize possible insomnia.)

My second choice is trazadone (brand name Desyrel), which like fluoxetine has few side effects except times of rather severe sedation which can pose a problem in aged patients. The initial dosage is 50 milligrams and the maintenance may go up as high as 200 milligrams daily.

Prozac: Is It Okay?

Dear Dr. MacInnis:

I have been taking an antidepressant drug called Prozac for over two months and am happy to say that my depression, which was considered by my doctor (psychiatrist) a major one, has completely cleared up. I could sense the improvement as early as three weeks after treatment.

I am disturbed by reports that Prozac patients have had some serious side effects, such as severe irritability and, in a number of cases, increased suicidal thoughts, with one case where the patient has taken the manufacturer to court. I would hate to see it taken off the market, for it did for me what no other antidepressant could do in the past—make me well again and that in short order. In your opinion, could it become unavailable?

Mrs. H.L., Avon, New York.

Answer

First of all there are some very positive things about Prozac. Over two million depressed patients (many like yourself) have been treated to date with this drug with no serious side effects except in a relatively small number of cases that you mention. It may owe its success to a profile of action different to that of other "depression pills": (1) It has generally fewer side effects than others; (2) it is, at least, just as effective as other antidepressants; and (3) the effective dose is only one pill a day. (This is very important for patient compliance.)

The celebrated case you mention (now before the courts) involves a female patient who within two weeks of starting Prozac showed irritability and assaultiveness to the point where she violently attacked her doctor, developed a suicide obsession (six attempts without previous history), and practiced self mutilation. Some other cases of suicidal ideation while on Prozac (but apparently not caused by depression) have recently been reported. (It should be remembered that suicidal ideation is often an element in major depressive illness.)

Re—your question: In my opinion, Prozac will continue to be available.

Exogenous Depression

Dear Dr. MacInnis:

My father (72) is a widower living alone. He recently lost all his savings due to the failure of a financial institution. He is quite depressed and is not responding to medication. In fact the medication, if anything, has made him worse due to the side effects. Is there anything else in the way of treatment available?

Mrs. J.K., Edmonton, Alberta

Answer

In two recent columns on depression, I mentioned two distinct types. The first is *endogenous* (coming from within) with no rational cause. The patient may be a millionaire, but he *knows* he's a pauper. He's also certain that there's no hope for him, and no amount of reasoning, cajoling, or counselling will change his mind. However, endogenous depression usually responds very well to anti-depressant medication. The second is *exogenous* (coming from without) depression. Here the cause is explainable and rational. It may follow bereavement (particularly of a spouse) or, as in your father's case, a financial loss.

A patient suffering from an exogenous depression usually responds poorly, if at all, to any form of medical therapy, for pills will not bring back a loved one or replace the loss of financial security.

I should point out here that an exogenous depression (like your father's) occasionally contains an endogenous element that may respond to antidepressant medication. In this case, a trial of anti-depressant medication would be helpful, if combined with skilful psychotherapy.

In most cases of exogenous depression, time is the all important member of the treatment team. Unfortunately, however, exogenous depression from a severe financial reversal in an elderly person carries a definite suicide risk and should be viewed seriously.

Specialists in suicide-prevention programs strongly advise against the overoptimistic you've-nothing-to-worry-about approach, because the patient, just to get rid of you, may act cheerful. The practitioner must always indicate by word and deed a strong empathy with the patient's mood. Only then will the patient emerge from his shell of despair and listen. This is what I meant by "skillful" psychotherapy.

To be helped, your father needs this special management and he should not live alone.

My Husband Is Strangely Sad

Dear Dr. MacInnis:

What are the main symptoms of depression? My husband is 66 years of age and appears to be depressed. Once an outward-going person, he is now strangely sad and does not show his usual sense of humor. His only complaint is fatigue, but I know he has lost his appetite and I have a strong feeling that he's depressed over the death of a dear friend recently. Have you an opinion?

Mrs. F.N., Ontario

Answer

If I can assume there's no physical or medical condition causing fatigue and loss of appetite, you may be on the right track. Depressed elderly people seldom come right out and say, "Doctor, I'm depressed." More often than not they will complain of symptoms such as fatigue, vague pains, or insomnia. If this arouses a suspicion of depression, and it should, the doctor follows up on it paying attention to body language, which can sometimes be quite revealing. The face is sad, the speech is slow, monotonic, and often devoid of personality.

At the appropriate time the physician can ask a few pointed questions such as, "Do things look gloomy to you?", "Do you find it difficult to smile?", etc., and then the clincher, "Do you feel you are depressed?" Nearly always the depressed patient will answer "yes."

Some doctors practice an elaborate ritual for "wringing a confession." My advice to you, the spouse, is to fill in the doctor privately with your suspicions so that he may gauge the patient's "body language" when confronted with possible causes. And there are many of them: living alone, recent financial loss, grief from loss of a friend (as in your husband's case), and forced retirement—just to name a few.

Diagnosing depression is not always a difficult task. It has often been said that if you let the patient talk long enough he or she will make the diagnosis for you. Probably in no area of medical practice can a doctor-patient encounter be so productive. And it must be thus, because there are no specific examinations, outside of psychological testing, to aid the doctor in diagnosis.

The Legacy of Loss

In my previous column I listed the more important symptoms of depression common to all age groups. Such mood disorders are characterized by marked loss of interest in anything pleasurable—food, work, sex, friends, hobbies, entertainment, and the like.

In the elderly the stress of loss is the prime motivation for depression. Common life stresses cited are death of a loved one (spouse or a close friend), failing health, dependency, loss of security, income and status, and sometimes a change of environment (from home to nursing home).

There are manifestations of depression peculiar to the elderly: apathy rather than sadness; fatigue (with special reference to body organs); confusion, hopelessness, "all is lost," and "hand-wringing" agitation are all more pronounced than in younger people.

Not infrequently the elderly depressed person voices only bodily complaints. Here's where the patient seeks medical help from a roster of caregivers and risks the chance of receiving over time a multitude of drugs for target symptoms, e.g., laxatives, sleeping tablets, pain pills, etc., which are not only useless but may intensify the depression. Such a patient may *act* demented, sometimes risking a diagnosis of Alzheimer's disease.

But the discerning practitioner (with always a high suspicion index for elderly depression) will question the patient specifically (see a previous column) and literally, in a few minutes, can either rule out or (more frequently) make a positive diagnosis of depression and treat accordingly, usually with success, for the old respond to antidepressants just like younger people. This is always a rewarding medical outcome for both patient and physician.

As I stated above, depressive illness in the elderly can be roughly divided into two groups: (1) exogenous or situational depression from something that's happened externally or "outside," and (2) endogenous depression, where there's no discernable "outside" reason but is caused from something chemical, mysteriously operating from "within."

An example of exogenous or situational depression is that caused by material loss of some kind (person or property), where an elderly person often suffering from a recent bereavement is transferred to a nursing home. In a situational depression like this, the treatment is not an anti-depressant drug but copious doses of social interaction on the part of family, nurses, doctor, social worker, and institutional clergy. It is a difficult but often rewarding challenge.

An example of endogenous (within) depression is where a wealthy man with everything in material comforts is totally convinced he is a pauper dying from some lethal disease. Though completely illogical, it can result in a devastating depression, which, if left untreated, can lead to suicide. Fortunately, endogenous depression in the majority of cases is eminently treatable with anti-depressant drugs.

But there can be exceptions—when a serious suicidal depression does not respond at all to drugs and psychotherapy and is fast regressing; or when the patient (usually elderly) steadfastly refuses and fights against all offered medication and nutrition, literally starving himself to death, a case of slow suicide.

These exceptions, in my view, call for immediate psychiatric consultation and intervention for lifesaving electroshock therapy (EST).

EST for an 85 Year Old

Dear Dr. MacInnis:

What is your opinion on giving electroshock treatment to an 85-year-old man suffering from severe depression? My father became so depressed when he was told he had cancer of the rectum that he lost all zest for living. He stopped eating and would only drink when he was forced to. The doctor had him admitted to hospital where he received anti-depressant medication without any benefit. The doctor referred him to a psychiatrist, who recommended a course of electroshock to bring him out of "slow suicide" from self-imposed starvation. As I write this they are feeding him by tube, getting him nutritionally prepared for the treatment. Please answer as soon as possible.

Mrs. M.Y., Toronto, Ontario

Answer

I answered Mrs. Y.'s letter by return mail and the following is an edited version of my reply. Unlike the state of affairs a decade or so ago when electroshock therapy (EST) was administered for just about everything with dubious or negative results in many cases, it is now mainly restricted to acute depression where there is a real potential for suicide. (Morbid postpartum depression and rigid catatonic states are two other indications for emergency EST.)

In such emergency situations time is of the essence and should not be wasted awaiting days or weeks for medication results. Here, electroshock therapy can be virtually lifesaving. Recently on my hospital service, an 84-year-old depressed male went on a hunger strike "to end it all" and was literally snatched from suicide in four treatments. He lived to age 90, enjoying a good quality of life.

I am convinced that many deaths from suicide could have been averted by the prompt intervention of EST. Anti-depressant pills and psychotherapy have their place but not for a morbidly depressed patient with a gun to his head.

I believe that your father's depression is being well handled and he should improve, as my patient did.

In a future column I will have the opportunity of dealing with EST and particularly EST in the elderly in more detail with all its indications and contraindications.

I'm against EST—It's a Barbarous Relic of the Past

Dear Dr. MacInnis:

I take strong issue against your glowing remarks about electroshock treatment for depression in the elderly. My father, age 76, came down with what was diagnosed as "depression and confusional state." After his first treatment he became further confused, but despite this, the doctors continued EST every second day for six more, since he became unmanageable. He's worse than ever now. Despite that "successful outcome" of yours (whatever you mean by "successful"), I maintain that EST is a barbarous relic of medical history and should be banned by law. It is not fit for any age, let alone a 78 year old.

Mrs. L.L., Ontario

Answer

Your story is so sketchy that it's difficult if not impossible to mentally visualize your father's clinical state when he received EST. If, as you say, he was both depressed and confused, then I'm not surprised he was more confused after treatment! This is because temporary confusion is a common side effect of EST, particularly in the elderly.

You refer, Mrs. L., to my "successful case." He was an 84-year-old severely depressed man who absolutely refused to eat a morsel of food or a drop of water and resisted gastric and intravenous feeding. He chose the path of slow suicide by starvation. Two weeks of anti-depressant medication was unsuccessful. After four EST treatments his depression lifted. As I said in that column, "He lived to age 90, enjoying a good quality of life." That, Mrs. L., is what I mean by the term "successful."

But as the saying goes, "One robin does not make a summer." Neither does one successful outcome constitute a panacea for depression in the elderly.

In my previous column on EST for morbid suicidal depression in the very old, I alluded to, but didn't comment on, numerous reports now appearing in the literature where EST has been lifesaving. In the July, 1990, issue of the *Journal of the American Geriatrics Society* there's an article titled "Electro-convulsive Therapy in Octogenarians," where thirty-nine patients all over 80 who received EST were compared to the results obtained with forty-two patients between 65 and 80. The studies were conducted in the section of Geriatrics, University of Miami School of Medicine, Miami, Florida, and presented at the annual meeting of the American Geriatrics Society, Boston, Massachusetts, May, 1987.

Without going into detail, there was "a somewhat less successful outcome in the 80 plus age group than in 65 to 80 year olds. As well, patients in the older group (80 plus) "had significantly more cardiovascular complications than their younger fellow patients."

To quote the conclusion of this trial: "This study confirms the role of EST as a relatively safe and *effective* treatment in *selected* depressed older patients. ('Selected' meant those in which medical treatment failed, where there was an adverse effect from medication, and where there was suicidal ideation and/or refusal to eat.) Prospective studies are needed to understand better the long term outcome and the morbidity and mortality in this frail high risk older group" (over 80).

To sum up: Despite the higher mortality and morbidity (illness) risk in very old, frail, elderly patients, I believe that in selected situations (cited above), EST should be tried for the compelling reason that there is yet no alternative therapy for the management of suicidal depression.

When He Felt His Best, He Took His Life

Dear Dr. MacInnis:

I know it is now too late to give advice, but I thought I would tell my story anyway in the hope it may be of help to others.

Two years ago my husband, age 56, came down with a major depression. The principal anti-depressant drug was amitriptyline, and it seemed to help him at the beginning as he began to improve. During a period when he was feeling his best, he took an overdose of the very drug that was helping him (amitriptyline) which killed him.

I hope that this experience with a major depression will serve as a warning that a depressed person can commit suicide when it's least expected, and anti-depressant medication should never be self-dispensed.

Mrs. L.H., Ontario

Answer

Thank you, Mrs. H., for that excellent advice from your personal tragedy.

It's a well known fact that a patient in the throes of a major depression may think of suicide, but is so retarded physically and mentally that he doesn't have the ambition to pull it off. But when recovering, the person's decision-making ability is improved, enabling him to go through with it.

It is important that patients suffering from a major depression be treated in a hospital, preferably on a one-to-one basis where the nursing attendants are fully aware of and prepared to deal with sudden changes in mood.

Side Effects of Anti-Depressants

Dear Dr. MacInnis:

My husband, age 66, was diagnosed as a severe case of depression. He was first prescribed Elavil, but he had to discontinue it because of severe side effects, namely, constipation, dry mouth, and urinary problems. More recently he was prescribed a drug called doxepin, which doesn't cause as much mouth dryness but makes him very sleepy. Do you know of any medication he could use that doesn't have such side effects? Both these drugs helped his depression but the cure is sometimes worse than the disease.

Mrs. M.E., Vancouver, B.C.

Answer

If I were asked what is the most prevalent reason for elderly depressed patients quitting their medication, I would, without hesitation, say the so-called anticholinergic side effects, some of which you mention. To dry mouth, constipation, and slowness of urination let me add blurred vision and a racing heart. These are the *external* or *peripheral* side effects. Now add to these the *central* side effects (arising from the brain)—delirium, confusion, impaired thinking, and excessive sleepiness—and the reader will have some idea why the depressed patient, especially the older patient, will often chuck it, even though the drug may be helping.

Clearly, your husband should see his doctor again, who will prescribe an antidepressant with minimal anticholinergic side effects. Two drugs come to mind. The first is trazadone (brand name Desyrel). This drug has few anticholinergic effects but strong sedative action, which may be acceptable if your husband has insomnia. The second drug has all the advantages of Desyrel without its sedative effect. It's called fluoxetine (brand name Prozac). The dose is 10 to 20 milligrams once a day and should be given in the morning.

It's Not a Pretty Tale

Dear Dr. MacInnis:

I have hesitated to write this letter as it is not a pretty tale. Early this year my mother died after a lingering illness. The day after the funeral, my dad killed himself. Dad was a devoted husband and all during Mom's last illness was a source of strength to us all. Even on the day of her death, he was under complete control—or so it seemed—much better than the rest of us. We were totally unprepared for this, as there were no telltale signs. Was there was nothing we could have done to prevent it?

Mrs. T.Y., California

Answer

As you tell it, Mrs. Y., I can assure you that there was nothing you or anyone could have done to prevent this tragedy. I have seen one case where the male spouse was so totally engaged in caring for his wife over many years that soon after her death he found his life devoid of responsibility and purpose and so ended it. This may have played a part in your father's case, but it's only speculation and the fact remains that you could not have read the future.

It is a grim statistic that the elderly (65 plus) make up 12 percent of the population but account for 25 percent of the suicides, a figure that is bound to increase with their ever-growing life expectancy. (Male suicide rates rise steadily with age and peak in the 80s; female rates peak between 55 and 65 years.)

Hopelessness, born of depression, is the main cause of suicide in old people. Many elderly people, particularly in large cities, live a lonely existence. I have often stated that when these people awaken in the morning, they look around and realize correctly that the world about them couldn't care a damn whether they got up or stayed all day in bed. Add to this, the long litany of losses expounded in previous columns, and we have all the ingredients of depressive illness.

Suicide pacts between elderly couples are becoming more frequent. Here's an actual scenario: The husband nursing his invalid wife who is totally dependent on him is himself stricken by a stroke that renders him also an invalid. So they make a pact in which death from a pistol shot is sure-fire and lethal. Other methods might be too chancy.

"Pretty tales" these are not, Mrs. Y. But it's happening out there and, however indelicate, it must be addressed. We're getting so conditioned to well-meant geriatric platitudes like the "Golden Years," the "Good Life," and the "Best Years" that we're blinded to that darker side in which many of the old, the lonely, and the depressed impatiently wait out what little time is left.

Home Alone

Dear Dr. MacInnis:

I feel I need help and I thought you could give it to me. It all started with spinal arthritis and I have become very depressed. I am 88 years of age and my walking has become affected to the point I'm afraid of falling. I haven't been outside all winter. I have thought of hiring someone to go out with me. I need an arm to hang on to.

All my relations and friends have died (from old age) and I'm alone in this apartment. I miss my two sisters who lived here in Toronto, as I spent a great deal of time with them but they are now both dead.

I am on Surgam (for arthritis) 300 milligrams, but I take it only when things get really bad. Should I take it every day?

I'm not getting enough sleep. It seems when I wake up, all I look forward to is "Meals on Wheels," and then I spend the rest of my time trying to get to sleep again.

What can I do to change the situation?

Sincerely,
Mrs. O.B., Toronto, Ontario

Answer

I get the impression, Mrs. B., from "reading between the lines" that you have been, and indeed are now, a very sociable person longing for companionship that doesn't come your way any more. Many of the elderly, secluded and frail, tell me (as you do) that their only daily company they depend on is their Meals on Wheels friends and they thank God for them!

Even though you are obviously depressed, you offer one glimmer of hope and that is in your intention of securing some help for getting out regularly for short walks and fresh air. You might ask your Meals on Wheels friends to arrange for a volunteer group to contact you. Failing this, and if you can afford it, hire someone yourself, as you have mentioned.

What many people like yourself have found comfort in is a cat or a small dog. In your case perhaps a cat would be preferable as it would not need to be walked and will always remain a constant and loyal companion.

As for your Surgam, I believe you should take it at least daily if you find it is effective. I suggest that you have someone take you to a physician who can sort various things out for you, including help for your depressed feeling. A start on a better life can begin right there for you.

The Four Stages of Grieving

Dear Dr. MacInnis:

I am a widow of only three months. Now that I see it in writing I still cannot believe it's me—that I'm the widow! A friend who is also widowed tells me that I am going through the normal grieving process and at present I'm still in the "disbelief" stage. When I asked her how long this stage lasts, she replied, "You think it never ends but it will." Some friends are encouraging me to get out, take a trip to "get away from it all," sell the house, and rent an apartment, etc., etc. But it's no use. I'm sure of that.

Most of the time I feel my mind is leaving me. I'm in terrible conflict. I still expect him to come in to the house any time, even though I know it's an irrational thought. But I can't help it. Please tell me if this is normal grieving and what does the future hold? I am 55 years old. My husband of the same age died suddenly from a heart attack.

Mrs. G.H., California

Answer

Your widowed friend is right, Mrs. H. You are in the first stage of your grief process—the stage of shock and denial. This was evident at the church, funeral, and grave services where you could be best described as a disembodied person watching yourself attend these functions for a bereaved friend but your husband never a part of it. That is why you often feel he didn't die and will return any day.

The second stage in the grieving process is that of anger and depression. Some surviving spouses in this stage often take it out on the doctors and nurses who are felt in some way to have been responsible for the death. Religious people may feel angry with God whom they feel "could have spared him." Even the deceased may not escape her anger, for in dying he's left a spouse defeated, dejected, and alone. This is also the stage of physical fatigue, bordering on exhaustion and probably explains why the grieving person simply cannot follow the advice of well-meaning friends. This again is normal.

After a variable period of time, three or four weeks perhaps, occasionally longer, the bereaved spouse enters the third stage—that of guilt. Here she feels that if she had done this or not done that on the day of his fatal heart attack, things would have been different. Maybe she should have talked him into staying home. Or if he died alone without her at the bedside, her self-censure could be overwhelming. Again normal.

The fourth and final grieving stage is that of acceptance of her spouse's death as a fact of life, for isn't death just an end of "life's final common path"? This in no way means that she's forgetting or has forgotten him. It simply indicates that she's getting to the stage where she feels as though life can and must go on without him, and she must necessarily adapt to this entirely new way of life where there will, at last, be a beckoning light at the end of the long dark tunnel.

This is the stage when I would advise a change of scenery, perhaps a short journey with an agreeable, understanding travelling companion. It also could be the appropriate time for rescheduling of new life activities.

But don't sell your house. Not yet. Grief counsellors tell us that life's big decisions (e.g., selling your home) should be deferred by the widow until two years after the death of her husband. This two-year time span is a rough rule of thumb in estimating the ultimate boundaries of the grieving process. These stages are never demarcated; instead, they insidiously meld into one another.

In rare instances grieving may be prolonged, languishing in the early stages of shock and denial. Here, professional counselling may be indicated.

(Note: The four stages of grieving, first described by Ida Anger, a Chicago United Charities social worker, are similar to Elizabeth Kubler-Ross's well-known stages in the dying process.)

Dear Dr. MacInnis:

Nine months ago I lost my husband after fifty-eight years of marriage. I am 81 and live alone. Most times I manage very well but once in a while I will awaken at night and start to cry and I can't seem to stop. It can go on for several days and nights. The only thing that helps is a sleeping pill. After these bouts I feel physically exhausted for a number of days. People tell me that time will heal, but it doesn't seem to help me much. I find it hard to talk about it. I can't discuss it with the family.

Is this abnormal? If so, should I seek medical help?

Mrs. D.P.

Answer

It's been truly said, Mrs. P., that the death of a spouse is the most traumatic emotional blow this world can inflict, for you lose not only a spouse but a lover, a companion and a friend, as well. It's hard to conceive that after fifty-eight years, such a void can even be partly filled, that your grief will ever abate. But in most cases it will and indeed, you're showing hopeful signs of recovery. I don't think you're seriously depressed, but you should see a doctor or a counsellor, or both, to help ease your burden and tide you over those dark hours of sleeplessness that leave you so miserable for the rest of the day. You're doing well by yourself but you need the added help of your family and friends.

A Happy Ending to a Long, Severe, Chronic Depression

Dear Dr. MacInnis:

Today in our Rochester (New York) Democrat & Chronicle, I saw a letter from the wife of a 61-year-old man about his experience. I'm 67 years old. My recent bout with depression has been helped considerably by Pamelor (nortriptyline)—10 milligrams at each meal and 20 milligrams at bedtime, a total of 50 milligrams a day. The only side effect I experience is dry mouth and I certainly can live with that when I consider the agony of the alternative—continually asking myself "Why am I here?" "Why don't my children and grandchildren call me?" "Nobody cares," "I might as well be dead," etc.

For the dry mouth I carry ice water to my work and chew sugarless gum quite often. In addition to alleviating the dry-mouth feeling, the moisture and increased saliva help keep my teeth and gums healthy. And guess what? I have now fewer problems with my previous stress incontinence. Also, I can now sleep. My depression and anxiety gave me much more mental confusion than any I might experience with Pamelor.

I feel like a person again! Yes, I am fortunate that the first medication my doctor prescribed worked for me. Also, I have learned that my many bouts with hysteria over the past fifty years have, in fact, been symptoms of depression.

You are in a unique position of telling your readers that there is a life beyond depression and that we are not weak characters just because our neurotransmitters (chemical messengers) don't always function correctly.

Mrs. D.S.M., Rochester, New York

Answer

Mrs. M.'s letter differs from my ordinary run of mail in that it's from a person admittedly previously depressed and who is now evidencing marked improvement, thanks to a wise (and perhaps fortunate) choice of anti-depressant medication by her doctor—something that Mrs. M is most thankful for. Contrary to popular belief, one antidepressant is *not* "just as good as another." That's because no two depressed patients behave the same. From Mrs. M's vivid portrayal of her pre-treatment, anguished thoughts, it's possible to discern a marked anxiety state along with insomnia. Since most tricyclic (anti-depressant) drugs might be equally effective in lifting the depression, it's a question of selecting one that has the least side effects. Nortriptyline (brand name Pamelor) has moderate sedative effects which would allay anxiety and help her insomnia.

More importantly, its side effects (dry mouth, constipation, urinary retention, blurred vision, and fast heart rate) are classified as "moderate." Mrs. M. reported that her previous stress incontinence was benefitted—and this from the usually undesirable side effect of urine slow-down from the antidepressant pill. Put another way, she's getting not only direct benefit from the antidepressive medication (lifting of her depression) but from one of its well known and usually bothersome urinary side effects!

I get the impression that Mrs. M. has suffered through the years from a recurrent chronic depression and has only recently received appropriate treatment for it with gratifying results. Now that she sees for herself "there's a life beyond depression," I would wish her the best and entreat her to follow well her doctor's guidance.

Anyone reading Mrs. M.'s letter will be impressed with her all-pervading optimism. She "treats" her constantly disagreeable dry mouth by sucking ice and chewing gum and even finding therein some positive feeling—they "help keep my teeth and gums healthy."

And to you readers who may be burdened with depression as Mrs. M. once was and are simply trying to "bear it through," take heed of her words, that it took her nearly a lifetime to learn that there *is* help out there for all of you.

Chapter 7

Disorders of Brain Circulation in the Elderly

Because the brain, especially the aging brain, is exquisitely sensitive to minute changes in its blood circulation, symptoms of brain failure can attack with dramatic suddenness from the mild and transient "dizzy spell" to the devastating onslaught of a hemorrhagic stroke.

Stroke can be roughly divided into two categories: (1) where the brain gets too much blood, as in cerebral hemorrhage, and (2) where it doesn't get enough, as in cerebral ischemia—a term meaning literally "anemia of the brain."

Over the past decade or so, the incidence, morbidity, and mortality of stroke has been steadily declining, thanks to better preventive measures and improved diagnostic methods like CT scans and other imaging techniques, enabling us to make an early and more definite diagnosis where medical or surgical intervention is most beneficial.

In this chapter I have attempted to describe some varieties of ischemic stroke such as the so-called transient ischemic attack (TIAs) where surgery has made a notable breakthrough in preventing a "completed" stroke, and where current advances have been made in anticoagulant preventive stroke therapy. In this respect, stroke prevention is following the lead of heart attack prevention.

For want of a better "home," I have included in this chapter two columns dealing with the pesky problems of "falls" precipitated by (amongst other things) postural changes affecting the brain circulation.

Stroke: Can We Predict the Outcome?

Stroke is the third major cause of death in the developed world. For those who survive, the majority face nursing home chronic care for the remainder of their lives. But we all know of people who recover well enough to resume their former occupations.

Is there any way to predict with some measure of certainty the outcome of a stroke? This is the first question put to the attending doctor by distraught relatives.

When a stroke hits with catastrophic ferocity as in brain hemorrhage, there is little room for optimism. The same applies to a sudden cerebral thrombosis (blood clot in a brain artery) accompanied by deep coma.

But these are exceptional modes of onset. Stroke presents itself many ways. Commonly, consciousness may be only slightly impaired. A speech problem severe at first may improve and sometimes completely clears up. But it also may get worse. The same applies to limb movements. Stroke is predominantly a disease of advancing age with the "aging" (65 to 79) usually faring better than the "aged" (80 plus).

With so many variations in presenting signs and symptoms, how then can the physician come up with a prognosis (medical outcome)? Unfortunately, this can never be done with certainty. Experienced doctors have, however, learned to be fairly good predictors by observing their patient's progress (or lack thereof) in the first few weeks of illness.

As medical school teaching on stroke prognosis is often fragmentary, I'm pleased to report on a scientifically conducted study addressing this important aspect of clinical assessment.

Researchers at the University College Hospital, London, England, have come up with an excellent compilation of early signs and symptoms having a bearing on prognosis. Their study titled "Who Goes Home? Predictive Factors in Stroke Recovery" was published in the January 1985 issue of the *Journal of Neurology, Neurosurgery and Psychiatry*.

The study involved 172 stroke patients. Of the 82 men and 90 women, 13 percent were between 45 to 60; 60 percent were in the 61 to 80 range and 27 percent were 80 plus.

They determined the significant clinical findings in the first two weeks of stroke and correlated them with the outcome after one year.

What second-week signs predicted a good outcome in one year? A high level of consciousness, normal speech, absence of visual disturbances, a positive mood, verbal learning ability, presence of isolated limb movements, presence of touch and joint position sense, upper limb sensory motor coordination (touching finger to nose blinded), ability to appreciate distance and space, and ability to perform personal and domestic activities.

And what second-week signs predicted a poor outcome in one year? Confusion, incontinence, perseveration (repetitious uttering of the same word or group of words), lack of tone in muscles, swelling of affected hand and/or foot, and pain in the shoulder.

Other variables predicting a good outcome were living with a partner, numerous social contacts, and previous independence. Signifying poor outcome was advanced age (over 80) and a stroke occurring during sleep.

Surprisingly, the authors found that "the amount of physiotherapy during the first two weeks . . . was not significantly related to outcome." However, from the sixth week onward, such treatment "became highly significant" in physical rehabilitation. And "motivation towards treatment was very significantly related to outcome at all stages."

Say "Stroke" and Be Done with It!

Dear Dr. MacInnis:

The doctor tells me my mother, age 75, has cerebrovascular disease. I wonder why he doesn't say "stroke" and be done with it! About a year ago she came down with paralysis on the right side, involving the arm and leg. Thanks to physiotherapy she's now able to get around with the aid of a walker and is able to feed herself. Would you please briefly discuss stroke. Can it be prevented? Does it run in families? What are the important risk factors?

Mr. B.M., New York

Answer

The term "cerebrovascular disease" refers to disorders of the blood vessels (usually arteries) supplying blood to the brain. Such an artery may fill up with plaque or blood clot, or both, much like a coronary (heart) artery does. And just as blockage of a coronary artery deprives heart muscle of life sustaining nourishment (blood), so may a blockage of a brain artery cause damage to brain cells. We are now dealing with a stroke from which, depending on the extent of brain damage, the patient may recover, be permanently paralyzed, or may die. Stroke also occurs when an artery ruptures and bleeds into a vital area of the brain. Commonly known as "brain hemorrhage," this is nearly always due to high blood pressure and the mortality rate is high. Chronic auricular fibrillation may cause "embolic" stroke.

Can a stroke be prevented? To answer this we must consider the risk factors concerned with stroke. Risk factors are the same as for heart disease. High blood pressure is perhaps the most important risk factor, especially for brain hemorrhage (hemorrhagic stroke). In addition, persons who drink alcohol excessively, are overweight, or have diabetes are at increased risk for developing stroke. So keeping your blood pressure and weight under control as well as making other changes in your lifestyle may help to prevent stroke. But despite a marked reduction in incidence, stroke still remains the third leading cause of death. Being male is also a risk factor for stroke, since it affects one and a half times as many men as women.

Transient Ischemic Attack (TIA)

Dear Dr. MacInnis:

I was diagnosed as having a "transient ischemic attack" about six months ago. The night I had my "little stroke," my speech became garbled, as I can best describe it. I was taken to the emergency and was immediately referred to a neurologist who confirmed the diagnosis of TIA.

He suggested one Entrophen (an acetylsalicylic acid [ASA] preparation) 325 milligrams once a day but did not order tests. He said, "If you were my mother, I would also say no to tests." I am 81 years old. My speech is not affected at the present time.

Do you think this will be progressive? I will appreciate your opinion.

Mrs. M.A., Penticton, B.C.

Answer

Transient ischemic attack (TIA), as the name suggests, is a stroke-like attack lasting from a few minutes to several hours (but less than twenty-four hours).

The patient may experience one or more of a number of subjective sensations, such as mental confusion, dizziness or clumsiness, or exhibit transient weakness or numbness in the face or an extremity, difficulty in speaking (garbled as you say) and in understanding speech, transient blindness in *one* eye, and other symptoms too numerous to mention here. It is sometimes called a "ministroke" because of its brief duration and is caused by a *temporary* loss of blood supply to a part of the brain (usually that supplied by the carotid artery system in either side of the neck). It can be regarded as a warning of an oncoming full-fledged stroke unless prompt treatment in instituted. TIAs can afflict people as young as 30, but it ordinarily happens to the middle-aged and elderly. Various clinical and special X-ray examinations of the carotid arteries help in the diagnosis but some of the tests (you make mention of them) can be of high risk in the elderly (especially 80 plus). This is why the neurologist spoke to you as he did.

You received prompt and apparently effective treatment with Entrophen (ASA) that helps prevent blood clots or "sludge" in your carotid arteries, considered to be a major cause of TIA.

Aspirin versus Warfarin for Stroke Prevention

Dear Dr. MacInnis:

My husband, 77, has been taking 2 milligrams of warfarin (blood thinner) every day for the past three years. This was prescribed after he suffered a stroke.

We are hearing a lot these days about aspirin being used to ward off heart attacks and strokes. I am wondering if it would be of value switching from warfarin to aspirin.

In your opinion, what are the merits of warfarin over aspirin or vice versa? I often wonder about the advisability of being on warfarin for long periods?

Mrs. T.L.

Answer

I must tell you, Mrs. L., before I write another word that I cannot give your husband specific advice regarding his treatment. Only his personal physician can do that. You do, however, ask a question of wide general interest and, as usual, I will answer it in a general way for the information of all readers.

One of the many dilemmas constantly besetting physicians is when to terminate anticoagulant (warfarin) treatment for stroke or coronary prevention, especially when the patient has remained free from attack and there have been no side effects. The patient's attitude is understandable. In effect it is, "Look, I'm doing fine; I haven't had another stroke; why stop it and risk another attack?" But the doctor may be having increasing difficulty maintaining blood thinning at a safe level. And if the patient is up in years, another dimension of danger is added. Frequently it has to be stopped.

Although the value of long-term blood thinning for the prevention of deep vein clots in the legs and lungs is well established, the same cannot with certainty be said about stroke prevention. Nevertheless, warfarin is often given, especially for the first few months after a stroke. And if it is not terminated in a certain time—pre-arranged by the doctor and made known to the patient at the beginning of the blood-thinning program—then it stands an excellent chance of being continued indefinitely (as in Mr. L.'s case). If there are no side effects and the patient is doing well, both patient and doctor are psychologically entrapped. And who can blame them? But the dilemma is always the doctor's—to stop or not to stop.

In the past decade, ASA (aspirin) has been extensively studied for its well-known blood-thinning effect. It does this by acting on the blood platelets (involved in clotting) by preventing them from sticking together and building up a clot in a brain artery leading in time to a stroke, or a clot in a coronary artery leading in time to a heart attack. Prevention of blood clotting is the rationale for using blood thinning agents, be it accomplished by heparin, warfarin, or aspirin.

(There's still some question about the "effective" daily dose of aspirin necessary to help prevent recurrent strokes and heart attacks. Dosages ranging from three tablets a day (975 milligrams) to a half "baby aspirin" (40 milligrams) daily, have been advocated. From a perusal of the current literature, I find a swing toward the middle road, i.e., one aspirin (325 milligrams) daily.

If warfarin is used in the long-term management of stroke, and the patient is easily controlled by regular prothrombin estimations (ideally maintained at 1.5 times normal) and if the patient is happy and the doctor is happy there's no good reason to discontinue warfarin and switch to aspirin. But if problems arise, one can always fall back on aspirin. No one really knows which one is better. For a new patient with stroke or suffering from that "herald" of stroke (transient ischemic attack), anticoagulant treatment with warfarin for three to six months followed by daily aspirin for an indefinite period would seem to be a reasonable treatment program. Warfarin therapy must be carefully monitored, especially in the aged.

He Knows What to Say but Can't Say It

Dear Dr. MacInnis:
My husband, age 56, came down with a stroke, which partly paralyzed his right arm and leg as well as severely affecting his

speech. He knows what he wants to say but cannot find the words. This makes him extremely frustrated and lately he is becoming depressed. He is still in the rehabilitation department and is making slow progress. His roommate has had a stroke too, which caused paralysis of the left arm and leg but his speech is okay. I have a couple of questions for you, please: (1) Since they both suffered a stroke, why can one talk and the other (my husband) cannot? (2) I read recently that there is a new drug being tested that if given soon after the stroke prevents or reduces the spread of paralysis, etc. Although this is too late in my husband's case, I'm wondering if you have any information on this treatment?

Mrs. T.L., Ottawa, Ontario

Answer

A stroke occurs when an artery supplying an area of the brain with blood is totally or partly blocked by a clot. If the artery was nourishing an area, say, on the left side of the brain, muscular power and feeling in one or both limbs on the *opposite* side of the body would be affected. Because the speech centre is located in the left side of the brain, the patient's ability to speak is often impaired (as in your husband's case). His roommate's left sided paralysis was caused by a blocked artery in the right side of the brain (where there's no speech centre), so speech was therefore not affected.

A stroke can be caused by a "wandering" blood clot, or embolus, originating in the heart (auricular fibrillation) and depositing itself in a brain artery, clogging it. Hemorrhage from a brain artery (often from high blood pressure) may also result in a stroke.

Strokes may vary in severity from the so-called transient ischemic attack, where there may be only a temporary speech disorder with fleeting paralysis, to a completed stroke with paralysis and coma.

On arrival in emergency the stroke patient normally receives oxygen and is given a blood thinner (heparin or warfarin) in an effort to revitalize the oxygen-starved area of the brain and to keep the clot from spreading. Nothing much more is ordinarily done, and we wait and hope that the stroke is transient and will not proceed to completion.

Neurological research has taught us that if brain cells are deprived of oxygen they die quickly, in four to ten minutes. Depending on the extent of oxygen depletion, brain cell death may spread, which explains why stroke symptoms such as paralysis and/or speech defects may worsen in the early course of the attack. Time, then, is of the essence and any measure to quickly prevent further irreversible brain damage would indeed be a breakthrough in management. And this, Mrs. L., brings us to the exciting new treatment you ask about.

The drug, tissue plasminogen activator or TPA, is not a new one. For several years it has been effectively used to open blocked coronary arteries in heart attacks, but only recently has it been proving its worth to liquify brain artery clots in stroke—initially in laboratory animals and followed by successful outcomes in humans.

The treatment of stroke is, in general, about twenty-five years behind acute coronary care as practiced in up-to-date cardiac centres today. What primary care physicians must learn is that acute stroke patients need to be managed exactly the same as coronary (heart attack) patients who are rushed to the hospital for immediate assessment for thrombolytic ("clot buster") therapy. As mentioned in a previous column, about 25 percent of acute strokes are from brain hemorrhage and the remaining 75 percent are due to thrombosis or clotting. Patients in the latter category may be candidates for brain arterial infusion with liquifying agents like TPA or streptokinase. Specialists in the field tell us that as in the case of coronary thrombolytic therapy, time is of the utmost importance and that the outside limit for brain infusion is six hours. Given beyond that time, the drug may cause a brain hemorrhage.

Impending Stroke

Dear Dr. MacInnis:

My husband, age 66, suffered several TIAs and the doctors have warned him of an impending stroke. He is on both warfarin

(to keep the blood from clotting) and aspirin for the same reason.
They told him that they may have to discontinue the warfarin,
because he is so difficult to keep under safe control (he sometimes
bleeds from the kidneys and quite often from the gums). I am
writing to you about surgery as an option to prevent a stroke. You
mentioned it in a previous column and stated that several large
trials were underway to determine if the surgical procedure is
beneficial. Any information would be greatly appreciated.

Mrs. T.Y., Toronto, Ontario

Answer

Maybe I should reiterate what I said about that procedure
and the rationale for its use in the prevention of a major stroke.
First of all, the cause of a stroke: When the blood supply to the
brain is halted due to severe narrowing of the carotid artery
(from clot and build-up of cholesterol deposits) that area of the
brain ceases to function, resulting in a completed stroke. I use
the term "completed" in contrast to a TIA, or "little" stroke,
that may last for less than twenty-four hours. This is what is
happening to your husband, and I appreciate your concern and
apprehension when the medical treatment he is receiving is becoming too hazardous to continue.

When I wrote that column you refer to, the prevailing treatment for the prevention of a completed stroke arising from TIAs
(transient ischemic attacks) or "little strokes," was an anticoagulant, usually warfarin and/or aspirin, along with management
of high cholesterol and hypertension when indicated.

Surgical "reaming" of the internal carotid artery blockage
(carotid endarterectomy) has been in vogue for many years and
has been performed worldwide. But results were so conflicting
that the operation was falling into disfavor. So to determine for
once and for all the effectiveness of this procedure, in January,
1988, a Canadian/U.S. study headed by Dr. Henry Barnett, president of the John P. Robarts Research Institute, in London, Ontario, and another in Europe, were initiated. The U.S./Canadian
trial involved six hundred patients with high-grade (70 to 99
percent) carotid artery stenosis, of which half received surgery

and the other half served as controls, receiving the aforementioned standard medical treatment. Both groups of patients in the trial suffered from symptoms of tight carotid stenosis. (See symptoms of TIAs in a previous column.)

The good news was announced in February 1991, at the annual stroke meeting of the American Heart Association in San Francisco. In effect, the announcement stated that the results of the Canadian/U.S. study indicated unequivocally that surgery was superior to the best medical treatment alone. The National Institute of Neurological Disorders (NINDS) that made the announcement, called off the Canadian/U.S trials so that the control group could also benefit from the surgery. Simultaneously, the European study was likewise stopped. A meeting's organizer put it this way, "It was a momentous announcement, seldom equalled in the career of anyone devoted to the problem of stroke."

So striking were the results of the Canadian/U.S. trials that they were sent by air express to a panel of expert reviewers whose conclusions would serve as an "emergency alert" to be sent out to medical organizations for relay to their members in both countries.

The researchers stress that the procedure (which consists of reaming out the blocked portion of the carotid artery) has been proven effective only when the carotid artery is over 70 percent blocked. The benefit of surgery in moderate narrowing of the artery (30 to 69 percent) is not proven but will be determined in a forthcoming second arm of the trial.

It would appear then, Mrs. Y., if your husband has more than 70 percent narrowing of one or both carotids he can approach this surgical option with confidence, if performed by a surgeon with the special skills required for the operation.

Falls in the Elderly

When primitive man forsook his fellow mammals and assumed the upright stance, he probably wasn't all that smart. True, his brain got bigger, he developed insight and judgment and learned to profit from experience. But as he grew upwards in stature, *Homo Erectus,* much to his chagrin, would experience falls—something unknown to that vast array of elder quadrupeds, from aardvarks to zorilas.

There are many well-documented studies attesting that control of posture is a function of maturity, i.e., from 16 to 60 years. After that, particularly in the 75- to 85-year range, falling is "the order of the day" from a diversity of causes—accidents, a drop in blood pressure, narrowing of the arteries feeding the brain, and the mysterious "drop attacks." It is convenient, then, to classify falls as due to (a) hazardous situations at home and (b) medical problems.

According to "Fact and Figures," National Safety Council (1978), falls are the leading cause of accidents in the elderly. In addition, it's the fifth leading cause of death in old people. And from the National Center for Health Statistics (1979), women, 75 and older, suffer more falls than men, but under 75, men outnumber women.

Hazardous situations predisposing to falls in the home include slippery floors; unsecured floor rugs, especially scatter rugs; high door sills; absence of handrails in bathrooms; and poorly lighted stairwells. Combine these household perils with failing vision and faulty balance and you have an accident just waiting to happen. But in many cases, such accidents are preventable. (See *Geriatrics,* May 1986, for Dr. Rein Tideiksaar's detailed listing of "Household Don'ts.")

The medical causes of falls in the aged are numerous. Limited space allows me only a brief listing. According to Sheldon's classic study on falls (*British Medical Journal:* 1685–1690, 1960), the "drop attack" is the commonest medical cause of falls. Here the fall is unexpected and instant. There are no warning signs or symptoms. The fall may occur with the patient walking, getting up quickly, turning around or rotating, or throwing back the neck. This last head movement gives rise to the hypothesis that it may momentarily deprive a part of the brain of blood and precipitate the fall. A serious feature of the drop attack is that it may, in some cases, cause the patient to remain helpless on the ground in a state of paralysis although fully awake.

Other causes of falls are dizziness—or vertigo—various drugs, disorders of the heart rhythm, heart block, and senile seizures; to these causes add such conditions as osteoarthritis of the hips and knees, Parkinson's disease, pernicious anemia, and orthostatic hypotension (drop in blood pressure on standing). Many of these causes are preventable or treatable.

Recently, I had the opportunity and pleasure of meeting with Dr. Rein Tideiksaar of the Department of Geriatrics and Adult Development, Mount Sinai Medical Center (in New York City). He is currently codirector of the Falls and Immobility Program at that facility. Dr. Tideiskaar believes that in spite of the popular perception that falls are inevitable in the aged, they are in most cases preventable. "They are best managed," he said, "by a team approach involving a physical therapist, a psychologist and a nurse practitioner supervised by a geriatrician." Dr. Tideiskaar's in-depth article, "Geriatric Falls" (*Contemporary Geriatric Medicine* 2 [1985], is the best on the subject.

I Can't Jump into My Pants Anymore

One of the commonest cardiovascular complaints I get from old people is dizziness on getting up quickly from bed or even a chair. And no less common is the feeling of faintness after eating a full meal, particularly breakfast.

Mr. A.N. (79) writes, "Gone are the days when I could literally jump into my pants on morning awakening. Now I have to get up 'by numbers': (1) I rise slowly and sit on bed, (2) I wait a minute and then rise to my feet, and (3) I get my bearings, preferably holding on to something. By being careful like this, I can usually make it to the bathroom. Ever so slowly the faint feeling leaves me and I'm able to dress up. But the same feeling often hits me again on getting up from the breakfast table. I've learned to overcome falling most of the time by getting up from the table, again, 'by numbers.' "

Mr. N suffers from "autonomic failure," a disorder where the blood pressure cannot adapt properly to quick changes in posture, for example, from a low level in bed to a higher level required for standing. If the blood pressure doesn't quickly rise, the brain doesn't get enough blood, hence, the dizziness. If, however, Mr. N. gives it time, the blood pressure adapts and the dizziness goes away. At breakfast, much of Mr. N's blood is required by the stomach and intestines for digestion, and it pools there and deprives the brain of blood. Had Mr. N. been a younger man his blood pressure system would have maintained adequate blood to the brain and he would have experienced no dizziness on getting up from the table.

I'm sure some readers of Mr. N.'s vintage will nod in recognition. Some with only "touches of it" and others, the whole bit. And all of you, like Mr. N., seek medical help.

Mr. N.'s "number routine" is a time-honoured one, especially good for morning rising and one I cannot improve on, and I have some good news for Mr. N. and fellow "fainters."

It's a well-known observation that caffeine raises blood pressure. With this fact in mind, scientists at the Autonomic Dysfunction Clinic, Vanderbilt University School of Medicine in Nashville, Tennessee, studied the effect of 250 milligrams of caffeine (equivalent to 2 cups of coffee) in reducing the fall of blood pressure after a meal in twelve susceptible patients. Their observations were published in the *New England Journal of Medicine* 313 (1985): 549–54.

Their findings: It worked on their group of patients. Their recommendation: Patients with autonomic failure with postural hypotension (low blood pressure on standing) should drink two cups of coffee with breakfast and abstain for the rest of the day.

So, Mr. N. and company, give it a try. And if you can afford the luxury of two cups of coffee in bed before rising, try that too. Even if it doesn't work you're still "livin' high"!

Dizziness

Dear Dr. MacInnis:

I wonder if you could help us with a problem of dizziness.

My husband is 79 years old and had a TIA (ministroke) a year ago. After two weeks the symptoms of pins and needles, weakness, etc., disappeared. He has been on Coumadin (a blood thinner) since that time. The only other medication he takes is a quinine tablet every night for leg cramps.

Dizziness is now his main complaint; it almost incapacitates him. He gets up, showers and shaves, and comes downstairs and is fine. But as soon as he has eaten and rises from the breakfast table, he gets dizzy. This has happened every day for the past two weeks. The spells can last anywhere from fifteen minutes to most of the day. He was fairly free from attacks during the months of January and February this year, but suffered a prolonged spell of dizziness last fall (1992) and it has returned. Our doctor does not understand why the dizziness always occurs after breakfast. (My husband's blood sugar was okay when last tested a year ago.) He has tried Gravol but it hasn't helped.

Any advice you could give me would be most welcome.

Mrs. S.A., Ontario

Answer

Please read my answer to Mr. A.N., who "can't jump into his pants anymore."

Carotid Sinus Problem

Dear Dr. MacInnis:

I am 62 and have enjoyed excellent health to date. I normally leap out of bed in the morning with no problems, but, recently, I spun right back into the bed with a quick dizzy spell. Once up, showered, and shaved, I had no apparent after-effects.

Upon retiring one night I was lying on my back when I jerked my head from one side to the other, which caused a sudden dizzy sensation. I now notice that if I take due care in getting up, I can avoid this sensation.

I would appreciate any comments that you might have.

Mr. J.A., Ontario

Answer

Although it is always difficult, if not impossible, to diagnose from "long distance," your graphic description of symptoms leads me to the feeling that you suffer from hypersensitivity of your carotid sinus. The carotid sinus is a plexus or nerve bundle situated in an area along the course of the carotid artery that runs up both sides of the neck. When this area is stimulated by pressure caused by a sudden jerking or twisting of the neck, a person with a hypersensitive carotid sinus may experience sudden dizziness, sometimes vertigo, and in severe cases, syncope, or fainting. It frequently happens when the patient is lying in bed on his back with his head twisted and he suddenly gets up. If this is what you've got, you've arrived at the right solution to your problem—getting up by numbers. And never, never try to quickly turn your head when wearing a tight collar!

If your problem gets more bothersome you should see a neurologist.

Three TIAs in a Year

Dear Dr. MacInnis:

My husband, age 68, has suffered three TIAs (ministrokes) in the past year. Each time the symptoms were the same, difficulty in speaking, mild confusion, and moderate weakness and tingling in the right forearm. The whole spell would last about ten minutes and then disappear leaving him perfectly normal. He was put on warfarin (a blood thinner) after the first TIA, but he had two spells after that at three-month intervals. The doctor feels that further examination and evaluation is necessary and is going to refer him to a neurologist. I would like you to tell me what sort of examination will be done and what it may show. Will an operation be necessary?

Mrs. K.L., Ottawa, Ontario

Answer

A transient ischemic attack (TIA) as the name suggest, is a stroke-like attack lasting from a few minutes to several hours, but not more than twenty-four hours.

The patient may experience one or more of a number of subjective symptoms, such as confusion, dizziness, and clumsiness, or may exhibit transient weakness or numbness in the face or an extremity on the same side or difficulty in speaking (as in your husband's case), temporary loss of sight in one eye, and a host of other sensations and physical symptoms. It is sometimes called a "ministroke" because of its short duration.

About one-third of TIA patients will proceed to a full-blown (completed) stroke, one-third will continue without suffering a completed stroke, and a third will, for reasons unknown, experience a full remission.

A TIA is usually caused by a temporary loss of blood to a part of the brain supplied by the carotid artery system on either side of the neck that becomes partly stenosed or narrowed, from cholesterol plaque and/or blood clot. If stenosis, or narrowing, of the left carotid is the culprit, then the physical symptoms appear on the right side of the body.

You were prescribed a blood thinning medicine (warfarin) in an effort to prevent blood clotting in the carotid artery, but evidently this measure, which is a standard initial medical treatment, has not been very successful.

A situation like this calls for further examination and evaluation, such as ultrasound, to determine the extent of stenosis of the carotid artery. Recent research (which I reported on in a previous column) has determined that if the carotid artery is stenosed (narrowed) more than 70 percent, the outcome for the operation (carotid endarterectomy) is good. A 90-percent stenosis predicts an even better outcome. An endarterectomy involves a reaming out of the blocked segment of the carotid artery.

Please bear in mind that the surgical approach (carotid endarterectomy) is done only in the light of ultrasound findings. If for instance, the carotid stenosis is found to be *less* than 70 percent, the chances for a successful outcome might be somewhat diminished. (On-going carotid endarterectomy research is tackling this problem and will in time provide an answer.)

What if an operation is not indicated? The patient will be continued on anticoagulant (warfarin/aspirin) therapy along with anti-hypertensive and anti-cholesterol measures when necessary.

These are matters that you will undoubtedly discuss with your neurologist, who, after evaluating your husband's condition, will come up with the best possible option under the circumstances.

Am I Going to Get a Stroke?

Dear Dr. MacInnis:

I am writing to you because the medical columnist in the local paper does not answer individual letters and I note that you offer a personal reply. As background, I am a retired Canadian spending six months every year in Florida. My problem is high blood pressure and my treatment seems to be very complicated.

My diastolic pressure seems to go up when I'm in bed. I take my pills at 6:00 A.M. At 8:00 A.M. my pressure is usually the highest of the day. Should I be concerned about having a stroke (which runs in my family) during the night? The other day my pressure was 159/105 at 7:00 A.M. and 139/96 at 8:00 A.M., then 120/79 at 11:00 A.M. If I were monitored for twenty-four or four-eight hours, could the doctors find the cause? Another day I had 170/107. If I were in Canada I would call my doctor. Should I be concerned?

I am presently on Vasotec twice a day and Lozide in the morning. I also take a thyroid pill. I have had several tests—thallium stress and an angiogram in Florida and an echocardiogram in Ottawa, and all show no coronary artery disease. I can supply additional details if you can use them.

Have you any suggestions?

Mrs. H.S., Port Charlotte, Florida

Answer

Should you be concerned about getting a stroke? You don't state your age, but there would be an added risk for stroke because of your family history. You evidence a rather labile hypertension with a tendency toward a diastolic elevation. This normally responds well to treatment.

There is far more to the treatment of hypertension than just the taking of antihypertensive medication with or without an added diuretic (water pill), which in your case is Lozide. Taking care of other risk factors, such as stopping smoking, treating obesity, committing to regular exercise programs, keeping cholesterol and its subgroups in check, and embarking on a low-sodium (half salt) high-potassium diet, should all be life-long commitments that are as equally important as taking pills for hypertension. If any of these apply to you, then take it to heart. (No pun intended.)

I'm enclosing a high potassium-low blood pressure diet program that you should adhere to as a way of life, and I believe that in the course of, say, six months to a year, you should notice a stable reduction in blood pressure and, as a bonus, you just might be able to reduce your daily drug dosage—who knows? And, yes, as a precautionary measure to prevent stroke you should start taking one aspirin (325 milligrams) every day.

Dear Dr. MacInnis:

My husband, going on 82, is receiving treatment for his high blood pressure (160/105) with a water pill called Diuril and is not taking to it very well. It makes him dizzy and often confused. I can always tell when he takes his dose because he becomes a different person. He also tells me he's no good sexually anymore and I guess I'll just have to believe him than look for proof. He went to the doctor recently, who didn't want to take him off treatment in case he gets a stroke. What do you think about his case?

Mrs. K.M., Ontario

Answer

The elderly are very sensitive to high blood pressure medication and the very old (over 80) exquisitely so. I have long been of the opinion in these columns that so-called treatment of high blood pressure in the very old (e.g., 82) with anti-hypertensive drugs (including thiazides) is getting perilously close to medical malpractice. My recommendation would be a palatable herb flavored diet, cutting back on salt, lots of fruit (oranges and bananas) and vegetables, a daily exercise (walking) program, cutting out smoking, and if you're too fat, trim that weight. This will lower the blood pressure.

My recommendation is that your husband see another doctor for a second opinion and seriously consider staying on his/her roster. You already have my opinion to which I can add that thiazides are notorious for causing impotence and could be the culprit (along with his age). To help prevention of stroke the best treatment is one aspirin (325 milligrams) daily or even a half of one, if it irritates the stomach.

"Mild Hypertension" Can Cause a Stroke

Dear Dr. MacInnis:

I am a male of 62 years and have what my doctor calls "mild hypertension," averaging 170 over 92. He gave me a pamphlet on blood pressure that advised treatment of even my mild type to prevent the possibility of stroke. Isn't this a bit extreme? I am well aware what very high blood pressure left untreated can do. My father had a blood pressure of 180 over 120 and was one of those people who was poor at following his doctor's advice and died from a stroke.

My question: Does mild high blood pressure like mine warrant treatment?

Mr. T.H.

Answer

Over the years there have been published reports suggesting that treating so-called mild hypertension prevented stroke, but since the number of patients involved in the clinical trials were small the results were not statistically significant. Consequently, doctors could not be on sure ground, and this is how matters have stood until recently. Now I am pleased to record some findings of Collins and colleagues in the April 7, 1990, issue of the British medical journal, *Lancet* (reported in *Canada's Medical Post,* April 24, 1990).

Collins and his group analyzed data from fourteen previous clinical trials of blood pressure drugs involving 30,000 patients with mild to moderate hypertension where treatment (mainly water pills and/or beta blockers) over a five-year period reduced the mean diastolic blood pressure by 5 to 6 points (mm hg.). Now with this very modest reduction in blood pressure determined, they followed the patients' progress and found that small as it was, it reduced the risk of stroke by 42 percent and coronary heart disease by 14 percent.

So there's your answer. But should we always treat mild to moderate high blood pressure with drugs? Many readers will recall my recent columns on the non-drug treatment of mild to moderate hypertension involving stress management, weight loss, daily exercise programs, sodium restriction, and moderation in alcohol. These simple lifestyle changes will not only make you feel better but will reduce your blood pressure to a modest degree. And to this I can now add with a greater certainty: You are reducing the risk of stroke and maybe a heart attack.

Is He Fit for Air Travel?

Dear Dr. MacInnis:

My husband, age 72, is making plans for an overseas trip for both of us. My general health is excellent but not my husband's. He has a problem with deficient brain circulation. It happens only occasionally, but when it does he seems to become confused, not knowing where he is. The spell (which the doctor calls

129

a transient ischemic attack) lasts only a minute or so and then he's okay.

I would appreciate your opinion as to his suitability for air travel with this condition. There's also a second problem. For over a year now he has been on an anticoagulant (blood thinner) called warfarin. He's had his (prothrombin) tests regularly every month and they're always fine. Would this be an added risk during a prolonged absence from home?

Mrs. T.L., California

Answer

Patients with cerebral blood deficiency problems, such as you describe, usually make poor air travellers. This is because of lower oxygen concentration in the pressurized aircraft. My opinion is that his condition poses a greater than ordinary risk for air travel, and an airline might request a medical escort in some instances. I believe that you should seek a second opinion from a physician who can examine your husband.

Your second question re blood thinner is simply answered. As long as your husband has been on a regular (unvarying) dose of warfarin with good prothrombin control for a period of six weeks prior to departure, there should be no problems. Prothrombin testing is available in most large medical laboratories abroad.

The International Health Guide for Senior Citizen Travelers, by Dr. Robert Lange of Johns Hopkins Hospital Travel Medicine Clinic, is a recently published 70-page wealth of information for the senior traveler as well as concerned doctors and nurses. (Available from Pilot Books, 103 Cooper Street, Babylon, New York 11702.)

Worried about a Brain Tumor

Dear Dr. MacInnis:

My father, age 84, is complaining of dizzy spells. When he gets these spells (on the average once a week), he always complains of headache and a feeling of numbness in one or both arms. I can't get him to see a doctor. He says he has no faith in any of them. Although I haven't mentioned it to him, I am worrying he may have a brain tumor so I would greatly appreciate your opinion.

Mrs. Y.L., Michigan

Answer

I believe you are overly concerned about your father's symptoms. Since as the old saying goes, "the commonest things happen the commonest," my educated guess from long distance would be that his little spells are "transient ischemic attacks," where an area of the brain is temporarily deprived of blood either through spasm of a cerebral (brain) artery or blood clot. In contrast to the poor outlook from a brain tumor, TIAs can often be prevented or reduced in frequency by the regular (daily) taking of an aspirin tablet or an anticoagulant like warfarin. (Of the two, and considering your father's age, I would favor the daily aspirin). I would strongly advise you to persevere in getting him medical attention despite his apparent built-in resistance.

Brain tumor has always been considered uncommon in the elderly and rare in the very old, that is, until recently, when a five-fold increase in the prevalence of brain tumor in the eighty-five and over age group became apparent in statistics. The increase began to manifest itself back in 1973, which coincides with the advent of CT brain scanning followed over the years by even more sophisticated brain imaging techniques. Authorities, then, believe that this apparent increase in brain tumor diagnosis is due not to natural causes but to better means of detecting something that has previously eluded us.

When You Can't Take Aspirin for TIAs

Dear Dr. MacInnis:
I am a male 65 years old. About a year ago I experienced what my doctor called "transient blindness" in my left eye. He

said it was much like a transient ischemic attack" (TIA) I had two years ago. This time a blood clot affected the eye, not the brain.

Although I have no symptoms now (it passed off in about a minute), it was quite frightening while it lasted. Here's what happened. One morning when I was shaving, I suddenly lost the sight in my left eye. At first I thought my left eyeglass (lens) was smudged with soap, but on examination it was okay. While rubbing my eye and wondering what to do next, something like a curtain or film lifted and I could see again as well as before. About two years ago, I had a "spell" of dizziness with clumsiness of my left arm that lasted in all about two hours. Because of these two attacks, the doctor sent me to a neurologist who found by ultrasound that I had a clot obstruction of my carotid artery but not enough to require a reaming out operation. I was put on one aspirin (350 milligrams) a day.

But I now have a problem with aspirin. It caused heartburn and a spell of bleeding from the stomach. As I needed a medicine like aspirin to help prevent the possibility of stroke, the doctor put me on a new drug called Ticlid. It's much more expensive than aspirin but I guess it's worth it if it can prevent a stroke.

D.L., California

Answer

The condition you describe is known as "transient monocular blindness," said to be caused by narrowing or clot in the "eye branch" of the internal carotid artery. (Another picturesque name for it is "amaurosis fugax" literally translated as "fleeting blindness.")

Ticlopidine (brand name Ticlid) according to two recent clinical trials may be somewhat more effective as an antiplatelet agent than aspirin but appears to have more extensive side effects. So much so, that the manufacturer (Syntex Laboratories) warns us that this drug should be "reserved for patients who are intolerant to aspirin therapy where indicated to prevent stroke."

Ticlid—its good points: Two important studies attest to its usefulness: (1) The Canadian-American Ticlopidine Study (CATS). This was a double blind placebo controlled trial involving over 1,000 patients. Result: Over a three-year period, ticlopidine reduced the risk of stroke by 24 percent compared with a placebo (inert look-alike pill). (2) The Ticlopidine-Aspirin Stroke Study (TASS) compared the efficacy of ticlopidine *versus* aspirin in preventing stroke or death in patients with a history of TIAs. Here over 1,900 men and 1,000 women were randomly picked and given either 250 milligrams of ticlopidine twice a day or 650 milligrams of aspirin (two tablets) twice daily. Result: The three-year rate of death or non-fatal stroke was 17 percent for ticlopidine *versus* 19 percent for aspirin. It is important to note that ticlopidine was effective for women as well as for men. (The value of aspirin for stroke prevention in women has been somewhat dubious.)

Ticlid—its not-so-good points: Both studies showed that Ticlid had, overall, a more serious side effect profile than aspirin, the most prominent being diarrhea—13.5 percent for Ticlid *versus* 5 percent for aspirin. But the most serious drawback for Ticlid was the occurrence of neutropenia (a low count of white blood cells called neutrophils) in 2.4 percent of patients on the drug. (For aspirin it was 0.8 percent.) For reasons not clear, it was found in controlled studies that neutropenia occurred from three weeks to three months after the start of therapy with Ticlid. Because of this, *all patients selected for ticlopidine therapy* (in place of aspirin) *must have blood counts for neutropenia every two weeks for the first three months of therapy*. If, after three months' monitoring, there is no evidence of neutropenia, "then blood tests need only be taken for patients with signs and symptoms suggestive of infection" (Syntex Laboratories, Inc.).

Systolic Hypertension: Can It Cause Stroke?

I am a 60-year-old male with what the doctor says is "systolic" hypertension averaging around 170 over 80. He advises treatment for the high systolic pressure to help prevent the possibility of a stroke. (My father developed a stroke when he was 70 years old.)

My question: Is this a special kind of high blood pressure, and what is the risk of getting a stroke from it, and what is the best treatment for somebody my age?

Mr. K.O., Ottawa, Ontario

Answer

First of all, a few words on the two different components of blood pressure. The *systolic* pressure is the blood pressure exerted by the heart at the peak of its activity in pumping blood throughout the body. It is recorded in terms of the height of a column of mercury that you can see on some blood pressure machines, and the normal averages out to about 140 (usually increasing as you age). The *diastolic* pressure is the pressure keeping the arterial walls from collapsing *between* beats. It is also expressed in milligrams of mercury and averages overall to about 75 or 80. A normal blood pressure reading is therefore expressed by the number 140 over 80. It should be remembered that the systolic component (upper number) fluctuates much more than the diastolic (lower number).

When both upper and lower numbers are *consistently* increased—for example, 210 over 110—it signifies what we know as arterial hypertension. In your case, which is not at all unusual for your age, only the systolic component is higher than the normal; hence, the designation "systolic" hypertension. (Your diastolic pressure is normal at 80.)

There is increasing evidence that this so-called systolic hypertension that increases consistently with age and once thought to be "benign," or "normal," can itself be a risk factor for stroke and heart attack.

A National Institute on Aging bulletin dated June 25, 1991, reported on a new study in the *Journal of the American Medical Association* (week of June 25, 1990) indicating that drug treatment can help prevent strokes in older people with systolic hypertension. According to the director of the National Institute on Aging, Dr. T. Franklin Williams, "This is the first clinical trial to demonstrate the possible health benefits of lowering iso-lated systolic hypertension in older people. The results tell us unequivocally that treating elevated systolic hypertension in this population reduces the risk of stroke, heart attack and other problems related to cardiovascular disease," Dr. Williams added.

Briefly, according to the study, drug treatment with low doses of a diuretic (water pill) chlorthalidone reduced the inci-dence of stroke by 36 percent and coronary heart disease by 27 percent. The authors of the *JAMA* article note that the treat-ment is "uncomplicated, inexpensive and causes very few side effects."

This was a randomized, double blind, placebo-controlled study conducted at sixteen clinical centers across the country. Nearly 500 men and women participated in the five-year study, the NIA bulletin reported.

Dr. Williams stated that systolic hypertension affects 7 per-cent of people aged 60 to 69; 13 percent of people aged 70 to 79; and 20 percent of the population 80 to 89 years.

There is a compelling reason for you to see your doctor about treatment, as your family history of stroke is an added risk factor.

Can Aspirin for TIAs Also Reduce the Risk for Colon Cancer?

Dear Dr. MacInnis:
I am taking one aspirin tablet (325 milligrams) daily to help stave off a stroke. I've had two TIAs minor strokes recently, but my neck artery (carotid) is not plugged enough for a roto-rooter job—at least that's what the doctor said. Well, here's my question. I've heard that taking aspirin regularly, like I am, can prevent the risk of dying from large bowel cancer. The reason I'm con-cerned about this is because my father died from colon cancer. It would be reassuring to know that the aspirin I take for stroke prevention may also reduce my risk of death from large bowel cancer. Am I taking enough aspirin for it to work both ways? I am 55. Thank you.

Mr. P.Y., New York

Answer

You may have heard about this from your doctor who is treating your transient ischemic attacks. I say this because it was reported in the December 5, 1991, issue of the *New England Journal of Medicine.*

The conclusion of this large well-conducted study was that white men and women who used aspirin regularly (for at least one year) had a reduced risk of death from colon cancer. (Professional caregivers wishing a reprint of this article should write to Dr. M. J. Than, Department of Epidemiology and Statistics, American Cancer Society, 1599 Clifton Road, Atlanta, Georgia 30329.)

Are you taking an adequate dose of aspirin for "double-barrel prevention"? Aspirin preventive therapy is so varied in its daily dosage—from half a daily "baby" (40 milligrams) aspirin to three regular (325 milligrams) tablets per day—all I can say is that your present dose is probably adequate. I fervently hope and pray that researchers will soon arrive at a *standard* preventive daily dose of aspirin.

And for others wondering if they should embark on a daily aspirin routine to lower the risk of colon cancer, my advice is that you follow the recommendation of your physician who is conversant with the research literature.

Again, on the subject of aspirin preventive therapy, I will briefly cite two very recent research studies.

(1) A Dutch study where the efficacy of 30 milligrams of aspirin daily was compared to 283 milligrams aspirin daily in preventing further "vascular events" in patients who suffered a TIA, or ministroke, within three months before entering the trial. The setting was sixty-three hospital clinics in the Netherlands. Results: In patients having had a TIA, or a ministroke, 30 milligrams of aspirin daily was no less effective in preventing vascular events (more TIAs or fatal or nonfatal strokes) than 283 milligrams of aspirin daily and had fewer side effects, such as gastric distress and bleeding (*New England Journal of Medicine,* October 31, 1991).

For a reprint, professional caregivers may write to Dr. J. Van Gijn, Department of Neurology, University Hospital, Utrecht, Box 85500 3508 GA Utrecht, Netherlands.

(2) A Swedish study where the efficacy of 75 milligrams of aspirin daily was compared to a placebo (dummy look-alike pill) for the prevention of stroke or death after TIAs, or minor strokes. Setting: sixteen clinical centers in Sweden. Result: Aspirin 75 milligrams daily lowered the risk for stroke or death in both men and women and increased the risk of bleeding (compared to placebo) (*Lancet,* November 30, 1991).

For a reprint, professional caregivers may write to Dr. B. Norving, Department of Neurology, University Hospital, S-221 85 Lund, Sweden.

Comment: Could these be indeed my "Answered Prayers"?

Chapter 8
Common Heart, Circulation, and Respiratory Disorders in the Elderly

Notable advances in the prevention, diagnosis, and treatment of cardiovascular disease over the past 25 years have reduced the overall mortality twenty-five percent. But despite this, in old people, heart disease is still the major cause of death and disability.

As I mentioned in the Introduction, heart disease usually presents itself differently in old people. For example, the often excruciating chest pain of myocardial infarction (acute heart attack) may be absent in the aged person, expressing itself instead by shortness of breath, heart palpitation, fatigue, confusion, or even by a stroke. This can be perplexing to the unsuspecting practitioner and may delay diagnosis.

In this chapter, I will be presenting some of the commoner manifestations of heart disease in the elderly, such as angina, myocardial infarction, disorders of heart rhythm, and congestive heart failure. There will be, in addition, a column on aneurysm of the abdominal aorta, which can become a true vascular emergency when it ruptures, and a "general utility" column featuring swelling of the lower extremities—its treatment and when not to treat.

But the "center-piece" of this chapter will be, I hope, the management of high blood pressure in the elderly where I emphasize their exquisite sensitivity to many, if not all medications routinely used in younger patients. I have long advocated the "no-drug" treatment in mild to moderate hypertension, indeed, at any age, and believe it should be given a fair trial before embarking on drug therapy. Longtime readers of "Senior Clinic" may also recall my almost pathological aversion to the unfortunate fetish of "getting the blood pressure down" in the "old old" at any cost. Several columns will attest to this nefarious practice, which in some cases is dangerously close, in my opinion, to medical malpractice.

******

What Is Angina?

Dear Dr. MacInnis:

What is "angina pectoris"? Is it the same as a heart attack? Can a heart attack cause a stroke? I guess I'm all mixed up. My doctor tells me the pain in my chest is angina. How does nitroglycerine stop the pain?

Mr. E.T. (60), California

Answer

This is a tall order but I'll try to be as clear as possible.

"Angina pectoris" literally means "pain in the chest." First of all, remember that the heart muscle, like a muscle anywhere, requires blood to keep it alive and functioning properly. And like an internal combustion engine, the faster the heart muscle pumps, the more "fuel" (blood) it needs to do this extra work. If there's not enough blood getting to the rapidly beating heart muscle, the muscle cries out in pain. This pain is usually felt behind the sternum (breast bone). It is the pain of angina pectoris.

To understand the mechanism of angina better, try this experiment on yourself. First, squeeze your left wrist as tightly as you can with your right hand, like a tourniquet. You have now cut off the two main arteries in your wrist supplying blood to your left hand. Now start opening and closing your left hand rapidly. In three or four minutes, sometimes less, the muscles

140

in your left hand will cramp and cry out in pain because they can no longer function without "fuel" (blood).

To ease the pain, you can slow your hand action or, better still, release the grip, allowing your left hand muscles to get their blood again and the pain completely disappears.

Now, to get back to your heart. The "fuel lines" that supply blood to your heart muscles are called coronary (heart) arteries with a bore of about one-half the diameter of a standard-size lead pencil. When these pipelines (arteries) are normal, they can supply the heart muscle with as much blood as it needs no matter how fast it beats (as when you're running). All is well, there is no pain. If, however, the fuel lines (heart arteries) become partly clogged from, say, cholesterol deposits, not enough blood gets to the hungry heart muscle when it has to work harder, and just like your left hand in the experiment, your heart muscle cries out in pain; the pain is referred to the mid-chest and may radiate down the left arm or to the jaws. You are now suffering from an attack of angina pectoris. (There is scientific evidence that coronary artery "spasm" of emotional origin, or entry of calcium ions into the artery wall, or both, can also cause angina.)

What brings on an angina attack? Anything that makes the heart work harder. As you may have guessed, the main cause is physical overactivity. Sometimes increased emotional activity will do it, but it can fool you by not coming on when you would normally expect it.

The angina patient feels the pain coming on during exertion or shortly thereafter—before the heart rate has settled to normal. Let me repeat, it's important; the chest pain typically radiates to the left shoulder, arm, and hand, and up the neck to the jaws, sometimes to the ears. Occasionally the radiation is on the right side.

What does the angina patient do in the face of this severe, sometimes excruciating, attack of pain? If at all possible, he stops in his tracks and stands perfectly still or sits down. This allows the heart rate to slow down. The heart muscle now requires less blood than before and the pain lessens. If he stands still or sits long enough, the heart rate will return to normal and the pain goes away.

Suppose the fuel lines (coronary arteries) could be opened up a bit. Then more blood could get through to the heart muscle. That is precisely how the drug, nitroglycerine, acts on the coronary arteries. When a nitroglycerine tablet is placed under the tongue, in less than a minute it is absorbed into the bloodstream and when it reaches the coronary arteries, dilates them, thus increasing the bore. More blood now gets to the heart muscle and the pain goes away.

I hope this explains just what angina pectoris is, its symptoms, and the action of nitroglycerine.

You ask, "Is angina the same as a heart attack?" No, the popular term "heart attack" refers to something more serious than angina—an extension of angina, if you will. When the bore of a coronary artery narrows from disease (atherosclerosis, or "hardening") to the point where it becomes clogged and is unable to transport sufficient blood to the heart muscle, that area of heart muscle deprived of blood softens, jellifies, and dies. The technical term for death of a muscle is "infarction," and since the heart muscle is involved, the medical term is "myocardial infarction." A coronary artery doesn't have to be completely plugged to cause a heart attack.

Again, as in angina, the pain of myocardial infarction (heart attack) is under the breastbone and the radiation may be similar. But the pain is usually more severe and does not respond to nitroglycerine. The patient may sweat profusely, become clammy, and may vomit. There may be a feeling of impending death.

If the heart attack is uncomplicated and responds to medication, recovery is the rule, and if there's no recurrence within six months the future outlook is good.

The two serious complications of a myocardial infarction (heart attack) are (1) congestive (pump) failure, and (2) failure of the heart's electrical system that controls its rhythm. The greater the heart area damaged, the greater possibility of these complications. Both require prompt medical attention. But of these two emergencies, electrical failure of the heart's conducting apparatus is the more serious and is the main cause of sudden death from a heart attack at home or in the ambulance on the way to the hospital. If it occurs in certain ambulances or in a hospital, it may be successfully treated with electrical counter-shock, providing treatment is immediate.

In the aged there is absence of pain in about 50 percent of myocardial infarctions (heart attacks). Often the most prevalent symptom is shortness of breath from congestive heart (pump) failure. And as before mentioned, sudden confusion or dizziness may be the only presenting symptoms, sometimes accompanied by pallor and clammy skin. Occasionally in the older person, the first obvious sign of a heart attack is a stroke.

You ask about the relation of a stroke to a heart attack. A stroke may occur as a result of severe heart muscle damage. Here the heart fails as a pump and less blood gets to the brain, an organ extremely sensitive to diminished nutrition. Another cardiac origin of stroke is when a blood clot becomes detached from the damaged heart muscle, proceeds up the blood stream to the brain as an embolus (travelling clot), and blocks an artery.

Aspirin Reduces Heart Attack
in Healthy Men over Fifty

In 1986 a group of healthy male doctors embarked on an experiment that has made medical history. It was a double blind, placebo-controlled trial involving 22,071 practicing medical doctors, whose principal mandate was to determine whether one ASA (aspirin) tablet of 325 milligrams taken every other day could decrease the number of deaths from cardiovascular disease. It was called the "Physician's Health Study."

I announced the start-up of this study, and about three years later gave a preliminary report indicating that ASA did indeed appear to reduce the incidence of fatal heart attacks in the group. But this optimistic finding was somewhat tempered by the disquieting possibility that the rate of hemorrhagic stroke appeared to be "slightly increased" in the aspirin-treated subjects.

Now the final report is out.

In an average follow-up time of 60.2 months the authors of the study found that there was a 44 percent reduction in the risk of myocardial infarction (acute heart attack). Better still, there was no statistically significant increase in the incidence of bleeding (hemorrhagic) stroke over the five-year period.

Some other highlights of the completed trial: The decreased risk of acute heart attacks was apparent only in those 50 or more years, particularly those with low cholesterol levels. No women were included in the trial.

Conclusion: ASA (aspirin) 325 milligrams every other day can reduce the incidence of myocardial infarction in healthy men over the age of 50.

As for patients with known heart disease, the authors state, "Given the available data, it now seems reasonable to advocate the use of ASA at a dose of 160 to 325 milligrams with clinical evidence of coronary disease if there are no specific contraindications, e.g., bleeding tendencies, present."

It is important to remember that ASA is only one of a number of measures calculated to decrease the incidence of coronary heart disease. These include weight and blood pressure control, stopping cigarettes, exercising regularly and reducing high cholesterol.

Update, July 1994: Preliminary studies indicate that up to one third of heart and stroke patients on aspirin may be "nonresponders." Check with your doctor.

He Can't Go on like This

Dear Dr. MacInnis:

My husband (age 80) has severe angina that now responds poorly to nitroglycerine or beta-blockers. The doctor doesn't recommend by-pass surgery, mainly because of advanced age. He is diagnosed as having "unstable angina." He can't go on like this. Should I get another opinion?

Mrs. L.M., California

Answer

Most doctors have been reluctant to advise coronary artery by-pass surgery on angina patients who are in the age category of your husband. But a report in the heart and blood vessel medical journal *Circulation* should serve as your "second opinion."

The study was conducted by Dr. S. H. Rahimtoola and co-workers from Oregon Health Sciences University and Heart Institute, Saint Vincent Hospital, Portland, Oregon. They followed 1,304 elderly coronary by-pass patients (65 and older) for ten years after surgery, coming up with five- and ten-year survival rates, which they compared with survival rates in a group of postoperative by-pass patients age 55 to 64.

The 1,304 patients were divided into two groups according to age. Group 1a was (65 to 74). Group 1b was (75 to 84). All had angina unresponsive to drugs.

Their findings: Operative mortality (death during or shortly after an operation) was similar (averaging 2.5 percent) in both groups. Five- and ten-year survival rates were 85 percent and 65 percent respectively, in the older age group and not statistically different from the younger age group.

Their recommendation: "That coronary by-pass surgery should be offered to the older members of our society for the usual indications." Personal Note: In November 1988, your dutiful scribe, at the age of 75, underwent successful open heart surgery for a mitral valve replacement with a coronary by-pass for an encore!

Which will serve, Mrs. M., as your "third opinion."

"Unstable" Angina Again

Dear Dr. MacInnis:

I have what the doctors call "angina pectoris." Lately it has been "acting up," as one of the doctors in the heart clinic put it. Because of this he has renamed it "unstable angina" and has brought up the possibility of by-pass surgery but wants to do tests first. At first my chest pain was predictable in that I could tell pretty well what type of activity would bring it on so that I could either avoid the activity if possible or would take nitroglycerine, which would usually prevent the chest pain from happening. Over the past three months the exercise-pain pattern has changed. For example, the pain can now occur when I'm at rest, and I'm now noticing that different forms of emotional stress can bring on the pain. It seems too, that the nitroglycerine is not quite as effective as it used to be.

I always thought there was just one kind of angina—the one I could always rely on! Would you please discuss further my new-found diagnosis?

Mr. R.Y., age 61

Answer

At the risk of being repetitious, I'll discuss angina again. Angina pectoris means literally "pain in the chest." And like any other muscle, the heart muscle requires blood laden with oxygen to keep it alive and functioning. And like an engine, the faster the heart muscle pumps, the more fuel (blood) it needs to perform this extra work. If there's not enough blood to meet the demand of the rapidly beating heart the heart muscle, as any muscle trying to work with diminished blood supply, cries out in pain. The pain is usually felt behind the breastbone. It is the pain of angina pectoris.

What brings on the pain of angina pectoris? Anything that makes the heart work faster, such as physical or emotional over-activity. This is called "stable angina," but even here it may occasionally fool you, coming on when you least expect it.

Sir William Osler, in his 1906 *Practice of Medicine*, describes a typical angina attack in his usual dramatic fashion: "The patient is seized with an agonizing pain in the region of the heart with a sense of constriction as if the heart was seized in a vice. The pain radiates to the neck and down the arm (usually the left) or there may be numbness in the fingers or in the cardiac region. The face is usually pallid and may assume an ashen-gray tint and not infrequently a profuse sweat breaks out over the surface. The paroxysm (of pain) lasts from several seconds to a minute or two. In severe attacks the patient feels that death is imminent."

What I have described is an anginal attack which may occur with more or less severity. When this pattern of angina occurs regularly and predictably and responds pretty consistently to nitroglycerine, it is called "stable" angina.

When the usual pattern and response to nitroglycerine goes awry and you don't know what to expect, your angina is becoming "unstable," just as you have so admirably described.

Yes, there just might be a by-pass in the cards for you with a very likely successful outcome.

Angioplasty versus Coronary By-pass

Dear Dr. MacInnis:

Would you please give us the facts as to what is the best treatment for what my doctor calls "chronic unstable angina"? The nitroglycerine tablets that I have taken for years with expected relief are no longer predictable and this applies to the nitroderm patch as well. My doctor has referred me to a cardiologist who tells me that I am probably at the "end of my tether" as far as medication is concerned and is faced with either doing an angioplasty (he does many of them at the hospital) or referring me to a heart surgeon for a bypass. My stress test is positive.

I am age 74 and in otherwise pretty good health. I have had an angiogram that showed partial blockage of two coronary arteries. As before stated, my nitroglycerine is finally failing me and I have pretty well decided to opt for either angioplasty or bypass. My wife and I have been reading up on the subject and would appreciate any further information on the merits of each procedure. Thank you.

Mr. K.Y., Toronto

Answer

When your coronary (heart) artery or arteries become fully or partially blocked with plaque (from cholesterol, fats and blood clot), severe chest pain may occur because the heart muscle is not getting enough blood for its own nourishment. Complete blockage can cause sudden death from a heart attack, but in slower partial blockage the heart can, over time, build its own collateral circulation, permitting it to function often imperfectly and requiring nitroglycerine to increase blood flow to its muscle. But quite frequently nitroglycerine may gradually lose its effect, as in your case.

In earlier times coronary artery by-pass surgery was the only option to remedy this blockage. Briefly, this open-heart major surgical procedure involves re-routing the blood around the blocked artery or arteries with a vein or artery harvested from another part of the body. Again, in brief, coronary balloon angioplasty consists in inserting a long, pliable catheter into a groin or armpit artery and threading it under special X-ray guidance up this vessel until it reaches the blockage in the heart artery. Next, the cardiologist inserts into this catheter an even thinner one tipped with a miniature (deflated) balloon, which again under X-ray monitoring is guided through the blockage. Now the balloon is inflated and then withdrawn, a procedure that compresses the plaque in the coronary artery and by enlarging its bore, results in increased coronary artery blood flow into the heart muscle.

Some pros and cons of angioplasty: It can work immediately with little or no physical after-effects. This is because it is "non-invasive" compared to that of major open-heart surgery required for a coronary by-pass. But despite its immediate effectiveness (in 90 percent of cases), after six months or so, reblockage of the coronary arteries may occur in about 35 percent of patients. Here the cardiologist may do a repeat angioplasty or opt for a by-pass depending on circumstances. Another advantage of angioplasty is the much less cost and more rapid recovery (about a day in hospital) compared to the more costly by-pass, often requiring more than a week in hospital.

Whether you should have a by-pass or angioplasty, I cannot of course decide for you (although from "long distance" I would probably favour a by-pass). But your cardiologist is the final arbiter and you're fortunate in having one who works out of a large metropolitan hospital and who presumably has had a lot of experience in performing angioplasties. The American Heart Association defines a *well-trained* cardiologist as one who performs no fewer than 75 angioplasties per year and receives retraining and updating in the procedure every two years.

Late Notes: The first successful treatment of blasting away a coronary artery clot with ultrasound waves was reported (in March 1994) from Hamburg, Germany. Although at this point only experimental, the procedure could in time replace balloon angioplasty, researchers say. Also, there's word out of Calgary, Alberta, that leaving a tiny mesh tube (stent) at the blockage will help keep the coronary artery open, and the Mayo Clinic researchers and others have shown that plaque blockage can be vapourized by a tiny laser beam.

Hail the Lowly Leech!

Dear Dr. MacInnis:

I am a retired physician who has always enjoyed your column.

Those of us who have studied history of medicine are aware that leech treatment played an important part in the therapy of practically every malady known to man. I can recall one of my professors in medical school reminiscing about how popular leech applications were in his day.

By the turn of the century, leech treatment virtually disappeared from our medical text books. About all the doctors of my time knew about leeches was that they secreted a substance called hirudin from their salivary gland that prevented blood from clotting. If this didn't help the patient it certainly did the leech, because it insured a supply of clot-free human blood in its belly. In other words, hirudin kept the blood line open for the benefit of the leech. Now I read that hirudin can help the patient with angina where its effect is similar to heparin without many of its serious effects. You most likely have heard of this, too, and I'm sure you have something to add to my remarks. Thanks again.

Dr. A.M., Winnipeg, Manitoba

Answer

Thank you for your admirable observations on the lowly leech. It has at long last become deserving of our respect!

Because natural hirudin is impossible to produce in large quantities, researchers have been able to produce it synthetically in the form of a 20-amino acid called "hirulog" and it has, as you say, the property to inhibit the production of thrombin in the circulation, and has been the most effective treatment for unstable angina. There is some research evidence from the Montreal Heart Institute that hirulog seems not only to be as effective as heparin in the treatment of unstable angina, but that it is much easier and less complicated to use as well as being safer and not any more expensive. It would seem to be the upcoming drug of choice for unstable angina. (Angina is deemed "unstable" when it deviates from its usual symptoms and does not react predictably to the usual anti-anginal medications.)

You're Okay, but Aren't You Just Lucky?

You waited till your angina became intractable and then had your coronary by-pass. Your operation was successful and, now, five years later, everything's still okay. Do you feel you're just lucky? The answer is unqualifiedly "no." You are still in that favourable 90 percent where after five years at least one graft was found patent and working, and in that 67 percent of by-pass patients in whom all grafts were found open after five years.

These are some of the findings of the European Coronary Artery Surgery Study (ECASS) involving 197 by-pass patients and published in *Circulation* (Supplement V), Vol. 71 (1985).

But what may happen some years later? In the same article are the findings of the Montreal Heart Institute. Their study showed that between six and eleven years there was a significant loss of graft patency. By the eleventh year only 60 percent of the grafts were open and half of these showed "relatively severe atherosclerosis" (hardening).

Commenting on this, *International Abstracts of Cardiology* reminds us that more than 5 percent now having by-pass surgery are repeaters and that this percentage will increase.

And repeaters will be happy to know that the mortality rate from the second operation is no higher than that of the first. However, only about 50 percent of repeaters are free from angina after five years.

But this could improve with elimination of such risk factors as obesity, hypertension, high cholesterol, and smoking, coupled with an ongoing exercise program and daily aspirin.

"Skipped" Beats

I get many letters from men and women (mainly men) in the over-55 age group complaining of "skipped" heart beats, and what they all have in common are "normal" hearts, so they have been told, not only by their family doctors but by cardiologists (heart specialists) as well.

So why do they write in? In most cases they have taken the word of their doctors that their hearts are okay, but are puzzled why a so called normal heart can act up so and cause them such anxiety, and why nothing more than just reassurance has been prescribed. Some are downright scared that the diagnosis is wrong and the skipping heart beats are the forerunner of more serious things to come. A few are totally convinced they have serious heart disease right now and their skipped beats are proof enough.

In this column I'll condense several of their letters, all telling pretty well the same story in a slightly different way. The common theme is perplexity and anxiety (with one case of thanksgiving).

Mr. A.L. (58) writes, "My health is good, my doctor assures me I have a good heart. But every night just as I'm trying to get to sleep my heart starts that infernal skipping! Sometimes if I stay perfectly still it will stop, but the moment I shift position away it goes again. I can predict it with certainty if I eat a late heavy meal. If I indulge in alcohol late at night, I can expect to awaken at 3:00 A.M. with a racing heart and skipped beats. Mostly it comes out of the blue. It's getting me down." (Caffeine from coffee or tea is also a common culprit.)

Mr. T.E. (62) awakens with skipped beats about 5:00 A.M. Like Mr. A.L., he tries to beat it "with total relaxation" but the moment he stirs "it's back." "It makes for a long day," he adds. Mr. L.L. (55) finds that if he gets a spell during the day, a short period of brisk exercise usually stops it. "I have the feeling," he says, "it's there quite a bit during the day and I don't notice it, but let things quiet down, then I begin to feel it—like throbs in the still of the night."

My final letter has a happy ending. Fifty-seven-year-old Mrs. M.B. writes, "After hardly a day in four years without it, it vanished, and that was two years ago." (A common occurrence, so travel hopefully!)

These four letters embody the main features of so-called benign ventricular premature beats which translated reads, "harmless extra beats originating in the electrical conducting system of the left or right ventricles." To qualify for this diagnosis, the heart must be judged as otherwise normal in structure and function. (The term "skipped beat" denotes that the heart has somehow "missed" a beat. What really happens is that the interposed extra beat causes the heart to momentarily pause while it regains its rhythm. The patient senses this pause as a skipped or missed beat.)

Should benign ventricular premature beats be treated? That depends entirely on the severity of the presenting symptoms. In tense, sensitive people even the mildest mannered skipped beats can cause an anxiety state sometimes requiring sedation. For more stoical persons, an explanation and reassurance may be all that is necessary.

If the skipped beats are frequent, that is five or more per minute on the average, then an arrhythmia drug (prescribed by your doctor) is indicated. This is to prevent the occurrence of more serious rhythm disturbances. Troublesome side effects are common with antiarrhythmia medication where there's dry mouth, constipation, and slow urination.

Skipped beats are quite common past middle life, increasing with age, and in the majority of cases are just never felt. Should an unsuspecting, "non-heart" patient ever then be told? My answer is personal. In forty years of "discovering" benign skipped beats, I've never told a patient.

And I've never had cause to regret it.

All about Swollen Legs

Dear Dr. MacInnis:

Will you please settle an argument. My wife is constantly bugging me to see a doctor about my swollen ankles, worse in the evening. She worries about everything and thinks I'm at death's door. I keep telling her there's nothing wrong. I'm 72 and never had a sick day in my life. Who's right?

Mr. E.L.

Answer

I think you are, but before congratulating yourself see your doctor to make sure your heart and kidneys are functioning okay.

Puffiness or swelling around the ankles and feet is very common in the elderly. It is due mainly to fluid seepage from the tissues, and fluid naturally accumulates in lower areas due to gravity. Sometimes blood tends to pool in the veins of the lower legs and ankles causing swelling and sometimes bluish coloration, particularly if the legs dangle for long periods.

Do not be mislead by well-meaning friends and relatives to take "water pills" for this type of swelling. They are not only useless but can be dangerous. This is something you can manage yourself by lots of walking and avoiding long periods of sitting.

Again on the subject of swollen legs, here's a part of a letter from an elderly lady who definitely has a problem and requires medical treatment. She is 74 and lives alone. She writes:

. . . About a year ago I began to have shortness of breath. I noticed it first on climbing even a few steps of stairs. I put it down

153

to "old age" and really didn't think much of it, but it gradually got worse. Now I'm short of breath walking on the level on very little exertion and my legs are swollen all the time. The skin around my ankles and my shins can be pitted with my fingers. I've gained about ten pounds although my appetite is poor....

                                                              Mrs. O.T.

Answer

In contrast to Mr. E.L.'s case, your leg swelling is associated with shortness of breath and overall fluid accumulation, which accounts for your gain in weight. You most likely have congestive heart failure (that responds well to treatment). Here is where the water pill comes into its own and can be a lifesaver. Digoxin will also be a part of the medical management. You should seek medical attention at once.

And another reader writes:

... About five years ago I was told by my doctor that the swelling in my legs and gain in weight was due to kidney trouble (he found albumin in my urine). I have been a diabetic for about twenty years and am fairly well controlled on pills. I used to take twenty units of NPH insulin every day.

I have been feeling fairly well and even though my legs still swell and pit on pressure, I am under pretty good control regarding my swelling and weight. I do not have shortness of breath unless I rush. The doctor is checking for poisons in the blood.

                                                              Mr. L.M. (65)

Answer

Deterioration of the kidney blood vessels involved in the urine filtering system can be caused by diabetes mellitus and long-standing high blood pressure, to name two.

Fluid accumulation in kidney disease can often be troublesome and requires meticulous medical management. Anemia, too, is a frequent complication and can be difficult to treat. You state that your doctor is looking for "poisons" in your blood. I think he is testing for uremia, caused by waste products accumulating in the blood due to the kidney's inability to perform normally as a filter. You are indeed fortunate to be receiving such good medical care.

There are, of course, many other reasons for swelling of the legs in the elderly but the three letters above illustrate the three commonest causes. Of the three, Mr. E.L. is the most fortunate because he doesn't require treatment. He should, however, see his doctor once a year for a heart and kidney checkup. Mrs. O.T.'s swelling, shortness of breath, and excessive weight from fluid retention usually respond well to treatment. Mr. L.M., whose leg swelling is caused by kidney disease, needs the most medical attention, which must be ongoing. He needs expert care and is getting it.

Horse Sense

The Reverend Stephen Hales, an Anglican priest (1677–1761), is better known for his remarkable experiments in vegetable and animal physiology than for his salvation of English souls. His most enduring legacy to modern medicine was his classic demonstration of blood pressure in his horse (published in his *Hemostatiks,* 1733).

By inserting a long glass cannula (tube) in the carotid artery of Aesculapia, his trusted mare, he could demonstrate that on every beat of the heart, the blood shot up the cannula to a point indicating what we now call the systolic pressure. Between heartbeats the blood column fell to a point we now recognize as the "resting" or diastolic pressure.

The Hales or direct method of measuring arterial blood pressure is often resorted to when the indirect cuff method gives a grossly inaccurate reading—usually on the high side. It is a fairly common hospital procedure. (In a previous column on hypertension, I commented on the "fat arm effect" where the usual cuff method invariably produces a falsely high reading.)

Now we have scientific evidence that blood pressure readings in older people may, in many cases, be falsely high, giving rise to a brand new medical term, "pseudo-hypertension."

The unfortunate thing about this false high blood pressure is that elderly patients are subjected to various types of anti-hypertensive drugs that, even in legitimate cases, may cause distressing, disabling side effects.

In the *American Journal of Medicine* 80 (1986): 906, the author, Dr. Franz H. Messerli (Department of Internal Medicine, section of Hypertensive Diseases, Ochsner Clinic, New Orleans, Louisiana) reports on twenty-five elderly patients considered as "hypertensive by the usual cuff method of determining blood pressure." However, when their blood pressure was measured by the direct intra-arterial (Hales) method, there was, in Dr. Messerli's words, "a striking difference." Cuff systolic (top) readings were found to be in a range of 10 to 54 (average 16) points *above* the true arterial pressure.

What causes pseudo-hypertension in the elderly? Over ninety years ago Sir William Osler provided a clue. He taught that if the radial artery (pulse) was compressed to obliterate the pulse and the artery could still be felt beyond the point of compression, it indicated "sclerosis" or hardening and thickening of the middle coat of the radial artery. (Nowadays, compression of the pulse is done by the blood pressure cuff.)

Osler suggested that this thickening of the radial artery accounted for the difference between direct arterial and indirect (cuff) readings. Elderly patients, then, with excessive "hardening" of the arteries (by Osler test) may be simply exhibiting pseudo-hypertension. Since almost half our senior population has been labelled "hypertensive," it is evident that many of them are being "treated" not only inappropriately, but are being subjected to potential or actual serious side effects of anti-hypertensive drugs, and all for naught.

My message to physicians: Always perform the Osler bedside test before diagnosing "true" hypertension in an old person.

Non-Drug Rx for Mild Hypertension

Dear Dr. MacInnis:
I am a male 67 years old with what the doctor calls "mild hypertension." My blood pressure runs pretty consistently at 160

over 100 when I'm relaxed and I have no blood pressure symptoms. There is, however, a positive family history. My problem is that the drug I'm taking causes bothersome side effects. Several of my friends with mild blood pressure seem to be doing well on a non-drug treatment. I was wondering if this would be the answer for me and would value your opinion.

Mr. B.W., Ottawa, Ontario

Answer

I have written on the non-drug treatment of mild hypertension on numerous occasions and have always believed it had merit. However, I was never able to back up my contention with scientific evidence. That is, until quite recently when I ran across the report of a study presented by a group of New Jersey researchers at the Fourth European Meeting on Hypertension in Milan, Italy.

Here, Dr. John Kostis of the Robert Wood Johnson Medical School, New Brunswick, New Jersey, presented data that clearly showed that in the treatment of mild hypertension the non-drug approach—which included diet, exercise, relaxation, and stress reducing techniques—was clearly superior to drug therapy.

Eighty-six men, all over 57 years, were involved in the study. They fell into the generally accepted category of "mild" hypertension with a diastolic level of 95 to 100 millimeters mercury and were randomized to drug or non-drug treatment. The anti-hypertensive drug chosen was the beta-blocker propranolol (80 milligrams twice a day).

I'll give you now the non-drug routine in some detail:

Dietary: A weight reduction diet (when indicated) with salt and alcohol restriction.

Exercise: (Non-drug) patients were enrolled in a triweekly organized exercise program.

Behavioral: All patients in the non-drug group were taught relaxation and stress reduction techniques by a clinical psychologist.

Results: Over a three-month observation period, the non-drug group showed an average drop in blood pressure of 13 mm systolic over 7.4 mm. diastolic. The propranolol group had an 8.2 mm. systolic over 7.0 mm. diastolic.

Admittedly, the non-drug group did only slightly better than the drug patients when only reduced blood pressure was considered. Where the benefits of non-drug therapy showed up was in improved exercise tolerance, believed by the researchers to be due to the drug side effects experienced by the propranolol patients.

There was a remarkable reduction in body weight (averaging ten pounds) in the non-drug exercising group. In contrast, the drug patients evidenced an average *increase* of three pounds. There was a "significant decrease" in LDL (low-density lipoprotein) cholesterol (the bad kind) and triglycerides. Both were increased in the drug group.

On psychologic testing the non-drug group did "significantly better" in cognitive (mental awareness) performance than the group receiving propranolol.

Which of the various modalities mentioned (weight reduction, calorie reduction, and behavioral programs) lower blood pressure the best? The National Institute of Health will be funding Dr. Kostis and his group to determine just that in a follow-up project.

I would suggest, Mr. B., that you discuss a possible change-over to non-drug therapy with your doctor.

She Lost the Will to Live

Dear Dr. MacInnis:

My 85-year-old mother was found to have "high blood pressure" (in the 180/90 range) while in the hospital with a broken hip. After hip pinning she was discharged to home in good spirits and was getting along quite well until her doctor (on the advice of the hospital specialist) put her on medication to "get the pressure down." After a few days she became giddy, anxious, depressed, and lost her appetite. She definitely was not her former determined self and began to lose the will to live. She continued this way even after the dose was cut in half, and it was not until another doctor from the same clinic took her off the pills entirely that she began to improve, and I'm happy to say that she soon regained her former spirit and is now walking well and glad to be alive. Is this an unusual reaction? Do you think she still needs some other type of medication to keep her blood pressure down?

Mrs. T.L., California

Answer

For the past ten years I've regularly responded to this question, and any reader following my column is well aware of my opinion. It's this: No elderly person in the "old old" age group (80 plus) should be given high pressure medication because of its almost totally predictable side effects. Most of the letters I receive relate to a previously healthy old person with no complaints, who for some reason (often at a driver's medical) is found to have a "high reading" on the blood pressure machine. Frequently, this is insufficient reason to initiate treatment "to get the pressure down." As I've mentioned in previous columns on this subject, there is some evidence that an elevated blood pressure in the "old old" is nature's way of maintaining adequate blood perfusion in the brain and may even constitute a life-extension factor. In my opinion, forcing the blood pressure "down" in this instance is meddling with nature and asking for trouble.

Aneurysm of the Aorta

Dear Dr. MacInnis:

My doctor has told me that I have an aneurysm of the aorta in the abdomen and I am worried. I felt this pulsating sensation when I pressed on my abdomen but didn't think much about it as I had never heard of such a thing. When my doctor discovered it on a routine checkup he immediately referred me to have X rays and sent me to a specialist who advised follow-up examinations every three months.

The book Old Enough to Feel Better *states: "If you are in good health and the aneurysm is of sufficient size, it is better to*

159

*have it removed before it leads to problems." I am 79 years old
and in very good health, very active, and look after myself.*

*Would it not be advisable to have the aneurysm tended to
now before it causes trouble? I shall be anxiously awaiting your
reply. Any advice will be appreciated.*

Mrs. L.P.

Answer

An aneurysm is a localized dilation of an artery due to a
weakness in the wall, which may be due to a variety of causes
including trauma from an accident or in older people from natural weakening of the aging wall. In a particularly weakened
area, which may be only a few centimeters in diameter, the
artery slowly balloons from the pressure of blood on its wall.
Those of us old enough to remember the bulge of a damaged
"inner tube" of an auto tire will get the picture.

Although aneurysms can occur in the arteries of the brain
or kidneys, the commonest site involves the largest artery of all,
the aorta, the main pipeline carrying blood from the heart and
running down through the back of the thorax and the abdomen
and hugging the spine.

Aneurysms involving the abdominal aorta are much more
common than those in the thorax. This is indeed fortunate because abdominal aneurysms are more easily repaired. Furthermore, the aortic type can often be palpated by the doctor in the
course of a physical examination. And often the patient can feel
it, as in your case, Mrs. P, long before symptoms of a leaking
aneurysm occur.

The size of the aneurysm is important in deciding management and this can be roughly determined by an ordinary X ray
but far more accurately by special procedures such as ultrasound. In an otherwise healthy middle-aged adult, an aneurysm
five or more centimeters in diameter should be removed surgically as an elective (foreplanned, non-emergency) procedure.
Here the mortality risk is 2 to 5 percent, compared to a death
rate of 25 to 50 percent if the aneurysm has started to leak or
has ruptured.

As you do not mention the actual size of your aneurysm, I cannot give you the specific guidance you ask for. But I can give you advice in a general way.

Even though you are, as you say, "in very good health," your age (79) would constitute a more than average surgical risk. Because of this, I would agree with the specialist who recommends periodic ultrasound examinations. If there should be an indication that the aneurysm is enlarging, then an elective operation can be planned. This, I believe, would be the more prudent course.

For the very old patient (but not you!) with severe associated medical conditions, such as hypertensive or coronary heart disease, there is a conservative surgical approach consisting of ligating (tying off) the aorta above and below the aneurysm and the placement of a by-pass (axillary/femoral artery) graft. This operation is described in the *American Journal of Surgery* 146 (1983): 93.

Non-Cardiac Chest Pain

Dear Dr. MacInnis:

I have a puzzling chest pain condition that many doctors immediately diagnosed as angina (heart pain), but when I was referred to a heart specialist for further investigation there was never anything found in the way of heart disease. I have always considered the pain to be "heartburn" because when it would awaken me in the night I would get up and take some baking soda and water and in a few minutes the burning chest pain would always go away and I could go back to bed and sleep again. But to complicate matters, the pain would sometimes come on when I indulged in heavy exercise and that's what influenced some doctors to call it "angina," even though I get no relief from nitroglycerine. My question: Is it possible to have heart disease without heart findings or could it be all due to "heartburn"?

I would be happier with a diagnosis of "heartburn" than angina!

Mr. B.L. (56), Ontario

Answer

If you suffer from ongoing mid-chest pain that awakens you in the middle of the night and is always relieved by soda or other antacid, the chances are that the pain is due to inflammation of the esophagus (food pipe) and caused by backflow (reflux) there of acidic juices from the stomach. The medical term is "reflux esophagitis."

I am assuming, of course, that heart disease has been definitely ruled out, even though your pain is sometimes induced, like angina, by exercise. (It is occasionally present in reflux esophagitis.)

Reflux esophagitis is very commonly the cause of so-called non-cardiac chest pain. In the *Annals of Internal Medicine 1989* 110: 6678, there is an analysis of 117 articles on non-cardiac chest pain published since 1979, where it was found that two out of three cases of such pain were due to reflux esophagitis.

If antacids are not effective for you, I would suggest a histamine blocker like Tagamet, Zantac or Losec under medical supervision. Drugs such as these are more curative than palliative. (Losec is my favorite.)

(It should be noted that reflux esophagitis can coexist with genuine coronary artery disease, in some reports as high as 50 percent.)

The Nitroglycerine Patch: How Good Is It?

Dear Dr. MacInnis:

You often advise nitroglycerine tablets for angina. Have you had any experience with nitroglycerine in the form of a skin patch where it is absorbed through the skin? My age is 61 and I experience chest pain (under the breast bone) after moderate exertion, such as walking briskly and climbing stairs in a hurry.

Mr. L.R., Sun City, California

Answer

Transdermal or "through the skin" nitroglycerine skin patch is the latest mode of delivery for this drug prescribed for anginal pain for nearly a hundred years.

But sometimes it takes that long to learn some surprisingly new things about nitroglycerine. How many of us (medical doctors included) have been aware that nitroglycerine delivered in any of its forms—by mouth, under the tongue, inside the cheek, by vein, and now by skin patch—consistently loses its effectiveness with continued use?

The July 13, 1989, issue of the *Medical Letter* (a medical advisory service for physicians) cites numerous recent research studies showing that "transdermal nitroglycerine patches rapidly become ineffective for treatment of angina if they are left in place for twenty-four hours and reapplied daily, and remain ineffective even if the dosage is progressively increased. Patches delivering 10 mg. or more can be effective if they are removed for ten to twelve hours daily (usually overnight)." In other words, the 10 mg. or more patch should be applied "during the day only, for ten to twelve hours," says the *Medical Letter*.

If you are thinking of changing from oral to transdermal nitroglycerine, you had better first consult a cardiologist.

Should My Husband Have Had a By-pass?

Dear Dr. MacInnis:

My husband, age 40, died from what was called a "massive heart attack."

Even though four years have passed, I still think of him many times a day and believe he would still be alive if he had been given a by-pass operation. Although his angina was pretty well controlled with nitroglycerine, he always feared a heart attack. He saw a number of doctors including a heart specialist who did special heart X rays, but no one advised the operation. Why didn't they do the by-pass anyway if it prolongs life in heart patients?

Mrs. T.T.

Answer

I hope, Mrs. T., that you get comfort in learning that a coronary artery by-pass operation is done specifically for the relief of severe angina (heart pain) that does not respond, or responds poorly, to medical management with nitroglycerine, beta-blockers, calcium blockers, etc. There is still no firm conclusive evidence that the operation will reduce the probability of further heart attacks or death from a heart attack except in a small but extremely important group of heart patients.

These are patients with angina who on coronary angiography (heart X ray) show obstruction or near obstruction at the origin of the left coronary or perhaps obstruction at the origin of all three coronary (heart) arteries. In such patients, the annual death rate is about 15 percent. A by-pass can reduce this mortality rate to about 5 percent.

Another candidate for angiography and possible by-pass is the patient whose heart attack is followed by, or complicated with, intractable angina.

It is obvious (from your letter) that your husband did not belong to the above-mentioned exceptions. Otherwise, I feel he would have been advised to have a by-pass.

It is also clear from your letter that his angina was under fairly good control, a situation where a coronary by-pass operation is not indicated.

Second-Hand Pacemakers: Are They Okay?

Dear Dr. MacInnis:

My question: Can a heart pacemaker be reused? I've often wondered about this when I see my deceased friends interred with a good working pacemaker implanted in their chest. I have a pacemaker myself and as a part of my will I have directed that at the time of my death my pacemaker be removed for the purpose of possible reuse at the discretion of my doctor or hospital. I have not discussed this matter with anyone yet (except my lawyer), so *would appreciate some up-to-date information on the subject in your column. I believe many others would be interested, too. My pacemaker, now a year old, cost $2,500.*

Mr. K.H, 62, Ottawa, Ontario

Answer

Heart specialists tell us that most modern cardiac pacemakers can be expected to function normally for ten or more years, which is considerably more than the remaining life expectancy of probably 50 percent of recipients. So your point is well taken and your question very valid.

Can a pacemaker be reused? The answer is yes, and they have been reused worldwide over the past fifteen years. The regulations governing reuse vary with different countries, but in general there must be medical proof available that there was no evidence of instrument malfunction causing death of the donor and that there should be at least five years of remaining life in the pacemaker. But many hospitals have a policy of not accepting a pacemaker that has been implanted for only two years. So I would advise you to speak to your attending physician to determine your hospital's attitude and policy toward the reuse and reconditioning of pacemakers.

The ethics of donating a cardiac pacemaker, at least in Canada, is the same as that governing the donation of any organ or organs at time of death. Permission, then, must be given by the donor before death, and in the case of a donor's known unwillingness to donate, the next of kin cannot give permission. However, in the case of implanted devices like pacemakers, the death certificate of the donor must be signed by two physicians, neither of whom has any vested interest in the reuse of the instrument.

I am in total agreement with your attitude towards the reuse of pacemakers when it conforms with medical and ethical considerations. In regard to the latter, I would advise that you ask your lawyer to determine the policy of your hospital on the matter.

Chelation

Dear Dr. MacInnis:

How come you never write anything about chelation? I have read that it is good for cleaning out plugged arteries in the brain, heart, and legs. The doctor tells me that my leg arteries are plugged up with hard blood clot and cholesterol, so much that my leg muscles are not getting enough blood when I exercise them by walking. I can now only walk about half a block before I get severe pain in by legs. If I rest my legs for a while the pain goes away, only to return when I start walking again. My doctor recommends a by-pass operation to give my legs more blood. But a friend of mine with the same complaints underwent a course of chelation and states he is much improved.

Would you please give me the latest information on chelation therapy, especially for the treatment of my condition.

Mr. T.G., Rochester, New York

Answer

The medical term for your condition is "intermittent claudication." "Claudication," meaning pain in the leg (usually the calf) is caused by reduction of blood to the muscles as a result of narrowing of the arteries. Here the muscles cry out in pain when they are required to exercise without sufficient fuel (blood) to nourish them. There is usually sufficient blood to nourish the muscles at rest, hence, no pain. This is why the claudication is "intermittent."

Over the years I have received testimonials from readers extolling the merits of chelation for the pain of heart disease (angina), as well as letters from satisfied patients with intermittent claudication like yours. I have often been impressed with the sincerity of chelation patients but my pat answer to them was that until scientifically controlled studies proved the effectiveness of chelation, it could never be accepted by the medical profession.

The first scientific study of chelation for intermittent claudication of the lower limbs is now completed with the conclusion published in the *Journal of Internal Medicine* (March 1992): 231–67.

Here is how the study was conducted in seven departments of vascular surgery in several Danish hospitals:

Objective of study: To assess the effectiveness of chelation with EDTA (ethylene diamine tetra-acetic acid) treatment of intermittent claudication—a double-blind, placebo-controlled study.

Design: Randomized double-blind, placebo-controlled trial with six-month follow-up after treatment.

Patients: Fifty-six women and 103 men over 40 years with stable intermittent claudication of over twelve months' duration.

Intervention: Patients were randomized to twenty intravenous infusions of Na_2EDTA. The duration of each treatment was three to four hours. Treatment took five to nine weeks. Vitamins, trace elements, and mineral supplements were given as one tablet daily during treatment period. Patients were given advice on diet, cessation of smoking, and exercise.

Main results: Pain-free walking distances in both groups (EDTA treated and placebo treated) improved in six-month follow up. What is interesting here is that the EDTA group improved 30 percent, while the placebo treated group improved 45 percent. This would indicate a strong placebo effect operating in this study. In addition, 50 percent of both groups indicated that they experienced benefit from the treatment.

Conclusion: EDTA chelation treatment was not more effective than placebo in treating intermittent claudication. (The placebo was an inert intravenous solution exactly matching the EDTA solution in appearance.)

I would like to credit the American College of Physicians, *Journal Club Magazine,* vol. 115 (July/August 1992), for this study information.

(Addendum: This study was severely criticized by many proponents of chelation as being seriously flawed. They maintained, for example, that it was not really conducted as a "true double-blind" experiment because many of the patients knew when they were getting either the EDTA transfusion or the placebo (dummy look-alike) intravenous. As far as I am aware, there has been no rebuttal from the authors of the study who apparently have taken the stand that their conclusion speaks for itself.)

Chelation Continued

Shortly after the above column appeared in newspapers, I received this letter:

Dear Dr. MacInnis:
I suffered my first stroke in the spring of 1988. In the next two succeeding years, 1989 and 1990, I suffered a mild stroke in the spring of each year. (I did not have a stroke in the third year.) Then in the spring of 1992, I had five mini-strokes (TIAs) and the fifth put me in the Royal University Hospital in Saskatoon. After one week of intensive testing, I was discharged by the head doctor in this department saying they had done "all they could." However, they did not offer any solution for my recurring strokes. They told me that I would have to live with my condition like everyone else. They attributed my strokes to "high cholesterol."
The reason for my problems was the main arteries (carotids) in my neck. They were found to be about 60 percent blocked, being confirmed by ultrasound.
When I got home I cut down on my work everywhere I could, and I accepted the fact that my working days were over. Then I talked to a friend who had some contact with chelation and EDTA and I called a doctor in the United States. I went and had a total of twenty-two treatments and I'm now told that my blockage is reduced to 4.7 percent (confirmed by a U.S. doctor).
I am feeling better than I have for twenty years and am doing my work on a full-time basis, including hunting, hiking, and whatever else I wish to do.
Mr. J.E., Saskatchewan

Answer

At the beginning of my column, I remarked that over the years, I have received numerous correspondence extolling the benefits of chelation. The above letter is a good example of what I mean and, as I stated before, I have often been impressed with many of them.

Apart from the Danish study of the effects of chelation treatment on peripheral atherosclerosis (narrowing and hardening of the femoral arteries), causing intermittent claudication, there have been no randomized, placebo-controlled, double-blind studies to determine the effects of chelation on patients with coronary (heart) or cerebrovascular (brain) atherosclerosis.

Chelation has been recognized in medicine for the past forty years as a means for removing toxic metals, as in lead intoxication and the excess iron in iron overload, from the body. The chemical agent used in chelation is EDTA (ethylene diamine tetra-acetic acid). It chelates or bonds with these metals and the resulting product is passed out in the urine. Since EDTA has a high bonding affinity for calcium, the modern proponents of chelation claim that since calcium is a component of the atheromatous plaque, plugging heart, limb, and brain arteries, chelation causes plaque disintegration resulting in alleviation of the pain in angina, intermittent claudication and the symptoms of stroke. It has been particularly advocated as an inexpensive alternative to coronary by-pass surgery. (A course of thirty chelation sessions costs about $3,000.)

These reported benefits, and there have been many, are basically subjective or anecdotal. There are also at least nine published studies (none using scientific methodology) on the effect of chelation therapy on coronary heart disease, all reporting mainly subjective amelioration of symptoms.

What's the solution to this perennial impasse between the medical establishment and the proponents of chelation? I suggest that the two parties get together amicably and rationally (for a change) and formally request the FDA in the United States or the Health Protection Branch in Canada, or both, to conduct a huge scientifically controlled study (there are plenty of subjects!) and decide for once and for all on the medical usefulness of what is currently a most controversial procedure.

Early Signs of a Heart Attack

Dear Dr. MacInnis:

Recently your column dealt with heart attacks. Is there any way I can tell when I am going to have a heart attack? I am a male executive, age 40, and have angina. A nitroglycerine tablet under my tongue is effective for the pain. In fact, I sometimes take it before anticipated exertion and can usually get through it without pain.

Mr. T.L., Ontario

Answer

Nitroglycerine taken before exertion can be quite effective. Many people with angina do this.

Can you tell in advance that you're going to have a coronary (heart attack)? Not precisely. But there are, I believe, warning signs: (1) Periods of unexplained tiredness which must be a new experience for you, (2) so-called indigestion or, perhaps, heartburn, and again this must be something new, (3) excessive sweating, (4) mild to moderate nausea without vomiting, (5) angina occurring from a lesser degree of exertion than previously, and (6) angina that no longer responds to nitroglycerine or to rest.

The first four signs may, of course, be signalling some other condition. But remember them and if you are the least bit suspicious see your doctor.

Can Angina Show a "Normal" ECG?

Dear Dr. MacInnis:
In your column about angina and heart attacks you didn't mention anything about an ECG. I have angina but the ECG always reads normal. How come?

Mr. C.T., Owen Sound, Ontario

Answer

The electrocardiograph is an instrument that picks up the electrical charge produced by the beating heart muscle and records these signals on a moving ribbon of paper. This record is called an electrocardiogram or ECG.

The ECG is exceedingly useful in demonstrating disorders of heart rhythm. In fact, there is often no other way of precisely diagnosing a heartbeat disorder.

If a heart attack (coronary) is suspected on clinical signs and symptoms, the ECG may verify not only the extent of heart muscle damage but its precise location as well.

There are many other heart conditions where an ECG is very useful, such as in detecting ventricle (heart chamber) enlargement from, say, long-standing high blood pressure or congenital (born with) heart defects. It may also be useful in diagnosing changes in blood chemistry affecting the heart muscle. In angina, the ECG may be abnormal in that it reveals certain areas in the heart muscle that may be anemic (due to the narrowed or "spastic" coronary [heart] arteries being unable to sufficiently nourish the heart muscle). If the patient exercises while having an ECG done (such as in a stress test), there is more likelihood of an abnormality showing up than with a resting ECG.

Unfortunately, most ECGs done in the doctor's office are of the resting type where the patient lies on a table during the recording. In such an instance, there is a good possibility that the electrocardiograph will not pick up any muscle anemia, as the heart in its "resting" state is now getting sufficient blood for its nourishment.

Here, then, is a situation where the ECG may be reported "normal" but where the heart is not—and yours is a case in point.

A Case of the "Silent" Heart Attack

I recently received a letter from the widow of a 78-year-old man who was seen in the outpatient department of a busy metropolitan hospital. She brought him there for examination and treatment of an acute confusional state of six hours' duration (he had been well before that). After a brief physical examination of the patient, the wife was told that her husband was indeed confused; an injection was given and he was sent home. His condition soon deteriorated and the paramedics were called and did a routine electrocardiogram that showed an acute myocardial infarction (heart attack). The patient died on the way to the (same) hospital.

If the patient had been a younger man, he most likely would have complained of acute mid-chest pain, which would have alerted the attending doctor to order an electrocardiogram that would have shown evidence of a heart attack. The elderly patient would then have received treatment that might have saved his life.

The so-called silent coronary in an elderly patient is not infrequently accompanied by a delirium or confusional state of sudden onset. Another fairly common sign is pallor and sweating, indicating a potential or an actual collapsing of the circulatory system.

Acute appendicitis in an elderly person frequently presents with few of the classical signs and symptoms found in younger people. This often accounts for a late diagnosis that may prove fatal.

The above two non-typical presentations of acute disease in the elderly are good examples of the difference between the practice of geriatric medicine and medical practice in general. Most doctors are becoming increasingly aware of the difference.

Pseudo-Hypertension

Dear Dr. MacInnis:

I was very interested in a recent article you wrote on a condition that I think you called "senior high blood pressure." I cut it out in order to give copies to my mother and her doctor. However, I'm sad to say that I lost it. My poor mother is 79. Her blood pressure when measured by a cuff is extremely high. Nurses and doctors start running around in sheer panic after taking it! The figures are often 250 over 110 and have been this way for over twenty-five years since she was involved in a motor vehicle accident. Medication makes her sick and does nothing to bring down the readings, even after lying down for half an hour. Medical personnel are always telling her she is lucky to be alive and that she could succumb to a stroke any minute. This does nothing to ease her anxiety. However, she ignores it as much as possible and leads a very healthy, normal life.

Two years ago she was hospitalized in order to study her condition and her blood pressure was measured by inserting something (a tube, I believe) into her vein or artery in her arm. Her reading was normal for a person her age. However, doctors seem to refuse to accept this as the more acceptable reading, and each year she has trouble with licence renewal. As well, doctors are always pushing her to take medication.

If memory serves me correctly, this condition was exactly what you described in your column. But I cannot find it and, worse yet, I don't remember when it was published. Could you please either let me know the date or send me a copy of that article. My mother and I would be so grateful.

Mrs. W.K.

Answer

I found the column and am sending you a computer printout. The heading in your newspaper read: "Blood Pressure Readings May Be Falsely High for Seniors." So you were not so far off. The subject of my column was "Pseudo-hypertension" or *"False* High Blood Pressure."

173

I feel I should comment on your mother's case. Two years ago, when your mother was found to have "a normal for age" blood pressure by the *direct arterial method,* that should have been the end of the matter, for this is the most accurate method of taking blood pressure that exists.

For the reasons outlined in my column (thickening of the radial artery or the "fat arm" effect, or both) abnormally high readings may result in high-dose medication in a frantic effort to "get the pressure down" at any cost, often resulting in a very sick patient.

Note: For further insight into pseudo-hypertension, please refer to my previous column titled "Horse Sense."

Cholesterol Levels in the Elderly

Democrat & Chronicle
55 Exchange Boulevard
Rochester, New York

Dear Editor:
I am writing in reference to a column by Dr. MacInnis which appeared recently in the Sunday edition of your newspaper.

Specifically, I refer to the good doctor's opinion on so-called normal cholesterol levels for various adult age groups, ranging from 225 to 265 milligrams per deciliter (m/dl).

According to various sources, three of which are listed below, the ideal *cholesterol reading for adults is 200 (or less) milligrams per deciliter. Some physicians have given the ideal figures as between 140 and 180 m/dl.*

1. *National Cholesterol Education Program. "U.S. Defines Cholesterol Hazards" by Philip M. Buffey,* New York Times, *October 6, 1987*
2. Circulation, *published by the American Heart Association, May, 1984*
3. New York Times *article by Jane Brody, March 29, 1987*

There are numerous adults who would be pleased if Dr. Mac-Innis' figures are accurate.

Very truly yours,
Mrs. A.M. Ithaca, New York

cc Dr. MacInnis

Answer

Here's how my cholesterol levels correlated with age should have appeared in your newspaper: In the age group 20 to 29 years the so-called normal cholesterol level is <200 m/dl, for 30 to 39 years <225 m/dl, 40 to 49 <250, and over 50 <265 m/dl. Note the "less than" or < symbol preceding each figure (omitted in most newspapers carrying my column).

It's unfortunate that when either "normal" or "ideal" cholesterol values are tabulated in the lay or medical press, age differences are never mentioned.

As I mentioned in a previous column, so called normal cholesterol levels should not be considered absolute but a rough reflection of North American (U.S./Canada) values. There's continuing debate as to just what is the "normal" range. Some feel the current figures for all age groups are set too high. And can you always trust your lab results? Laboratory readings throughout the country are far from consistent. In 1985, the American College of Pathologists prepared a standard blood sample with a cholesterol content of 263 milligrams per deciliter (m/dl) and sent it to 1,000 laboratories. Although the majority clustered in the 222 to 294 area, the general range was 197 to 397!

In my medical references, I am reading less and less about total cholesterol levels and more about low density lipoprotein (LDL cholesterol), the "bad" kind that predisposes to coronary heart disease, and the "good," or high-density lipoprotein (HDL cholesterol), that tends to protect us from coronary heart disease.

Probably the best source of cholesterol information is the *International Lipid Information Bureau Newsletter (ILIB)*, 1775 Broadway, New York 10019. Every issue contains a bewildering array of cholesterol information dealing with lipoproteins, HDL and LDL cholesterol, with their protein fractions such as Apo-lipoproteins. I do not recommend this newsletter to the lay reader with no knowledge of biochemistry, but it certainly keeps one up-to-date on the vagaries of what is becoming an exceed-ingly complex area of laboratory and clinical medicine that only specialists in the field are truly familiar with.

Before you begin dozing off, let me tell you I came across an interesting item, meaningful and—more importantly —understandable, which I quote directly from an *ILIB* Newslet-ter. "In the Framington study follow-up (of thirty-two years) those with low total cholesterol plus low HDL run a higher risk for heart disease." The reason for this seeming contradiction is that a very low HDL can pull down the total cholesterol level and illustrates the importance of knowing what the HDL and LDL blood levels are before determining the risk of heart disease.

Although total cholesterol readings are the most often re-quested blood levels for elderly patients, they are in fact even poorer indicators of coronary risk than in younger adults. And here again, the HDL and LDL fractions are important—at least in the "young old" (60 to 75)—to determine future risk for heart disease, and if treatment is warranted it should be along the lines of restricted dietary fat and not by cholesterol-reducing drugs.

In the "old old" (75 and up) there has been remarkably little research done and prognosis has been derived almost exclusively from extrapolation of data from research on younger age groups, which questions its validity.

Nevertheless, the "old old" are remarkably preoccupied and some pathologically concerned with their cholesterol levels if the correspondence I receive is any indication. Although their fears are totally unwarranted, I feel there's a positive side to it, for it often keeps them watchful and alert to the ever-increasing cholesterol hype bombarding them from all directions, which in the end may make them more sensible eaters than their often obese, fat-addicted parents!

High cholesterol should never be considered solely in terms of a single number but as one of the many risk factors for actual or future heart disease, and these are obesity, hypertension, cigarette smoking, lack of exercise, being male, and having a family history of heart trouble. This applies to all ages, but as we reach the venerable age of 80 plus such generalizations have less and less validity, and this particularly applies to "high" cholesterol. At this age "low" cholesterol associated with chronic debility and malnutrition is commonly a predictor of approaching death.

When Cholesterol-Lowering Drugs Fail

I've received letters from numerous readers claiming that their blood cholesterol remained unchanged after several months of treatment with various cholesterol-reducing drugs. Most said that they followed prescribed dosage but none of them offered any "excuse" for their so-called therapeutic failures. All tended to blame the drug itself and many well known cholesterol-lowering agents were incriminated. No mention was ever made about the possibility of lifestyle and other factors being at least partly responsible. Without such information I wasn't of much help to them.

At a recent lipid conference in Edmonton, sponsored by the pharmaceutical firm of Merck, Sharp and Dohme, this question of treatment failure was discussed at some length. Here is a list of reasons given for poor therapeutic response:

1. Failure to lose weight. If the patient is obese, weight reduction is extremely important.
2. Non-compliance on the part of the patient. Although my readers assured me that they followed their doctor's order to the letter, many patients apparently do not.
3. Inappropriate medication. Here the doctor may prescribe a cholesterol-lowering drug that is not the most appropriate given the patient's overall lipid profile.
4. Excessive alcohol intake. This is a clear-cut prescription that virtually guarantees failure!

177

5. Interaction with other drugs. Make sure your doctor is aware of any other drugs you may be taking.
6. Diabetes mellitus, hypothyroidism, and kidney dysfunction may all antagonize the beneficial effects of cholesterol reducing drugs.

It is therefore incumbent upon the patient and even more so on the attending physician to make sure that if a cholesterol-lowering drug is the management of choice, that (1) the appropriate drug is used, and (2) the drug is not necessarily in itself a means to an end. The patient's overall medical state and lifestyle should always be kept in mind.

With cholesterol so very much in the news I have devoted many columns to the subject. One continually recurring complaint I receive from readers is that the expression of cholesterol levels can be confusing, particularly for my Canadian followers who derive much of their information from U.S. sources. The problem is that each country uses a different chemical expression. U.S. patients are conversant with the expression in milligrams per decilitre (m/dl), while their Canadian cousins declare their levels in millimols per litre (mmol/l).

For your scribe who writes for both U.S. and Canadian papers, I am continually beset with this problem. My only solution is to give the two references and for the umpteenth time I will proclaim for the sake of better international understanding that always elusive conversion factor—0.02586.

Example: To convert a cholesterol level of, say, 200 m/dl (American reference) to the new Canadian reference, *multiply* 200 by the conversion factor 0.02586, which is 5.17 mmol/l. To convert 5.17 mmol/l back to the American *divide* 5.17 mmol/l by 0.02586. Eureka! 200 m/dl.

At the aforementioned Edmonton lipid presentation one speaker, on the subject of low-density lipoproteins (LDL, the "bad" kind), cited the desirable level to less than<130 m/dl (<3.36 mmol/l) and high risk level—anything greater than >160 m/dl. Note to Canadian readers: Armed with your redoubtable conversion factor, please carry on with your evening's homework.

High Blood Pressure in the Elderly

Dear Dr. MacInnis:

I am a male, age 70 years, and feel fine. The doctor tells me my systolic (upper figure) pressure is high at 170 but my diastolic (lower figure) pressure is normal at 60.

My question: Should I have treatment with my lower figure normal?

Mr. L.K., Utica, New York

Answer

Before addressing your question I would like to ask you one. Are you sure your systolic blood pressure is 170 milligrams? Did you, for instance, have a *baseline* blood pressure reading established? Here your doctor takes the *average* of three readings in two or three occasions preferably two days apart and will try to make you relaxed and used to the foreboding clinical surroundings, not forgetting the "White Coat Syndrome"! The discerning physician will also get several standing, sitting, and supine readings, and if there was a marked blood pressure drop on standing, it may indicate postural hypotension, something the doctor must keep in mind when or if you're put on an anti-hypertensive drug.

So okay, your blood pressure is 170/80 and you're *sure* of it. Should you now have the treatment you ask about? You have a special type of high blood pressure. It's called isolated systolic hypertension (without the usually increased diastolic component). It is said that systolic hypertension is associated with a higher morbidity (hypertensive-related illness, e.g., stroke) and mortality (death) than from a predominately diastolic elevation. But there are as yet no controlled comparative studies to support this contention. (See page 133 for recent update.)

What we do know is that there are several large randomized trials all attesting to the benefit of anti-hypertensive therapy in the elderly who had both diastolic and systolic hypertension. All studies however were beset with bothersome to severe side

179

effects that often necessitated cessation of drug treatment. Exquisitely sensitive were the elderly hypertensives who exhibited the aforementioned postural hypotension (on standing from the supine or sitting position).

I would treat you as any elderly hypertensive, with great caution and discernment, beginning with the relatively mild diuretic (water pill) and if at all possible staying with it. The doctor must always weigh any benefits of treatment against side effects with its reduced quality of life. I would be hard pressed indeed to continue any kind of drug therapy after the age of 75 and in very rare circumstances on reaching 80.

I recently received a letter from the son of an aged patient who was clearly the victim of a frantic compulsion to "treat" a blood pressure reading rather than the whole person. Here it is (in part):

Dear Dr. MacInnis:

Back in March 1989, my sister in Rochester, New York, sent me one of your columns dealing with treating high blood pressure in the very old. At the time my father was on 10 milligrams of Vasotec and 20 milligrams of Procardia daily for high blood pressure and Desyrel, 50 mg. (presumably for agitated depression). . . .

I took him to another doctor who agreed that he should be taken off the high blood pressure medication and prescribed a water pill (25 mg. hydrochlorthiazide per day). This change in medication appears to be helping him . . . also for the past five nights he has not taken the Desyrel. . . .

So I am optimistic at the present that at last my father will get some relief from the headaches and dizziness that have been plaguing him. Now if I can just convince him that he has reached the age of 91 and should stop expecting that he should be able to work as well as he did before all his health problems started four years ago!

Answer

This letter is typical of what happens when patients of great age suffering from side effects are taken off their offending medication. It's more than likely that stopping the Desyrel may have helped the headaches and dizziness, both side effects of this drug.

Are Old Patients with a Heart Attack Getting "Short-Changed"?

It is well known that the elderly are more vulnerable for fatal heart attacks than younger age groups. But despite their greater risk, "they receive," according to Montague and co-workers from the University of Alberta Hospitals, "significantly less aggressive, investigative, and therapeutic attention than their younger counterparts with acute myocardial infarction" (acute heart attack). Their findings were published in the *American Journal of Cardiology* 68 (October 1, 1991): 843–47.

The researchers studied 402 consecutive admissions treated for acute heart attack (myocardial infarction) between July 1, 1981, and June 30, 1989. Of these 402 patients, 132 were 70 years and older and the remainder, 270 patients, were below the age of 70.

They concluded that older patients tended to be treated less aggressively than younger patients with acute myocardial infarction. A good example is immediate clot lysis therapy—TPA (tissue plasminogen activator) or streptokinase—used in 28 percent of younger patients and in only 4 percent of older patients in the study. Special tests to assess risk for a repeat attack were performed less frequently in older than in younger people. For example, exercise tolerance (stress tests) were done in 54 percent of younger patients compared to 22 percent in the senior group, and special X rays of the heart arteries (coronary arteriography) were ordered on 51 percent of the younger *versus* 20 percent of the older group.

As would be expected, in-hospital mortality rate was 27 percent in the older age group against 8 percent in younger patients.

It is difficult to escape the conclusion that older patients with acute heart attacks have been "short-changed" in the way of specialized diagnostic and therapeutic procedures afforded to younger patients. But there's probably more here than meets the eye. As an accompanying editorial in the journal points out, the bulk of current research in this area of cardiology has been directed to the younger patient, and since attending physicians are not sure of the possible adverse reactions to procedures and therapy in older patients, they are often reluctant to go "full out" as they might tend to do in their younger patients.

So it looks as though most seniors will continue to be treated "differently" for their acute heart attacks until further research in this area of geriatric cardiology gives the green light, which is somewhat "iffy."

Heart Pain: Do Women Get Short-Changed, Too?

Dear Dr. MacInnis:

I am fully convinced that women, on the average, get "short-changed" compared to men when they see a doctor or go to the emergency department complaining of chest pain. Why do I say this? I speak from personal experience. I am a 45-year-old man who last year saw my doctor because of a dull, sickly pain in my chest that he diagnosed as a heart attack, and within an hour I was in the hospital where the diagnosis was confirmed and emergency (clot buster) treatment initiated.

Quite recently, my wife, age 42, went to the same doctor with chest symptoms similar to my case, but apparently, it did not impress him, for she was given a prescription for Tagamet to try out for a few days in case it was "just heartburn." Well, it wasn't "just heartburn," for that same night she was rushed by ambulance to the same hospital where tests showed she had suffered an acute myocardial infarction (heart attack)—something the heart specialist there found hard to believe—all because she was a woman it would seem. She did receive treatment, but twelve hours late, when it really didn't have to be when early treatment is so important.

*Fortunately, everything turned out okay. But it got me think-
ing. What might have happened if we hadn't rushed her to the
hospital? Since then I have read a magazine article which stated
that since women my wife's age are "hormone protected," they are
not so inclined to turn up with a heart attack as frequently as
men. My question: What is your opinion on this?*

Mr. T.F., Florida

Answer

I would agree with you in principle. Just recently, a group
of researchers from Harvard University found that women were
less likely to receive surgery to clear coronary artery clot (angioplasty) or to by-pass blocked heart arteries. A second study
(also at Harvard) found women were less likely than men to be
transferred from small local hospitals to larger medical facilities
to obtain the most advanced diagnostic services and treatment.

While it's true that women *before* menopause are not so
susceptible as men to heart attacks because of their "hormone
protection" as you say, some doctors don't have the high index
of suspicion that they do with men. *After* menopause a woman's
susceptibility gradually increases so that by age 55 or so her
risk for a heart attack is about the same as for a man.

Is Alcohol Good for the Heart?

Dear Dr. MacInnis:
*I have some questions for you regarding heart disease. (1)Are
men more likely to develop heart disease then women? (2) Is alcohol good for the heart? (3) How does cigarette smoking affect the
heart?*

Answer

1. There is a lower incidence of heart disease in women up
to the menopause. After that (50 to 55) they become equally
susceptible to heart disease when their protective female sex
hormone level drops.

2. Recent research has indicated that about two cocktails per day regularly can increase the level of HDL cholesterol (the good kind) and there is a lower incidence of heart disease in people with elevated HDL. It should be kept in mind that alcohol in large amounts is a cardiac poison that can depress heart function. So easy does it.

3. Cigarette smoking increases the heart rate as well as the blood pressure, both predisposing to heart disease in later life.

Heart Valve Replacement

Dear Dr. MacInnis:

My husband had a mitral heart valve replaced at the age of 76 three years ago. The doctors told him that there were two kinds of heart valves. There was the mechanical type, which lasted longer on average than the live tissue pig valve but caused clotting problems requiring a daily anticoagulant (warfarin) for the rest of his life. Because my husband reacted badly to anticoagulants previously, he chose the pig valve and has done well over the past three years with it.

My question: Could you tell us the long term results of both kinds of valves? In your opinion, considering his age, did my husband make a good choice by choosing the pig valve?

Mrs. K.N., Toronto, Ontario

Answer

Your doctor's evaluation of the two valves at the time of your husband's surgery three years ago was correct as it was prophetic. Up to that time there were no compelling long-term comparative studies available to cardiologists who based their opinion only on five-year results that indicated no statistical differences in survival.

Now it appears we have the answer. A large study called the Edinburgh Heart Valve Trial involved 541 patients randomly assigned to receive either a synthetic (mechanical) valve or a porcine (pig) valve. (Valves were both mitral and aortic.)

Results: After *twelve years* 37 percent of the pig valves needed reoperation *versus* only 8.5 percent with the mechanical valves. As for survival, the study revealed that patients with the mechanical valve survived statistically longer than patients with pig valves, with the most significant difference in mitral valve replacement—mechanical 42 percent *versus* porcine 24 percent.

Now to answer your question: I believe your husband made an excellent choice in choosing the pig valve for the following reasons: (1) he has not needed daily warfarin for anti-coagulation, something he would have required with the mechanical valve with perhaps catastrophic results; and (2) since year twelve appeared to be the critical time period for the porcine valve, the question should be who on the average survives longer, the elderly patient or the valve? This is answered by the authors of the study who suggested that porcine valves may be considered for older patients whose life expectancy at time of operation would probably not exceed that of the valve (approximately twelve years).

Another finding of interest to senior patients: The survival rate of the porcine valve in the elderly appeared to be longer than in younger patients, for reasons not clear.

Heart Transplant Survival Rate

Dear Dr. MacInnis:

My wife and I would like you to settle an argument between us. It's about heart transplantation. She says that it is still an experimental procedure and the survival rate is uncertain. I maintain that it is the generally accepted treatment for heart disease that has reached "the end of the line" and that the survival rate is quite good. Who is right?

Mr. E.L., Toronto, Ontario

Answer

You are, of course. Heart transplantation, as you say, is the treatment for "end stage" heart disease.

Over the past decade there have been tremendous strides made in the survival rate after heart transplantation, thanks to the anti-rejection properties of cyclosporin and steroids—the all-important factor in postoperative management. Also, periodic heart muscle biopsies are more refined and are employed to act as a monitor for the slightest hint of rejection.

In the United States, the three-year survival rate is 92 percent. (Meaning that three years after their heart transplantation, 92 percent of patients are alive.) The five-year survival rate is approximately 90 percent.

The term "end stage" heart disease means that the patient is totally incapacitated and is not responding to regular cardiac treatment and is failing rapidly. In such a case, without transplantation, even the one-year and perhaps the six-month survival rate would be near zero. And the age limit: Ideally, under 60 and without other chronic debilitating illness. But there are always exceptions.

Sick Sinus Syndrome

Dear Dr. MacInnis:

What is the heart condition called "sick sinus syndrome"? This is what the doctors said my husband (age 74) had when he suffered a fainting spell that came right out of the blue. After a long series of tests they fitted him with a heart pacemaker. That was a year ago and he hasn't had a spell like it since. He is now in good health in every way. The doctors didn't explain this condition in a way I could understand it, although I guess they tried.

Mrs. K.L., Webster, New York

Answer

First, a brief lesson in heart anatomy and physiology. Situated in the right atrium (upper chamber) of the heart is a miniature electric power station called the sinus node that initiates the heart beat. When something affects this nodal power station, various kinds of rhythm disturbances can occur—from spells of slow heart beat (bradycardia) to fast heart rate (tachycardia), from rapid, irregular heart beats (fibrillation) to spontaneous sinus "arrest" with momentary cessation of the heart beat. In addition, sick sinus syndrome (SSS) is a common cause of cerebral embolism in older people where a clot from stagnant blood in a poorly functioning heart chamber travels to the brain causing a stroke. (In a group of one hundred patients with SSS, sixteen suffered from wandering clots, or emboli, of which thirteen travelled to the brain.)

And what is this "something" that may affect the sinus node rendering it "sick?" By far the commonest "something" is degeneration from the aging process. That is why a myriad of rhythm disorders, some mentioned above, occur mainly in the elderly and the commonest disorder is recurrent slow heart beat (often as low as 30 per minute). At that slow rate the heart cannot pump sufficient blood to the brain, so giddiness and even fainting can occur. Paramedics, called to the scene of a fainting attack, are usually the first to note the often slow heart rate, and this finding can provide the first clue in diagnosis.

A pacemaker is the treatment of choice for a "sick" sinus node causing such conditions as sinus arrest, sinus pauses, and, as in your husband's case, prolonged bradycardia (excessively slow heart rate)—all which may result in giddiness, dizziness, or fainting spells.

I am sure many readers have heard of cases of sudden cardiac death occurring in athletes during strenuous physical activity. The *Annals of Internal Medicine* 67 (1967): 1013, reports on the sudden death of young athletes caused by the spontaneous formation of a clot in a tiny artery nourishing the sinus node and thus crippling the heart's electrical power station. This is an example of an *acute* sick sinus syndrome causing sinus arrest with sudden death.

I Have Varicose Veins—and Bad!

Dear Dr. MacInnis:

I am a female, age 56, with varicose veins that are pretty bad. The doctor says I should get them stripped and cure them for once and for all. I don't look forward to that kind of surgery and was wondering if injecting them would do the job. The doctor said, "No, they're just too big for either injection or laser." I guess there's nothing much more to ask about but would like your opinion anyway. They cause swelling of my legs but that's not the reason I want treatment. Those "worm bags" on the inside of my knees, calves and ankles are so disfiguring.

Mrs. K.P., Winnipeg, Manitoba

Answer

Did you know that hemorrhoids, or "piles," in the anus and rectum are also bona-fide varicose veins? But mere mention of the term "varicose veins" invariably conjures the image of an irregular, tortuous ballooning of the long and/or short saphenous veins ascending inside of both legs from the ankle to the groin Rarely visible in its normal state, these two superficial veins normally drain venous blood from the "skin-deep" leg areas back to the heart and lungs for oxygen. It should be remembered that the bulk of venous blood draining the legs is carried by the larger deep femoral veins. So if the saphenous veins become varicosed (ballooned and obstructed) and rather useless as a blood carrier, it's no big deal, for the deep femoral vein can carry the venous load. And this explains why both varicosed saphenous veins can be removed surgically without compromising the blood circulation in the legs.

Varicose veins are very common, occurring in about 15 percent of adults in the 30 to 60 age group. Women are four times more susceptible than men. They do not occur overnight. They develop slowly over years.

What causes them? Let's concentrate on that long saphenous vein. As we age, the walls of this vein become less elastic. When the walls weaken they bulge or balloon. Inside the walls of the saphenous veins are valves that help to keep the column of blood moving up against gravity to the heart. But if the wall of the saphenous vein becomes weakened and stretched, the valve fails and can no longer hold up the blood column, resulting in pooling and stagnation. The veins now show up as the blue colored "worm bags" you so aptly describe.

Your legs may ache from varicose veins, especially if you stand for long periods. The skin area over the veins can become itchy and inflamed. Ulcers may form in severe cases and sometimes they may bleed when accidentally banged. But what probably brings most patients to the doctor is that nasty disfigurement, particularly on the inside of the knees and down the legs to the ankles in varying degrees of ugliness.

Treatment, too, varies with severity. In mild cases progression may be delayed by a daily walking routine and remembering to elevate your legs when sitting or lying down several times a day (the oftener the better) for, say, ten minutes. And never sit in one position too long. If you're car driving get out every hour or so and take a short walk. If you're overweight, slim down; it reduces pressure in the veins. Low pressure stockings are often helpful.

If your varicose veins were mild to moderate, Mrs. P., your doctor might have injected a sclerosing agent into the affected vein or veins causing them to close down and, in many cases, disappear.

Only about 10 percent of varicose veins require surgery (stripping) where a plastic (stripper) wire is passed up the saphenous veins from the ankle to the groin and the vein is stripped or pulled out. The procedure requires general anesthesia and takes about half an hour.

Over the past two decades the treatment of varicose veins has become much more conservative. Only in selected cases, mainly where a venous valve or valves have failed, is surgical stripping usually done.

The "White Coat Syndrome"

Dear Dr. MacInnis:
Every time I have my blood pressure taken at the doctor's office, I have the feeling my pressure shoots up! Just thinking of seeing the doctor makes my pressure elevate and heart go fast.

He's no heart-throb. He's as gruff as can be and that's what makes him scary. I've been seriously thinking of buying a blood pressure machine to check myself, so as to get a more realistic reading than at my doctor's office. I've read that there are good digital devices out that are quite accurate and easy to operate. Would you kindly give me the names of some that are approved and the approximate price.

Mrs. K.N. (56), Sun City, Calfornia

Answer

You are a victim of the "White Coat Syndrome" a well-documented nervous response to having your blood pressure read or just awaiting it. The person in the white coat may be your doctor, your nurse, or the receptionist. It doesn't happen to everyone—mainly to hyper, tense individuals who are always expecting the blood pressure to be "higher than last time" and are seldom disappointed. Susceptible patients have told me that then can feel "a surge" of blood pressure and heart throbbing on entering the doctor's waiting room.

It's easy, then, to understand why some initial blood pressure readings are falsely "high." No discerning physician would ever think of making a diagnosis of hypertension and prescription treatment on the first visit. The experienced doctor will sense the patient's anxiety and will use various means to allay his or her fears. In some cases of hypertension, however, the emotional element is so prominent that many doctors request some patients to self-record their blood pressure in the quiet privacy of home to establish a normal baseline. Yours, Mrs. N., is a case in point, except that you've beaten your doctor to it! Congratulations.

It can be very difficult for any untrained or even, in some cases, a trained patient to accurately use the mercury or aneroid blood pressure machines usually found in the doctor's office. They require the use of a stethoscope that takes considerable experience to operate accurately.

It is not surprising, then, that most patients opting for self-measurement choose, like yourself, one of the many digital devices on the market.

The *Canadian Consumer* magazine (February 1987) rates a number of digital devices as *good:* Astropulse 78, Homecare 2740, Lumiscope 1060, Marshall 85, Nissei DS-115, and Tycos 7052.

Digital devices range from the ultra-sophisticated that you pay through the nose for (over $300) to much cheaper but entirely adequate products that average $100. One authority recommends the "oscillometric" device over the widely advertised "microphone" instrument.

Contrary to lay opinion, digital devices that record a seemingly "exact" reading of, say, 137 over 77 can be deceiving. Recent tests have shown that the best available electronic digital devices give the majority of blood pressure levels within 5 millimeters of mercury on the standard machine found in your doctor's office. But sometimes there may be unexpected variations that require repeating. Digital devices should be checked periodically against standard machines.

No hypertensive patient should embark on a self-measuring blood pressure routine without undergoing training in the doctor's office. Most doctors would welcome patient participation in selected cases, particularly where the basic blood pressure level can only be established by "home readings," as in your case, or in other situations where the patient wished to play a more active and personal role in self-care.

But first of all talk it over with your doctor.

Pneumonia Vaccine

Dear Dr. MacInnis:

Could you please answer my questions about a vaccine to prevent pneumonia? Is it given the same way as the yearly flu vaccine? When is the best time of the year to get it? And does it cause any bad reactions. I am a male, age 67, and have had a by-pass operation for heart disease. Thank you.

Mr. M.B., British Columbia

Answer

With fall approaching we should start thinking about flu vaccination and as I have done without fail for many years, I'm again advising everyone 65 or older and anyone with chronic lung and heart disease regardless of age *to take the pneumonia vaccine as well.* And if you happen to reside in a nursing home there's all the more reason to "double up," because the flu bug and pneumonia can run wild, with a high mortality, in such a setting.

The pneumoncoccal vaccine protects against the pneumococcus germ, the commonest cause of bacterial (pneumococcal) pneumonia. The pneumonia vaccine is Pneumovax a product of Merck, Sharp & Dohme. Pneumovax affords protection against the 23 most prevalent strains accounting for 88 percent of all cases of pneumonia in Canada and the United States. It does not protect against viral pneumonia or pneumocystis carinii (the pneumonia commonly associated with AIDS). Reaction? No different from flu vaccine. There's usually soreness at the needle site lasting 24–48 hours.

Surprisingly, few people even know that there's such protection against pneumonia. It is estimated that only about 20 percent of people ask for it like they do for flu vaccine, and practically no one knows that, unlike flu vaccine, which has to be given annually because of changing strains, Pneumovax needs only be given *once in a lifetime,* a fact that always inspires my perennial bit of doggerel:
You take your flu shot every fall
But Pneumovax JUST ONCE—that's all!

Need Help for Your Asthma? Read This

Dear Dr. MacInnis:

My husband, age 55, suffers from severe bronchial asthma. As he wanted to learn as much as possible about this disease, he asked his doctor to suggest a good book on the subject. Unfortunately, the book he recommended is very difficult to read, requiring a medical degree to understand! We were wondering if you

*could suggest something on the subject that a layman can under-
stand and appreciate.*

Mrs. J.N., Souris, P.E. Island

Answer

Asthma Update, a Newsletter for People with Asthma is an
excellent source of information. Subscription: One year (4 issues)
is $10.00 in U.S. funds. Address: Asthma Update, 123 Monticello
Avenue, Annapolis, MD 21401. (Please check for *current* yearly
fee before ordering.)

In case you didn't see my recent item on Denver's National
Jewish Center for Immunology and Respiratory Disease and
their toll-free Lung Line service, here it is again. If you have
questions about lung diseases (such as bronchial asthma,
chronic bronchitis or emphysema) or allergies and diseases of
the immune system, call their toll-free number, 1(800)222-5864
and specially trained nurses will answer. (Canadian callers
please phone 1[303]355-5864.)

I have learned (from the Spring 1990 issue of *Asthma Update* that the above-mentioned national Jewish Lung Line telephone service has come out with a new audio cassette tape titled
Living with Asthma, where you can hear the answers to 100
questions the Lung Line staff nurses are most often asked about
asthma. Side 1 deals with understanding the nature of asthma,
what triggers attacks, the role of allergies and the physical as
well as the emotional effects of the disorder. Side 2 covers treatments, describing each of the currently used drug groups, the
role of immunotherapy and various preventive measures. Interested readers can procure this *Living with Asthma* tape by sending U.S. $7.60 (which includes postage and handling) to
BIOCOM, P.O. Box 20021 Columbus Circle Station, New York,
NY 10023. Telephone: (212) 481-7430. (Check current availability and price of tape before sending your order.)

A Bad Case of Sinusitis

Dear Dr. MacInnis:
*I am having problems with chronic sinusitis. For the past
five years it has been intermittent. I have been able to go for*

193

perhaps a week without any symptoms and then I may have it for a week straight. Usually I have been able to obtain relief by using an over-the-counter oral decongestant. I have also had nasal congestion with pain in the sinus cavities over my face.

I have not experienced any nasal drip, teary eyes, etc., accompanying the sinusitis. It is not associated with season change, although it seems a trifle worse when the temperature is low outside. I had a related X ray done four years ago and it was normal.

In the last six months, though, the pain from the sinusitis has been unrelenting. I visited an M.D. because I could feel pressure in my ears. That appears to have been relieved with Vibramycin. I am now concerned because even the oral decongestants have ceased to be effective. I have now started using nasal drops, which relieve the congestion in the nose but does nothing for my pain. My house is humidified and I have no allergies except for penicillin and Bactrim. I feel miserable at work and at home with this constant dull ache over my face.

Please help if you can. Any advice you can muster up would be gratefully appreciated. I am a registered nurse, so I will understand your terminology.

Mrs. N.B., Alberta, Canada

Answer

The sinuses are air spaces in certain paired bones of the skull that give them their names—frontal (forehead), maxillary (cheekbone) and sphenoid and ethmoid (behind base of nose). They empty their secretions through a narrow and rather inefficient drainage system into the nose. Because of this faulty runoff, sinus secretions easily dam up and become infected. Maxillary sinusitis is the commonest infection in adults, followed by frontal sinusitis. In children, the ethmoid sinus is most commonly involved. In severe cases, all of the sinuses become infected, a condition called pan-sinusitis. When fluid or pus in the sinuses replaces air, the well-known symptoms of acute sinusitis occur—headache, usually frontal or around the eyes, regardless of which sinuses are affected, and the intensity of headache depends on the degree of blockage.

In chronic recurrent sinusitis, which is probably the type you have, Mrs. B., the mucus lining in the sinus becomes thickened and ladened with pus along with nasal and postnasal discharge and bothersome headache. Blocked drainage can be caused by a deviated nasal septum or polyps (easily seen with a nasal speculum) and allergies and rhinitis (inflammation of the lining of the nose). A cold can sometimes lead to nasal congestion and sinusitis.

The treatment for acute sinusitis is a nasal decongestant, an analgesic (painkiller) and an antibiotic. If this does not help, then the patient is frequently referred to an ENT specialist for drainage of the sinuses. The extent of sinus infection can usually be determined by X ray or, better still, a CT scan which gives a clearer picture.

For chronic recurrent sinusitis that defies the usual antibiotic routine, the thickened lining of the sinus involved may have to be surgically removed and effective drainage established.

There is a brand-new upper respiratory infection antibiotic that I would recommend for chronic sinusitis (when others fail). It is called Clarithromycin and is said to be the most quickly accepted antibiotic of its class in Canadian medical history. It has a much wider spectrum than other related antibiotics, such as erythromycin, and is more potent. Furthermore, it has exhibited an impressive lack of gastro-intestinal side effects so characteristic of erythromycin. Check with your doctor.

"Constantly Stuffed Nose" A Real Problem!

Dear Dr. MacInnis:

I have a constantly stuffed up nose. It is clear in the morning after I sleep with a cool air vaporizer on my face. But once I raise my head, my head and nose get stuffy.

I have no allergies and no physical abnormality of the nose. The allergist describes it as "nerves gone to sleep." The pills and nasal sprays he prescribed are useless.

Can you suggest any treatment? The problem is very debilitating at work or at home. The condition has worsened over about a year.

Mrs. M.W., Edmonton

PS. I have consulted medical specialists in the appropriate disciplines.

Answer

From your letter, it looks as if your medical consultants have covered most aspects of your case and have come up empty-handed. This leaves me with little room to even speculate on your problem—especially since I'm interrogating you from "long distance."

Are you satisfied that your upper nasal passages (including your sinuses) are not harboring a nest of *chronic infection* to which you are "allergic"? Allergic rhinitis complicated by *chronic infectious sinusitis* can cause a persistent nasal stuffiness. As well, the symptoms of the so-called "perennial rhinitis of unknown origin" can occur with changes in temperature or humidity or when one is exposed to irritants or air pollution. (Please refer to column on chronic sinusitis.)

Even though I may seem to be "grasping at straws," I hope my comments may be of interest to you.

Postnasal Drip

I frequently hear from elderly people complaining about troublesome secretions from the back of the nose trickling into the throat—the so-called "postnasal drip." Here is a excerpt from a typical letter:

. . . I'm always bothered with this sensation of something in the back of my throat . . . I cough and it goes away, but usually within a few minutes it's back. My doctor tells me that I'm producing "excess mucus" but can find nothing wrong. Is this common condition and is there any remedy for it?

Mr. M.N. (74), Ottawa, Ontario

Answer

Before answering your questions let me explain what "post nasal drip" is. Readers will be surprised to learn that the nose of an average adult normally produces as much as a quart of mucus every 24 hours to humidify the upper respiratory tract (nasal passages, windpipe and bronchi). Once the upper respiratory system is adequately moistened, any excess mucus drains down to the back of the throat, where it is coughed up and spit out or swallowed.

Some people, and maybe you're one of them, have oversensitive throats and cannot tolerate the presence of anything "foreign" in that area, hence the constant hacking. This is not to be confused with a condition called "rhinitis" (inflammation or allergy affecting the nasal passages), causing an overabundance of secretion. In case this is your problem, you can relieve the symptoms with an antihistamine nasal spray. But use only for a few days as it loses its effectiveness over time or may even aggravate the problem. Other types of sprays (steroid or plain saline solution) may be recommended by your doctor.

Please remember that "post nasal drip" is usually a normal, natural process and is not associated with aging. In fact, it is commoner in younger people.

Chapter 9
Disorders of Movement: Cerebral, Articular, and Muscular

In this collection of columns dealing primarily with movement disorders, I have deviated from the strictly textbook format of attributing them exclusively to cerebral origin, classically found in Parkinson's and Huntingon's disease. But, loosely speaking, movement disabilities arising from joint and muscular disease, like arthritis and "rheumatism," are very real problems, too, so I have included them in the group. Most of my readers will remember the awful scourge of poliomyelitis in the fifties and sixties followed by its almost total eradication, thanks to a very effective vaccine. But no one expected the emergence of a "second stage" of the disorder, called the "postpolio syndrome" affecting our senior population after a dormant period of twenty to forty years. This new muscular disorder syndrome will also find its rightful home in this chapter.

The "Shaking Palsy"

In 1817 an English surgeon, James Parkinson, published his *Essay on the Shaking Palsy*. Here he described in minute detail the signs and symptoms of a progressive movement disorder arising in the brain, which we now call Parkinson's disease. In the 1960s research scientists achieved a tremendous breakthrough in medicine by determining not only what was lacking in the brain (dopamine) to cause the symptoms of Parkinson's disease but came up with up with a treatment (levodopa) that replenishes what Parkinson's patients lack and what has been the mainstay of medical treatment since 1963. Briefly described, levodopa combines with a chemical called carbidopa that prevents the transformation of levodopa into dopamine in the body (where it can become an undesirable hormone) and allows levodopa to cross the blood-brain barrier to become dopamine, the "nerve messenger-transmitting" chemical, that can benefit to some extent some of the more important symptoms of Parkinson's disease. The combination levodopa-carbidopa has for many years been marketed under the brand name Sinemet and comes in varying proportions of carbidopa and levodopa, depending on the needs of the patient.

I should emphasize at this point that although Sinemet has over the years been a godsend for many Parkinson's patients, it is by no means a cure-all and, indeed, the time may come when it is of little or no use and may have to be assisted by other drugs, such as bromocriptine (Parlodel) and more recently by Eldepryl (the subject of an upcoming column.)

What I would like to stress in the remainder of this column are the symptoms and signs of Parkinson's disease, a condition that afflicts well over a million Americans and Canadians, the majority of whom are past middle age. It would seem that every debilitating disease in later years has its own peculiar tragic twist. Parkinson's disease, more often than not, attacks its victim at the tail end of what's often a highly productive life with expectation of many good years ahead.

The four prominent symptoms of Parkinson's disease are tremor, weakness, and rigidity of muscles, combined with a characteristic gait and attitude.

The tremor is usually marked in the hands, often exhibiting the so-called pill-rolling action of the thumb and forefinger; it comes on slowly, very slowly and insidiously, and may be accompanied by a continuous feeling of fatigue that's hard to account for. The patient may "feel" there's something wrong but cannot "spell it out."

And the signs and symptoms always advance over time. The tremor may become evident in the ankle joint but much less in the toes than in the fingers. Shaking and nodding of the head is infrequent, which serves to differentiate it from the very common "senile tremor" that has no relation to Parkinson's disease. (An upcoming column on senile tremor will further distinguish it from the tremor of Parkinson's.)

Muscle rigidity may occur early in the disease and is expressed as a slowness and stiffness in voluntary movements. As the disease progresses, every movement seems to be "deliberate." The head is bent forward and the back stooped. The arms are held away from the body and are often flexed at the elbow. The gait is shuffling with the patient giving the appearance of falling headlong over his center of gravity. The face becomes expressionless and masklike, giving rise to the expression "Parkinson mask." In late Parkinson's the voice is characteristic, often "shrill and piping." The initiation of speech is often hesitant, then bursting into a staccato "explosion" of words.

The early writers on Parkinson's disease were of the opinion that dementia was not a feature of the condition. This may have been so before the advent of levodopa. I share the feeling of others that such modern therapy merely extended the life of the Parkinson's patient, allowing signs of dementia to emerge. It is now thought that dementia is present in about 10 percent of cases.

Suggested Reading for Relatives of Parkinson's Patients

David Grimes, M.D., Peggy A. Gray, and Kelly A. Grimes, *Parkinson's Disease: One Step at a Time* (Ottawa, Ontario: Parkinson Society of Ottawa-Carleton, 1989). Problems and answers for patients and health professionals, Ottawa Civic Hospital, 1053 Carling Avenue, Ottawa, Ontario K1Y4E9.
Dwight C. McGoon, M.D., *Parkinson's Handbook* (New York: W. W. Norton, 1990). An inspiring, practical guide for patients and their families by a former Mayo Clinic surgeon with Parkinson's disease.

Familial Tremor

Dear Dr. MacInnis:

Three family members, my brother, my sister, and myself, all over 60, have been bothered with a troublesome hand tremor that several doctors thought at first was Parkinson's disease but later diagnosed it as "essential tremor." In all our cases, the condition began slowly in our mid-thirties and has progressed very slowly over the years, and has only become bothersome and to some extent disabling in the past five years. We all experience difficulty in lifting a cup of tea to the lips, and it's embarrassing when we sometimes spill it! Any voluntary hand motion can cause a tremor. In fact, even intending to perform a certain hand motion can initiate a tremor. All of us have difficulty in handwriting and one of us (brother) has lately acquired quite a noticeable nodding of the head. Our father suffered from some type of "palsy" in his later years. We are all on a drug called Xanax. It is very helpful but has one drawback; it causes drowsiness and if the drug is reduced in dosage the tremor starts up. Can you recommend any other drug for essential tremor?

Mrs. L.Y., Ontario

Answer

Essential tremor (ET) is often called "familial" tremor, if there is a family history of the disorder, as in your case. The tremor must be differentiated from that found in Parkinson's disease. Familial tremor is an action tremor that is initiated during the maintenance of a static posture, such as outstretched hands, or during fine manipulation, such as handwriting or pouring liquid from one test tube to another. Head nodding is frequently alone or is an associated movement disorder. About 50 percent of the million or so estimated cases in the U.S. is familial.

This so-called action or intention tremor is not usually found in Parkinson's disease. A person with Parkinson's usually has no problem lifting a cup of tea as you do, Mrs. Y. Again, in Parkinson's, the finger movement at rest is a rotary motion involving the index finger and thumb, the so-called "pill-rolling" movement (when pills were rolled by hand).

Essential or familial tremor can begin at any age, although the incidence increases with age. As in your case, the tremor begins insidiously and most often affects the hands. It can be occasionally associated with other movement disorders.

Once the condition is diagnosed and differentiated from Parkinson's disease, and is not physically disabling, the patient should be told of the benign nature of the disorder. In the rare case of severe disability a brain operation called "thalamotomy" is recommended.

The drug of first choice for ET is propranolol, preferably the long-acting kind, in dosage of 240 milligrams daily. Alprazolam (brand name Xanax) is often quite good, too, but (as in your experience) can cause bothersome drowsiness. However, its sedative property can be beneficial in cases where anxiety precipitates the tremor. Another drug called primidone is sometimes successfully used but may produce troublesome side effects, such as dizziness and light-headedness.

Long-acting propranolol has recently been found beneficial as adjuvant therapy in Parkinson's disease. Ten Parkinson's patients on treatment (Sinemet) and with tremor as their most predominant symptom were treated randomly with either long-acting propranolol, clonazepam (an anti-convulsant) or primidone, brand name Mysoline (also an anti-convulsant).

It was found that long-acting propranolol "caused marked improvement, decreasing tremor more than the other two agents tested."

Propranolol would seem then to be the drug of choice both for essential (familial) tremor (like yours) and in cases of Parkinson's disease where the tremor is not adequately controlled with Sinemet.

Reference: *Archives of Neurology* (1987): 921–23.

Deprenyl* for Parkinson's Disease

There's good news for patients with early Parkinson's disease, a progressive neurological affliction affecting nearly a million people in North America.

"Patients diagnosed with early Parkinson's disease may now be able to substantially delay the onset of disabling symptoms by taking a drug called deprenyl* (or selegiline). This (preliminary) finding reported in the November 16, 1989, issue of *New England Journal of Medicine* is the result of the largest controlled clinical trial ever conducted for Parkinson's disease" (University of Rochester, [N.Y.] Newsletter, November 14, 1989).

It is a most exceptional departure in a research study to modify a trial because of a drug being so beneficial. But that is exactly what has happened. In this ongoing study of 800 patients the original protocol has been aborted, so that from now on all participating subjects will be taking deprenyl until completion of the study in 1992.

According to the University of Rochester's Dr. Ira Shoulson, principal investigator of the twenty-eight study sites in the United States and Canada (begun in 1985), "The decision to release preliminary findings in 1989 was based on the remarkable statistical information analyzed from the data collected from our various study sites. Our monitoring procedures detected clear and powerful evidence that deprenyl delays the onset of serious symptoms. We just didn't expect so much so soon," he explained.

And Dr. Anthony Lang, director of the movement disorders clinic at the Toronto General Hospital and Canadian spokesperson for the trial, was equally exuberant. "We're ecstatic," he told a press conference. "Our results are striking and expected to provide tangible benefits for patients with Parkinson's disease, especially those in the early stages of the disease," he added (reported in Canada's *Medical Post* (November 28, 1989).

---

*Also known as selegiline and marketed in Canada and the U.S. under its brand name, Eldepryl.

Here is an excerpt of the original protocol: Eight hundred subjects with early signs of Parkinson's disease were enrolled between September 3, 1987, and November 15, 1988, and were randomly assigned to receive: (1) deprenyl, (2) tocopherol (vitamin E), (3) deprenyl and tocopherol, or (4) placebo (dummy pill). The subjects were systematically evaluated at approximately three-month intervals and followed to the "end point," where their illness became so severe that levodopa was indicated. Because the study was "double blind" neither patients nor investigators knew which treatment was being administered.

Space limitations here will only allow one of numerous beneficial results: Of 158 subjects *not* taking deprenyl and who were employed full-time, 39 (25 percent) had to discontinue full-time employment during follow-up while of 134 taking deprenyl who were employed full time, only 20 (15 percent) ceased working because of their disability.

Tocopherol (vitamin E) may protect cells from damage due to the formation of so-called "free radicals." The potential benefits from tocopherol will be analyzed at the termination of the study in 1992.

Since Parkinson's disease results primarily from degeneration of the dopamine-producing cells in the brain, it is thought that deprenyl acts by protecting these cells from damage by certain toxins and may also exert an anti–free radical action similar to tocopherol.

Seventy-five percent of Parkinson's disease patients are in the 50 to 65 age group. Not all patients initially have tremor. They often consult a doctor because of balance problems, such as stumbling and having the sensation of falling forward. Diagnosis is difficult at this stage but, if possible, this should be the ideal time to start deprenyl. And all we now know is that it definitely "buys time."

In January 1989, deprenyl was cleared by the (U.S.) FDA as an adjunct to levodopa in the treatment of Parkinson's disease. At the time of writing it has just been okayed by Canada's Health Protection Branch, the equivalent of the U.S. FDA.

Is Parkinson's Disease Inherited?

Dear Dr. MacInnis:

I've read a lot about Parkinson's disease because my mother has it, but nowhere have I found that the disease runs in families. Have you any information on the subject?

Mrs. T.H., Kelowna, British Columbia

Answer

Until quite recently there has been little evidence that genetics played an important role in the causation of Parkinson's disease. Indeed, in one survey of forty-three monozygotic (one egg) twins published in *Neurology* (1983), only one pair evidenced the disease. But a 1990 report from the Robert Wood Johnson Medical School showed a familial connection. This study traced forty-one cases of Parkinson's back through four generations and concluded that a child with one parent having it had a 50-50 chance of contracting the disease.

In October 1991, researchers from the University of Southern California School of Medicine reported at the international symposium of Parkinson's disease in Tokyo that they may have identified an inherited form of the disease. In their study, they followed one family with a history of nine cases of Parkinson's over a span of five generations. Dr. Cheryl Waters, a USC assistant professor of neurology and one of the researchers, feels that genetics may play an important role in Parkinson's although the specific genetic defect in unknown. "A genetic defect," says Dr. Waters, "may predispose certain people to being harmed by environmental factors" (and develop Parkinson's).

So to answer your question, there is some evidence that there may be an inherited form of Parkinson's disease but much more research is needed to prove this hypothesis.

Dopamine to Brain Transplantation

Dear Dr. MacInnis:

My father, who is now 70, has suffered from Parkinson's disease for the past eight years, and for the last six years has been fairly well controlled by Sinemet. That is until lately when it is starting to lose its effect. He began to develop sudden periods of shaking that would just as suddenly change to stiffness, and he would look as if he were frozen all over with a fixed face. This would make him very anxious and frightened. The doctors at the clinic tried many changes in dosage and even added another drug called Parlodel. This has helped a bit but he is definitely going downhill.

I read about the transplantation of fetal cells right into the brain and wondered if you could enlighten me as to its value. It's an operation that was first done in Mexico and that's about all I know about it. Is it done here in the U.S.? Thanks for any help.

Mrs. J.L., Florida

Answer

The well-known signs and symptoms of Parkinson's disease are caused by the loss of a specific group of brain cells situated in a tiny area in the brain stem. These cells produce a hormone called dopamine that is absolutely necessary for the control of normal muscular movement. One writer has picturesquely put it this way: "without dopamine, we'd all be stiff as a board and unable to move so much as a finger."

One of the great medical breakthroughs of the sixties was the discovery of levodopa for Parkinson's disease. In effect it replaced what was missing in Parkinson's (levodopa is the major ingredient in Sinemet). Unfortunately, Sinemet does "wear off," which prompts your question re the transplantation of fetal dopamine-producing cells into the brain. The operation was first performed in Sweden and Mexico in the early eighties with controversial results. In 1988, researchers at the University of Colorado performed the first dopamine to brain transplantation in a severely afflicted 52-year-old Parkinson's patient. After three years, the patient has maintained his initial improvement on only half his Sinemet dosage. The second patient, similarly afflicted, also showed marked improvement but the third man in the series showed no improvement. It is interesting to note that the two successes both exhibited "on-off" symptoms (as described in your letter). The third had responded poorly to Sinemet.

Serious Side Effects of Sinemet

Dear Dr. MacInnis:

My husband, age 65, has Parkinson's disease and has been on Sinemet for the past three years. Over the past six months he has exhibited more than ordinary sexual interest and activity that is definitely becoming abnormal. I have hesitated to bring this to the attention of his doctor who is a personal friend. Can this be caused by Parkinson's disease or the side effect of treatment?

Concerned in Toronto

Answer

More than likely it is a side effect of Sinemet, which is a combination of L-dopa (levodopa) and carbidopa. Hypersexual activity is not confined to Sinemet, however. It has been reported with the use of other anti-Parkinson drugs, such as bromocriptine, pergolide, and deprenyl. The incidence is relatively small, approximately 2 percent, in several recent studies. Manifestations include increased masturbation, incessant sexual demands on the spouse, and, in some cases, extramarital sexual activity. There have also been reports of deviant sexual behavior and exhibitionism.

Reducing the dosage of the anti-Parkinson drug (in your husband's case, Sinemet) has been found helpful in some cases where the dosage has been excessive.

I would strongly recommend that you discuss this matter with your husband's doctor.

If You Have Parkinson's, It's Early

Dear Dr. MacInnis:

I'm a woman in my 60s and my doctor tells me I have Parkinson's disease. I was first put on medication last year—one capsule of Symmetrel twice a day and one capsule of Eldepryl (one-half tablet twice a day). Due to swelling of my ankle, the doctor took me off Symmetrel and put me on two tablets of Eldepryl daily.

The reason I went to him was that my left hand seemed to be stiff and weak with my right hand not quite as bad. I still have a problem buttoning clothes, peeling potatoes, rolling dough into loaves, washing my hair, signing cheques, etc. My doctor really believes in exercising, so he gave me a program I have to do everyday. I am checked by the physiotherapist every six weeks. I seem to get tired easily.

What do you think of my medicine and general program?

Mrs. B.K.

Answer

If you have Parkinson's disease, it would appear to be in its early stage. I say this because your handwriting, which is often the first skill affected, is quite normal, in fact it's exceedingly fine penmanship.

It's impossible for me to comment any further on your improvement, if any, since you began treatment, as you do not mention it one way or another. (I do have a hunch it may be working since your attending physician has not changed it.)

Amantadine (brand name Symmetrel) is an antiviral drug used for Type-A influenza. Some years ago Russian researchers observed that Parkinson's patients given amantadine for their flu showed improvement, not only in their flu but in their Parkinson's symptoms as well. It was later found that amantadine stimulated the brain to make dopamine (the neurochemical deficient in Parkinson's). It is now used as one of a number of supplementary drugs for Parkinson's.

Another one is Eldepryl, (brand name for the generic drugs selegiline and deprenyl. Readers will recall that I have written many times on the benefits of Eldepryl, particularly in early Parkinson's, where research has indicated that it can in many instances delay for a number of years the need for Sinemet (levodopa and carbidopa), the mainstay treatment for Parkinson's disease.

What do I think of your medicine and general program? Well, if my assumptions are correct—that you have early Parkinson's, that you are on a daily exercise program, and that you're improving on Eldepryl—then my conclusion is that you are receiving world-class treatment right where you are.

Selegiline, Again!

Dear Dr. MacInnis:

My husband, age 67, has Parkinson's disease and has been on Sinemet three times daily. Lately, the third dose has been wearing off too quickly. I recently read about a new drug called selegiline, which is supposed to improve the action of Sinemet.

Could you please give me some information on this drug. If it appears to be promising, I will make it a point to see his doctor about it. Thank you.

Mrs. M.J., Sun City

Answer

Selegiline (brand name Eldepryl) has been shown to supplement the action of Sinemet in the treatment of Parkinson's.

Besides enhancing the effect of Sinemet, it will most likely play an even more important role as initial medication in early Parkinson's, where it has been shown to slow the onset of debilitating symptoms, thus delaying the necessity of using Sinemet (levodopa and carbidopa).

This was the result of clinical trials conducted in twenty-eight medical centers in the U.S. and Canada and published in the *New England Journal of Medicine* (November 16, 1989). (See a previous column on page 204.)

Of eight hundred patients with early Parkinson's disease, half were treated with selegiline and half with a placebo (dummy pill). The selegiline patients took one and a half years longer than the controls to develop debilitating symptoms requiring the use of Sinemet.

Late Note: A 1992 analysis of these trials indicated that the effect of vitamin E alone and with selegiline was no better than selegiline acting alone.

Bromocriptine for Parkinson's Disease

Dear Dr. MacInnis:

My husband, age 72, has been taking Sinemet for his Parkinson's disease for four years now but it is getting less effective lately. For instance, instead of one dose lasting for about four hours, the effect begins to fade after three hours. The doctor put him on several other drugs to help out the Sinemet but without much success, as he was not able to tolerate them. I don't have the names of the drugs.

Have you any suggestions? Thank you.

Mrs. J.M., New Brunswick

Answer

There are several drugs that enhance the action of Sinemet. They are called agonists (the opposites of antagonists). One is bromocriptine (marketed under the brand name of Parlodel), which I will briefly describe here. It can help relieve many of the symptoms of Parkinson's such as slowness of movement, rigidity, and tremor. Its most beneficial use, however, is when combined with Sinemet. Here it may prevent the "wearing-off" effect of Sinemet that you describe in your husband's case. As bromocriptine has many side effects it must be started in low dosage (less than 30 milligrams a day) and then slowly increased. As the bromocriptine is increased it may be necessary to lower the dosage of Sinemet. This is something that requires careful titration of both drugs, something you must do under the supervision of your doctor.

Although sometimes a godsend for the Parkinson patient, bromocriptine, alone or in combination with Sinemet, has several prominent side effects, usually dose related. Orthostatic hypotension (low blood pressure on standing) with nausea is a common complication that can be avoided by increasing the dosage slowly.

Again I stress, always consult your doctor for advice on this drug.

Should Sinemet Be Started Early or Not?

Dear Dr. MacInnis:

My husband, age 68, has Parkinson's disease and has been on Sinemet (levodopa and carbidopa) since his condition was first diagnosed about five years ago. For the first two years there was a remarkable improvement in both the muscle rigidity, tremor, and his ability to initiate movement. But now he's not responding well, and I'm wondering if what I read recently was true—that when levadopa is started early in the course of the disease, it may actually in time, hasten the deterioration. What is your opinion?

Mrs. L.K., FL

Answer

It is not at all unusual for levodopa to lose its hold over time, requiring dosage manipulation that is not always satisfactory. One thing stands out with levodopa. There is no standard dosage we can depend on. We must tailor the dose schedule to the patient's response, which may in time become unpredictable. This is the natural progressive history of Parkinson's disease and should not be blamed on the early initiation of levodopa treatment.

According to a report from the American Academy of Neurology, French researchers recently monitored the treatment of 185 patients with Parkinson's disease to determine if the early use of levodopa accelerated the course of the disease and caused increased side effects, an opinion expressed by other researchers in the field.

The conclusion of this large French study was that "early treatment with levodopa does not cause nerve damage nor does it cause increased side effects when administered in proper dosage. . . . It is the consequence of a more severe case of Parkinson's, not a result of the medication," explained the researchers.

Adrenal Gland Transplant for Parkinson's Disease

On several occasions I have reported on the surgical treatment of Parkinson's disease where the patients received a transplant from their own adrenal glands into their brain. You may recall the dramatic news out of Mexico City where Dr. Ignacio Madrazo presented miraculous surgical results in his two patients.

Since the report was published several years ago, physicians in the United States, Canada, and other countries have performed more than a hundred adrenal transplants in an attempt to replicate Dr. Madrazo's published results *(New England Journal of Medicine,* April 2, 1987).

Some of these doctors reported on their operations at the annual (1989) meeting of the American Academy of Neurology (AAN) in Chicago.

Although a few patients experienced some improvement after adrenal transplant, none showed anything like the dramatic results obtained by Dr. Madrazo. In fact, some serious post-operative complications, such as confusion, disorientation, and reduced (former) efficiency of anti-Parkinson's medication emerged.

Said Dr. Abraham Leiberman, professor of neurology at New York University, "Our study indicates that the operation can influence the course of Parkinson's disease; however, the results are inconsistent and the risks are high."

And Dr. Ray Watts, director of the Movement Disorders Program at Emory University, concurs: "We have seen mild to moderate improvements in some of our patients for up to one year," he said, "but further study is needed to determine if the benefits outweigh the risks."

Such less than enthusiastic reports prompted the AAN to issue a position statement, urging "great caution" in expanding the practice of adrenal tissue transplantation and calling for more testing of the procedure in highly specialized research centers.

Huntington's Disease: A Tragic Roll of the Dice

The tragedy of Huntington's disease in itself is only surpassed by the frightful years of suspense it inflicts on the patient's family.

This is because the condition doesn't usually manifest itself until the parent's adult years, when it may have already been passed on to the children who must now await the verdict of genetics since each one of them has, at birth, a 50 percent chance of inheriting the disease.

The havoc wreaked on a family by Huntington's disease is eloquently expressed in a letter from Mrs. M.T., the wife of a victim.

Dear Dr. MacInnis:

. . . When we married neither my husband (24) nor myself (23) knew there was Huntington's in his family. Would we have married if we did? We were in love enough to, but God only knows.

For fifteen years we enjoyed a happy married life blessed with four children—two boys and two girls. Then we began to see the change. He was 40 when we noticed what we now know to be the early symptoms of the disease, which progressed slowly over two or three years. He became just "different." His personality gradually changed little by little for the worse, and then there appeared tremor of the hands that in time grew to jerking movements that spread to the arms and legs and face. Speech became difficult and, in the end, he couldn't be understood. He walked like a drunken person.

The disease took fifteen years to reach its peak. By that time he was in a chronic hospital, bedridden, exhausted from his constant writhing, and totally demented.

When my husband died at the age of 55, it was the merciful end of one chapter of Huntington's disease and the beginning of another—this time for the four children now age 30 to 36.

Over the years they received what is called genetic counselling and are well aware that each one has a 50 percent risk of going the way of their father, and their time is getting short. . . . .

Answer

The hereditary nature of the disease was first noted over a hundred years ago by Dr. Huntington, a general practitioner of

East Hampton, Long Island, New York. Huntington's father and grandfather and other physicians of the time had treated the disease in previous generations of the family he described.

Since that time, the genetic basis of Huntington's disease (formerly called Huntington's chorea) has been fully established in that every child, male or female, of a Huntington's parent runs a fifty-fifty chance of getting the disease. Between 35 to 45 years it commonly begins, and the long vigil is over.

The cause of Huntington's disease, striking about one in ten thousand of the white population (much lower in blacks), is a defective gene on chromosome 4 that targets a well-defined brain area, ultimately destroying it. This defined area (mainly the corpus striatum) normally produces certain enzymes that serve as transmitters of nerve impulses responsible for muscular function and cognition (mental awareness).

This slow but relentless "genetic" destruction of these highly specialized brain cells produces over time the well-known signs and symptoms of Huntington's disease.

The current medical management for Huntington's disease is symptomatic. Haloperidol and chlorpromazine are both useful in controlling the more serious physical and mental (dementing) problems.

In 1983, Gusella and co-workers at the Massachusetts General Hospital (using DNA technology) discovered a genetic "marker" they identified as being linked with a defective gene on chromosome 4.

This notable discovery made it possible for identification (by a blood test) of the defective gene in relatives of Huntington's victims. Some limited testing began at Johns Hopkins in Baltimore and the Massachusetts General Hospital in Boston on selected patients, but the results of the tests have not yet been reported (1986).

Addendum: In 1988, a new marker, reported to be much closer to the defective gene than to the previous one, was discovered by a team of scientists at the University of British Columbia (UBC) and the University of California (Irvine). According to Dr. Michael Hayden of the UBC, the new marker "will significantly improve diagnosis and will advance the search for the Huntington gene itself."

In March 1993, Dr. Hayden's prediction was realized. The Huntington gene was found, a discovery that has made genetic testing for the disease not only much simpler, but virtually 100 percent accurate.

How will the children of a Huntington parent react to knowing, often years in advance, the outcome of such an accurate test? Before the first limited (and imperfect) testing was done at Johns Hopkins and the Massachusetts General Hospital in 1986, about 70 percent of those enrolled in the study said that they would take the test when it became available. But when 300 were eventually notified to present themselves for the actual test, only 70 (23 percent) turned up. This reaction illustrates the terrible dilemma confronting the children at risk—to test or not to test, to know or not to know, questions still haunting the more than fifteen thousand of them here in Canada and 10 times that in the United States.

In Canada there are now 14 genetic testing centres (founded by Dr. Hayden as a research project) operating across Canada and an integral part of this program is to give ongoing psychological support services to all, with special counselling to those carrying the Huntington gene.

There are active Huntington societies in Canada and the United States and all are as close as your telephone. While most of you at risk are already registered, there's always the possibility that some of you are not or may not be sure. So my advice to you is to contact your nearest Huntington society for up-to-date information, including their genetic testing program.

Arthritis: The Big Three

I receive a lot a correspondence from readers—middle-aged or better—complaining of arthritis. Now if you will allow me to get a bit technical, there are more than a hundred kinds of arthritis. And all this time you may have thought your kind was the one and only!

But as the old medical maxim goes, "The commonest things happen the commonest." So let's pare them down to the "big three"—rheumatoid arthritis, osteoarthritis, and gout. For now, let's concentrate only on these.

Let me briefly describe each type. Rheumatoid arthritis: About ten million people (U.S. and Canada) have this type. It occurs at any age but is most prevalent in early middle age and occurs more frequently in women. Although it can affect any movable joint, the commonest sites are the joints of the hands, wrists, and feet (roughly in that sequence). Rheumatoid arthritis is an auto-immune disease, where the body's immune system goes awry, attacking its own protein in the cartilage of joints and eventually destroying them.

Osteoarthritis: This is "old people's arthritis" and is by far the commonest. About twenty million elderly Americans and Canadians suffer from some degree of osteoarthritis. The joints most frequently affected are those of the hands, feet, knees, hips, neck, and back.

Gout (gouty arthritis): Gout causes the severest joint pain and tenderness of all, but fortunately it's not nearly so common as the previous two and usually affects the main joint of the big toe. Senior readers particularly, will recall ("Bringing Up Father") where Mr. Jiggs' periodic bouts of acute gout were blamed by Maggie on his secret tippling!

This begs the question: Is gout associated with chronic alcoholism? Historically, yes. My old medical textbooks leave no doubt. Here is a brief passage (excerpted) from Osler's 1906 text book *Practice of Medicine*. "Alcohol is the most potent factor in the etiology (cause) of the disease. Fermented liquors favor its occurrence much more than distilled spirits and it prevails most extensively in countries like England and Germany which consume the most beer and ale. The lighter beers used in this country (U.S.) are much less liable to produce gout than the heavier English and Scotch ales. Many cases occur in bartenders and brewery men."

But my modern-day medical reference *(Scientific American Medicine)* is not so sure. In fact it cites one study where "gouty attacks were no more prevalent in heavy drinkers than in non-drinkers." But like Osler, it believes that "populations having a high proportion of heavy drinkers have had a high prevalence of gout." Its overall conclusion: "It is unlikely that moderate alcohol consumption affects the frequency of gouty attacks."

Treatment: Some general principles in management of both rheumatoid or osteoarthritis: (1) Alleviation of pain, and (2) as far as possible, restoration of joint function. This can be achieved by rest, weight control, exercise, heat therapy, and drugs. (Note: All drugs effective for both rheumatoid and osteoarthritis may have serious side effects and should always be supervised by your doctor.)

Rheumatoid arthritis: ASA (aspirin); corticosteroids, such as prednisone; disease-modifying drugs like gold compounds (oral auranofin and Myochrysine by intramuscular injection); and immunosuppressant drugs like Imuran and Methotrexate.

Osteoarthritis: NSAIDs (non-steroid anti-inflammatory drugs) are the most commonly used treatment for osteoarthritis. Brand-name examples are Voltaren, Motrin, Feldene, Orudis, and Advil, to name a few. And again, all may produce side effects such as inflammation of the stomach and sometimes gastrointestinal bleeding that can be particularly serious in the elderly. Note: Most NSAIDs are prescription drugs. An exception is Advil which is available "over the counter" and has recently been found to aggravate pre-existing kidney dysfunction.

Gout: The mainstays of treatment are colchicine and allopurinol. Both are effective but often have distressing gastrointestinal effects, particularly colchicine. Again, consult your doctor.

Worried about Advil

Dear Dr. MacInnis:

I have been taking a drug called Advil for painful arthritis. I found it quite good and have noticed no side effects. Recently I read that it can be dangerous to take it if your kidneys are not functioning well. As far as I know I have nothing wrong with me but the arthritis. I was told by my doctor not to worry. What is your opinion?

Mrs. T.E., Calgary, Alberta

Answer

If your doctor can give you a clean bill of health (apart from arthritis), I would agree that you have nothing to worry about.

But if a patient has even mild kidney dysfunction and takes the generic drug ibuprofen (brand names Advil, Medipren, Nuprin and Motrin IB) in high dosage over several weeks, there's a one in four chance the impairment will worsen. Researchers at Johns Hopkins University made this discovery which was published recently in the *Annals of Internal Medicine.* On the optimistic side, kidney dysfunction returned to pretreatment level when ibuprofen was discontinued. Because all NSAIDs increase body fluids, they should not be given to arthritic patients with congestive heart failure. In such cases I would recommend aspirin or Tylenol, but check with your doctor.

Patients with diabetes or high blood pressure often have kidney trouble, so it would be prudent on their part to have a kidney function test before trying out over-the-counter brands of ibuprofen.

I would also advise *healthy* patients on ibuprofen for extended periods to have periodic kidney tests. So see your doctor.

Over the counter brands of ibuprofen contain 200 milligrams per tablet and are widely used not only for arthritis but are popular for the pain of headache and menstrual periods. (As this is written another popular NSAID, Voltaren, is being investigated by the FDA for similar kidney side effects.)

Methotrexate for Severe Resistant Rheumatoid Arthritis

Dear Dr. MacInnis:
I am a woman 64 years old who has had severe rheumatoid arthritis for ten years. I have taken just about "everything in

the book," including gold therapy, without much benefit. Just recently, when I was about to give up, I saw a program on TV that was highly supportive of a new treatment for rheumatoid arthritis with a cancer drug whose name escapes me.

Have I given you enough information for you to identify this drug? If so could you tell me a little more about it in the treatment of rheumatoid arthritis.

Mrs. L.J., Toronto

Answer

The drug you refer to is called Methotrexate, a well-known anti-cancer medication. About a year ago in these columns, I mentioned Methotrexate for the treatment of resistant rheumatoid arthritis and that it had been approved by the Federal Drug Administration in the United States and was then available to doctors in that country. I'm pleased to state that it has now received the green light from Canada's Health Protection Branch, making it available in your pharmacy on a doctor's prescription.

What you probably heard about was the report from a Canadian Arthritis Society research group at the Montreal General Hospital where fifteen severely afflicted rheumatoid arthritis patients were given a megadose (1,000 milligrams) every two weeks for 6 months and then followed with a regular dosage schedule (7.5 to 20 milligrams) weekly. This regimen was similar to that given to cancer patients. Results: According to Dr. John Esdaile, director of the research team, Methotrexate is "the most amazing drug" for rheumatoid arthritis. (Previous research showed that Methotrexate in much smaller doses, e.g., 10. milligrams per week, was only effective in mild cases of rheumatoid arthritis.)

Again, according to the director, the study group had been told prior to their entry that very little could be done for them, "but," said Dr. Esdaile, "the effect was so dramatic—similar in impact as the first use of penicillin on meningitis."

Readers should be aware that Methotrexate is a toxic drug, where rheumatoid arthritis patients sometimes suffer liver, mouth, and gastrointestinal side effects similar to cancer patients taking the drug. It should therefore be given under strict medical supervision and please note that **it is absolutely contraindicated in pregnancy, where it has caused fetal deaths and congenital abnormalities.**

Rheumatoid Arthritis versus Osteoarthritis

Dear Dr. MacInnis:
What is the difference between rheumatoid arthritis and osteoarthritis?

Mr. V.K., Sun City

Answer

Rheumatoid arthritis: About ten million people in Canada and the United States suffer from this type of arthritis. It occurs at any age but is most prevalent in early middle age and is commoner in females. Although it can affect any movable joint, the commonest sites are the joints of the hands, wrists, and feet (roughly in that sequence). Rheumatoid arthritis occurring in the elderly more commonly hits the larger joints.

Osteoarthritis: This is the so-called old people's arthritis and by far the commoner. About twenty million Americans and Canadians suffer from some degree of osteoarthritis. The joints most frequently affected are those of the hands, feet, knees, hips, neck, and back.

Auranofin for Rheumatoid Arthritis

Dear Dr. MacInnis:
As a sufferer of long-standing rheumatoid arthritis, I was pleased to read in one of your recent columns about a gold medication that could be taken by mouth. Over the years I've taken gold by injection with some benefit but nobody wants to take needles if at all possible. My question is how does gold by pill compare in effectiveness with gold by injection? How expensive is it?

Mrs. A.B., Regina, Saskatchewan

221

Answer

The oral gold product you refer to is auranofin (brand name Ridaura) and is marketed for the treatment of rheumatoid arthritis unresponsive to non-steroid anti-inflammatory drugs like Indocid, Motrin, Feldene, Orudis, and the like. It compares favourably with injectable gold in effect. Like other gold compounds, it may modify rheumatoid activity but does not cause remission of rheumatoid arthritis.

Although the manufacturer states that it has fewer side effects than injectable gold (Myochrysine), this claim doesn't appear to be verified by one study that reported a 47 percent occurrence of diarrhea and associated abdominal disturbances—only rarely found with Myochrysine *(Scandinavian Journal of Rheumatology,* 12 [1983]: 254). Another study found it less toxic to the kidneys and producing a lower incidence of skin rash than Myochrysine.

The cost? Based on the usual dose of 3 milligrams twice a day, the cost for a month's treatment is U.S. $34.20 to the pharmacist. The monthly cost for Myochrysine (based on 50 milligrams per week) is approximately U.S. $20 to the pharmacist. (You can expect a retail markup plus a dispensing fee.) (NOTE: The above-mentioned price comparisons are only valid in a relative way, as they were compiled several years ago.)

Both Myochrysine and Ridaura should be administered by a physician experienced in gold therapy.

Addendum (September 1993): A team of Harvard University scientists have reported in the journal *Science* a marked decrease in joint pain and swelling in rheumatoid arthritis patients fed collagen extract derived from chicken cartilage. In contrast to the often severe side effects from the aforementioned rheumatoid arthritis drugs, the collagen-fed patients suffered no ill effects. Taking advantage of the so-called "oral tolerance," where the immune system does not recognize ingested food as "foreign material," the researchers, in effect, tricked the immune system into believing that the collagen (given in orange juice at breakfast every morning) was indeed food in the hope that it would "go easy" not only on the ingested collagen but on

collagen elsewhere in the body—specifically in the joint cartilage. The ploy worked. Of the sixty patients taking part in the
study, half received the chicken collagen and the other half a
look-alike placebo. Results: The collagen-treated patients
showed improvement in their arthritis after one month while
the group given the placebo went further downhill. The study
will continue with other medical centers participating.

Fibromyalgia and Polymyalgia Rheumatica

Dear Dr. MacInnis:

*I read your column regularly but do not recall you writing
about fibrositis.*

*Could you please explain the causes of this ailment, the rec-
ommended treatment to relieve the extreme pain it causes, and
whether there is a local or self-help group who share information.
I am 81 years of age and am also suffering form chronic osteoarthritis.*

Mrs. H.W., Rochester, N.Y.

Answer

The term "fibromyalgia" has replaced "fibrositis," as there
is no scientific evidence of inflammation present at the various
sites of pain and tenderness so characteristic of this disorder.
The cause of fibromyalgia is not well understood, but there are
several features of your ailment that distinguish it from other
joint and muscular disease. Patients complain of severe pain,
particularly in the shoulder and hip muscles but the pain may
be anywhere. Many patients with a severe form of the disease
give a history of disturbed sleep that makes them fatigued the
following day. But the most important diagnostic sign is the
presence of exquisite tenderness in scattered muscular sites induced on deep pressure by the doctor's thumb.

There is no specific treatment for fibromyalgia. The usual
painkillers used in arthritis (NSAIDs and prednisone) are singularly useless. However, tricyclic anti-depressive medication

should always be given a trial. This is administered in much smaller dosage than for clinical depression and, when effective, some improvement can occur, often in a few days. Some rheumatologists (arthritis and rheumatic specialists) have reported benefit from courses of aerobic exercises, and other experts have reported good results from biofeedback training.

But even though notable improvement may occur with various managements, fibromyalgia tends to be a chronically progressive disease. Fibromyalgia self-help groups do exist. You should check your telphone directory.

I would recommend a consultation with a rheumatologist.

Dear Dr. MacInnis:

Have you got any information you could forward on "polymyalgia rheumatica"? Is there any similarity between this condition and "fibrositis"? My symptoms seem to fit the latter condition but I've recently heard from a friend who has PMR and I'd like to be informed before seeing my doctor.

Mrs. J.M., Ottawa, Ontario

Answer

First, read previous column.

Polymyalgia rheumatica (PMR) differs from fibromyalgia (FM) in the following respects: PMR attacks females over 50 years old. FM attacks males and females with equal frequency in a broad age range of 30 to 60 years. The multiple muscle areas revealing intense tenderness on deep pressure so characteristic of FM are not found in PMR. The intense pain of FM occurs most frequently in the shoulder and hip muscles whereas in PMR it usually strikes the distal muscles of both extremities. The fever and elevated blood sedimentation rate found in PMR are not present in FM. And PMR responds often dramatically to prednisone, which is ineffective for FM. Finally, PMR is a much more common condition than FM.

Polymyalgia rheumatica is very frequently associated with an inflammation of the arteries of the neck and head, most commonly the temple arteries, where it is known as temporal arteritis. A serious complication of temporal arteritis is extension into the branches of an ophthalmic (eye) artery causing one-eye blindness. Other symptoms of temporal arteritis are headache, tenderness over the affected temporal artery, and often lower jaw pain. As in the case of PMR, there is a high blood sedimentation rate. The diagnosis can be confirmed by biopsy of the affected artery. The treatment of temporal arteritis is prednisone, where it is highly effective. In the case of PMR occurring without temporal arteritis high dosage nonsteroid anti-inflammatory (NSAIDs) drugs can be used effectively, **but if there is the slightest sign of visual complications, Prednisone treatment should be instituted immediately.**

Postpolio Syndrome

Dear Dr. MacInnis:

My wife, now age 60, suffered from severe poliomyelitis thirty years ago, from which she eventually recovered. About two years ago she began to develop undue fatigue and tiredness in her leg muscles, the ones that were affected by the original polio. She is now quite incapacitated and fears she is going to get worse. I have read that there is such a thing as a "flare up" of a former polio attack and I wonder if anything can be done about it. Several doctors have told me that very little can be done. I would like some more information on this condition.

Mr. T.T., Alberta

Answer

The disorder you refer to is called "postpolio syndrome." It is estimated that of the approximately one million victims in the U.S. and Canada of the poliomyelitis epidemic in the early fifties, about 25 percent have come down with progressive aching pain and tiredness and fatigue in muscles or muscle groups—the same muscles afflicted by the original polio attack—and it's only natural that these "old" polio victims become fearful of a second attack coming on. This is not so, for it's rather a second stage of the condition coming to light after a dormant period of twenty to forty years.

225

You wonder "if anything can be done" about your wife's disorder. Rehabilitation specialists in the neurological field would say yes. They have devised special therapy programs, such as non-resistive exercises, energy conservation, muscle supports, and pain management whose objective is to prevent further deterioration of the muscles. Most medical practitioners are not too conversant with the management of poliomyelitis, particularly those who began practice after the early fifties in Canada and the U.S., which means the majority of them. But with the rash of postpolio syndrome cases emerging over the past few years, most of them are seeking counsel from the few skilled postpolio specialists in the country, and you, Mr.T., are fortunate to live quite near one of them. I refer to Dr. Rubin Feldman, chairman of the Department of Physical Medicine and Rehabilitation at the University Hospital in Edmonton. I would therefore recommend that you arrange an appointment for your wife at his clinic.

(Thanks to a most effective vaccine, developed by Dr. Jonas Salk in 1954, the scourge of poliomyelitis (infantile paralysis) has been "wiped off the map" in North and South America, with the last case reported in Peru in 1991. But worldwide, it still annually attacks over a hundred thousand people, mostly children. This year (1993) there was an outbreak of poliomyelitis in the Netherlands with a reported sixty-eight cases of adults and children, with several deaths. The victims of this outbreak all belonged to religious sects who, on principle, refused immunization.)

My 80-Year-Old Neck

Dear Dr. MacInnis:
What can I do about my poor neck now age 80 years and full of arthritis? My problem is trying to get it resting free of pain on the pillow at night. I twist and turn it every which way for comfort and even try to roll up the pillow between my chin and shoulder for support. Sometimes I hit it right and off to sleep I go. But most times I have to take a sleeping pill. Any advice?
Mr. M.B.

Answer

This is the commonest complaint from "old arthritic necks," and for forty years I listened to their tales of woe and could do little more. But now, that I've joined the club myself, my personal "research" has come up with at least a partial remedy—one that I can live with or, more specifically, one that I can sleep with.

My prescription? Throw away that second pillow. Two pillows can put too much crook strain on your already painful cervical (neck) spine. One pillow tends to keep your neck bones straighter with less strain and pain.

Now people are going to write in and swear testimony to all sorts of contraptions, the commonest, I'll bet, being commercial neck rests or supports whose main function, also, is to keep the neck straight. That's fine, stick to whatever helps you best. Mine happens to be *one* pillow. I can always shape it to my liking and because of this, I find it most effective, and of course it's much cheaper than commercial devices.

Another beef I'm going to hear is, "I've trouble breathing on one pillow." I concede that in advanced congestive heart failure, two or even more pillows may be necessary. However, more often than not, raising the head of the bed can take the place of that extra pillow.

While I don't expect a Nobel prize for this "scientific breakthrough," I believe that many in the past have been nominated for achieving much less. A red ribbon in molecular physics is great, but it's the pits for what ails me tonight.

Like the pain in my neck.

I'm 70; Should I Have a Hip Replacement?

Dear Dr. MacInnis:

I have suffered from chronic right hip pain for over five years. The doctor says the X ray shows "advanced" osteoarthritis in both hips. He advises a hip replacement operation on the right one that's giving me the pain. Since the symptoms have not improved much under so-called conservative treatment—heat, rest, special exercises, and various drugs, it looks like I'll have to take the operation.

If you were my age (70) with a hip like mine would you go for the operation? How about an "osteotomy" instead? My nephew, age 40, with osteoarthritis is very pleased with his.

Mr. M.N., Indiana

Answer

I bounced your question off an experienced orthopedic surgeon who agreed in principle with your doctor that you would indeed benefit greatly from a total hip replacement. So go for it.

If you were twenty years younger (like your nephew) and your hip degeneration was *not too far advanced,* an osteotomy might be just the thing for you. (The following remarks are directed to younger patients.)

This hip operation, called a "valgus osteotomy," involves cutting the thigh bone (femur) just below the hip joint and re-aligning the way the bone fits into the joint. The joint is thus rebalanced by changing the tilt of the joint's ball (head of femur) within the socket.

According to Dr. Frank Gottchalk, assistant professor of orthopedic surgery at the University of Texas Health Science Center at Dallas, "The re-balancing gives the hip muscles a better mechanical advantage while alleviating the pain, since now the femoral head is rotated to a new position where there is still good cartilage.

"Our goal is to buy as much time as possible. . . . By providing several years of good joint use . . . we try to delay total joint replacement as long as possible, especially for patients under 50, because of problems when artificial joints loosen," explains Dr. Gottchalk. (In the older, less active patient, the artificial joint doesn't commonly loosen.)

Zostrix for Arthritic Pain

Dear Dr. MacInnis:

I recall a column you wrote on the use of a "hot pepper derivative" to treat the severe prolonged pain that often occurs at the site of acute shingles (herpes zoster). What is the actual name of the drug and is it in the form of an ointment or cream to apply to the sore area? Is it used only for post-shingles neuralgia?

Mr. M.N., 75, Ontario

Answer

I have written numerous columns on capsaicin (brand name Zostrix) for the treatment of post-shingles neuralgia. Over the past four or five years it has enjoyed popularity mainly because it is the best we have to offer for this bothersome complication of acute shingles. Its active ingredient is, as you say, hot peppers, and it appears what it does for post-shingles neuralgia it can do even better for the pain of arthritis.

There's research going on at the University of Wisconsin on the effect of capsaicin on both osteoarthritic and rheumatoid arthritic pain and initial results are encouraging. Twenty-one patients with painful arthritis of the hands (fourteen with osteoarthritis and seven with rheumatoid arthritis) were treated with 0.075 percent capsaicin ointment applied to their painful joints four times a day. Result: Pain was reduced by 49 percent and tenderness by 30 percent.

In another study reported by *Clinical Therapeutics,* 101 patients with painful arthritis of the knee (seventy had osteoarthritis, thirty-one had rheumatoid arthritis) received either the commercial product Zostrix (0.025 percent capsaicin cream or a placebo (inert dummy) cream four times a day for four weeks. Results: Ninety-three patients completed the trial. Of these, 69 percent of the patients on topical Zostrix reported pain improvement from 21 percent after the first week to 57 percent pain reduction in four weeks.

Chapter 10
Stomach and Bowel Disorders; Surgery in the Aged

As a columnist in geriatric medicine, I probably receive more reader correspondence about bowel problems than on any other subject. It is strange but true that readers don't write in when they or a family member is acutely ill or in the terminal stage of chronic illness. What prompts them to write are the common, run-of-the-mill disorders of the digestive system that beset us all: flatulence—or gas—constipation and the like. It would seem that readers live with their condition for a long time and when things begin to go wrong and they are "getting nowhere" with the treatment, they write as a "last resort" to see if there's "anything new."

This chapter on stomach and bowel problems will not follow the usual textbook format, but will feature the more common day-to-day gastrointestinal maladies of the multitudes.

I thought it would be convenient in this chapter to include some columns on surgery in the aged, as the most serious major surgery in the old-age group is gastrointestinal. In addition there will be a column on anesthesia in the aged and a few ancillary topics.

Flatulence, or "Gone with the Wind"

What causes flatus? There are two main mechanisms. First, air swallowing while eating. This air is never entirely belched and "goes down" becoming rectal gas—oxygen and nitrogen—mainly the last mentioned.

The second and by far the most common cause is undigested or partly digested food entering the colon (large bowel), where it becomes what is scientifically called a "substrate" and is acted on by bacterial ferments. The result: hydrogen and carbon dioxide gases.

For example, baked beans (one of the so called musical groups of foodstuffs) contain a special carbohydrate substance (polysaccharide) that just cannot be digested in the stomach and upper gut and enters the colon where it ferments mainly into hydrogen gas, and plenty of it!

Some people cannot digest the gluten portion of bread made from certain flours and must eat gluten-free wheat-flour bread to avoid excessive flatus.

And then there are people who are deficient in an enzyme called lactase, necessary for the digestion of lactose in milk and milk products. A patient with lactose intolerance suffers from a continuous, bloated, gassy feeling, cramps, excessive flatus, and sometimes "explosive" diarrhea. Management of lactose intolerance involves cutting down or completely eliminating milk and milk products from the diet and taking lactose enzyme powder or LactAid milk at mealtime.

It would appear, then, that most cases of excessive flatus are caused by faulty digestion of certain foodstuffs, mainly carbohydrates. If the offending foods could be identified and then eliminated from the diet, this would go a long way in reducing large bowel gas and relieving of flatulence.

I will now present an abbreviated history of a 28-year-old man suffering from extreme flatulence (partly from lactose intolerance) who, after consulting seven physicians without relief, took matters into his owns hands. He developed a method of recording every belch and passage of wind from the high-frequency "squeaker" to the low-frequency "puff," seldom heard but invariably felt by this intrepid researcher. Every food was subjected to this test. In all, over a period of five years, 130 different foods were laboriously tested by his method of "flatographic" recording, the first in medical history!

From this he produced a food list that reduced his rectal gas passages from an average of thirty-four times per twenty-four hours to seventeen (normal, twenty-four) passages per day.

Writing under the pen name "L. O. Sutalf" ("flatus" spelled backward) and in collaboration with Dr. Michael D. Levitt, associate chief of staff, Research Service, Veterans Administration Medical Center, Minneapolis Missouri, his unique in-depth study was published in *Digestive Diseases and Sciences,* vol. 24, no. 8 (August 1979). My thanks to Digestive Services, Inc., for permission to reprint.

Normal flatus-producing foods: (Nineteen or less gas passages per day):

1. Meat, fowl and fish
2. Vegetables—lettuce, cucumbers, broccoli, peppers, avocado, cauliflower, tomato, asparagus, zucchini, okra, and olives
3. Fruits—cantaloupe, grapes, and berries
4. Carbohydrates—rice, corn chips, potato chips, popcorn, and graham cookies
5. All nuts
6. Miscellaneous—eggs, non-milk chocolate, Jell-O, and fruit ice
7. Water, probably the safest of all consumables

Moderate flatus-producing foods (twenty to forty gas passages daily): Pastries, potatoes, eggplant, citrus fruit, apples, and bread.

Extreme flatus-producing foods (greater than forty gas passages per day): Milk and milk products (patient was lactose intolerant), beans, onions, carrots, raisins, bananas, apricots, prune juice, pretzels, bagels, wheat germ, and brussels sprouts.

Note: It should be remembered that this classification applies to the food intolerance of Mr. Sutalf and may not apply exactly to you.

However, I believe that with some individual modifications, it should have wide general application for the thousands of people afflicted with flatulence.

An Aeolian Symphony

Dear Dr. MacInnis:

Your column on flatulence was just great. It's reassuring to have an expert on "musical foods" like you around. Your diet is really working. For years I've tried everything with not even a whiff of success.

Now I'm happy with a few high-frequency beeps. Gone forever are those crashing crescendos of an Aeolian Symphony.

J.C.M., Kelowna, British Columbia

Answer

Thank you. Mr. M.'s "Aeolian Symphony" refers, of course, to the thunderous commotions of the mythical Aeolus, Greek god of the Winds.

They're Arguing over Flatus

Dear Dr. MacInnis:

My wife and I are having an argument about flatus. She claims it is gas regardless of how it leaves the body, be it up or down. My feeling is that it's a passage of rectal gas only. I recall a column you wrote on flatus a few years ago, where you gave a list of the so-called musical foods to avoid if at all possible—at least if company's coming. The list has mysteriously disappeared and there are rumblings that someone in greater need than us blew off with it.

I'm sure many fellow windbreakers would enjoy experimenting with that list again.

Mr. J.M., Olds, Alberta

Answer

You win the argument. But your wife's confusion is understandable, for the term "passage of flatus" is often misapplied. So I'm pleased to report that the ungainly expression "Flatus

Advanced by Rectal Transport" is now replaced by its time honored acronym by most discerning men of letters.

Hernia Operation at 82?

Dear Dr. MacInnis:

I am a man 82 years old and my problem is a lump or bulge in my left groin that is present when I am standing but disappears when I lie down. The only time it bothers me is when I cough or strain. The doctor says it's a rupture and wants to fix it.

The reason I'm writing is to ask your opinion on a person my age having an operation. What about a truss? A friend of mine wears one and seems to get along okay.

Mr. T.Y., New York

Answer

Should you have it fixed at 82?

If your rupture (hernia) is really hurting you, then go for it whether you're 82 or 102. The surgeon can do the repair under local anesthesia allowing you to be up and walking right away and out of hospital in a day or so. This is a far cry from years ago when a hernia patient had to "rest" flat in bed for up to two weeks to give the surgery a "chance to heal." This led to all sorts of complications—especially in older people who often developed pneumonia and/or blood clots in the lungs and legs. And the leg muscles? That two-week period of inaction rendered them virtually useless, requiring that one had to learn to walk all over again.

A truss is a supportive device placed in the groin that's supposed to restrain the rupture from popping out. Although it has enjoyed popularity with elderly folk from time immemorial, its effectiveness in "holding in" an inguinal hernia is questionable. And a current view is that a truss can "impede blood flow not only from the involved section of the protruding bowel (rupture) but also to surrounding healthy tissue which the surgeon must utilize to repair the hernia" (*Mayo Clinic Health Letter,* July 1989).

The fact that you are concerned about your problem is indeed a healthy sign, for many elderly people tend to be secretive about the appearance of physical defects and tend to let them progress to an advanced state when they may be difficult to treat. It is not at all unusual for an aged patient to finally reach the emergency department with a strangulated hernia requiring immediate surgery, where the bowel may have to be resected, with its attendant increased mortality. (These elderly patients will often tell the doctor that they had this "rupture" for years, but it never bothered them much except on straining, coughing, or heavy lifting.) And then that night the excruciating lower abdominal pain awakened him. The bulging rupture was quite evident to the doctor who tried to "reduce" it (get it back into the abdomen), but it had swollen so much it was impossible. By the time he got to the operating room the bowel had strangulated and gone dead.

The above scenario is a good argument for the early detection and possible surgical treatment of hernias on an "elective," or planned basis. Or the doctor may take what is called "the expectant surgical approach." Here the patient or a responsible family member is thoroughly briefed on the various symptoms signalling early incarceration or "imprisonment" of the bowel in the rupture. The doctor is immediately notified when suspicious signs or symptoms arise.

What I have briefly discussed in a very general way is the inguinal or groin hernia, occurring more frequently in men than women (where femoral hernias are commoner). I should mention here that very frequently in elderly males an inguinal hernia may co-exist with an enlarged prostate (prostatism) and occasionally both may require elective treatment at the same time.

Umbilical (belly button) hernia occurs frequently in the aged and often becomes incarcerated. Repair should be done if at all possible on an elective basis. Huge scrotal hernias filled with bowel are not uncommon in the aged and can be successfully treated surgically if the patient is deemed mentally and physically fit to undergo the operation.

Hiatus Hernia

Dear Dr. MacInnis:

I read your column all the time and would like to see more on hiatus hernia. I've been to quite a few doctors and they all

*said I have a bad one. But no one has been able to help me deal
with the situation very well. Beyond elevating the head of the bed
and taking antacids at bedtime, that was all in the way of help
I received.*

*And even when I did those two things, once in a while I
would awaken in the night with a mouthful of acid anyway, even
when I'd taken four big Gaviscon (antacid) tablets at bedtime.*

*I don't need to tell you the unpleasantness of it all—the taste,
the smell, the burning. It seems to me that in this day and age
there should be some help for my condition. It doesn't happen
every night, but even several times a year is too often. The last
time it happened to me was in August this year (1989) and I
coughed for two days—phlegm and small amounts of blood, some
of which got into my lungs.*

*I would appreciate any advice or whatever (literature, book-
lets, etc). How do others handle the situation?*

Mrs. E.

Answer

I receive so many requests for information of hiatus hernia
that for the past several years I've been sending readers a copy
of a column I wrote on the subject in 1982 and absolutely nothing
has changed in the management of this common and troublesome gastric disorder since that time.

So I am forwarding to you, Mrs. E., my old column, and for
the benefit of new readers I will now condense the subject matter
without sacrificing medical accuracy.

What is hiatus hernia? "Hiatus" means an opening, referring to the opening in your diaphragm where the esophagus
passes through to join the stomach. This so-called esophagus-
stomach junction is right at the diaphragm where the weakness
leads eventually to an enlarged opening in the diaphragm
through which the stomach (usually only a part of it) slides into
the chest cavity and is easily visible on X ray. How much of
the stomach slides into the chest depends on what increases
abdominal pressure, such as lying down after a meal.

This upward protrusion of the stomach can cause a backflow
or "reflux" of stomach juice and acid into the esophagus and

often right into the back of the throat, causing the symptoms Mrs. E. so vividly and accurately describes.

Hiatus hernia is extremely common in the elderly, particularly in elderly women. In a 75-year-old woman, the chance of a hiatus hernia showing up on a routine X ray is about 70 percent. But only a small percentage of these stomach protrusions into the chest cause symptoms such as heartburn, "indigestion," bloating, belching, coughing and vomiting of acid reflux, and even bleeding sometimes.

Diagnosis is made by barium X rays of the stomach and direct visualization of the esophagus with a lighted instrument.

Treatment: Nearly always medical. If you are obese, weight reduction is a must. Small frequent meals of a bland nature (but never before retiring) are the mainstay of management. The head of the bed should be elevated to help prevent the stomach sliding up into the chest. Your doctor will often prescribe antacids or histamine antagonists like Losec, Tagamet or Zantac to treat the acid reflux. Sometimes stomach "sedatives" like Librax are helpful.

What about surgery to repair the hernia? Very rarely is it necessary, probably in 2 or 3 percent of cases where strict medical management doesn't work or where the hernia is very large and is causing intolerable suffering. Is the operation serious? Yes, at any age and in the elderly all the more. And there's always the possibility of recurrence after operation.

Diverticulosis: What Is It?

Dear Dr. MacInnis:

After my doctor performed a routine abdominal X ray, he told me I had a condition called diverticulosis of the large bowel. He assured me it was a very common X ray finding, especially in people over 60 and as a rule they rarely caused symptoms. I've been worrying about this for several years now, and am wondering if you could give me some information on diverticulosis. For instance, I would like to know just what it is, what causes it, can

*it lead to something serious and is there anything I can do to
prevent it getting worse?*

Mrs. T.D., 68

Answer

The term "diverticulosis" is used to describe the presence
in the outer wall of the colon (large bowel) of one or more out-
pouchings or diverticula. They are found in nearly 50 percent
of people 60 years or older. This is in sharp contrast to a 5
percent incidence fifty years ago. It is rare in rural areas of
Africa and India, where the diet contains a high percentage of
roughage causing bulky stools. In more highly industrialized
countries (headed by America), the diet is far more refined containing much less fiber. It is a result of "modern civilization."
Even rural Africans have developed diverticulosis after moving
to urban areas where the food is more refined with less roughage.
At least thirty million people in the U.S. and three million in
Canada currently have diverticulosis. Diverticula usually range
in size from 1 millimeter to 5 centimeters or more in diameter.
By far the greatest number of out-pouchings develop in the distal
end of the colon (sigmoid colon).

It is difficult to definitely correlate abdominal symptoms
with the presence of diverticulosis. However, about 2 percent of
cases are complicated by bleeding when a blood vessel in a pouch
ruptures. In such cases care must be taken to eliminate other
causes of bowel bleeding before attributing it to diverticulosis.
Diverticular bleeding is more frequently found in the older patient. It is comforting for you to know that a bout of diverticular
bleeding usually stops spontaneously and doesn't occur again. If
it should continue, then surgical intervention may be necessary.

You ask if diverticulosis may lead to something more serious? Apart from the rare occurrence of bleeding, inflammation
in the interior of a pouch, especially a narrow-necked pouch,
may lead to diverticulitis with symptoms of appendicitis. But
since diverticulitis originates in the left lower colon, it is often
called "left-sided appendicitis." Diagnosis can usually be confirmed by barium enema and carcinoma of the colon can usually

239

be ruled out. In difficult cases, colonoscopy may have to be performed to differentiate diverticulitis from carcinoma.

As for treatment of diverticulitis, two-thirds of cases can be treated conservatively (non-surgically) and the patient will not experience another attack. However, if the first attack is successfully treated medically but later followed by recurrence or by repeated occurrences, surgical intervention is necessary with subtotal colectomy (partial resection of the colon).

Are preventive measures such as the long-term use of a high fiber diet worthwhile? Although there is some evidence that increasing intake of fresh fruits and vegetables, whole wheat bread, carrots, oranges, and apples may be of immediate benefit, it's controversial that such dietary measures can actually reduce the occurrence of additional diverticula. Metamucil is a good added supplement.

But patients with diverticular disease (both diverticulitis and chronic recurrent diverticulosis) should avoid irritating laxatives.

How I Beat Constipation

Dear Dr. MacInnis:

I thought your readers suffering from constipation would like to hear of how I successfully beat it without using harsh chemical laxatives. First of all I drink eight or more glasses of water every day. I now eat a lot more fiber than I used to. My fiber comes from fruits, whole grains, and vegetables. If I ever have to take laxatives, I choose the "vegetable" type that I make from psyllium seeds. I got the recipe from Prevention *magazine: Two parts of ground psyllium seeds with one part of flax and one part oat bran. Mix all in water and take it as a little mash every night around nine o'clock. As for exercise, I walk a brisk mile every day, rain or shine. I am happy to state that my constipation is now a thing of the past.*

Mr. T.W. (71), Sun City, California

Answer

I too am a subscriber to *Prevention* magazine and found your recipe in its supplement "Prevention's Book of Home Remedies." Here are a few more gems of interest taken from this booklet. "Crushed psyllium seed is a 'super-concentrated' form of fiber which, unlike chemical laxatives, is non-addictive and generally safe even taken over long periods." But a word of caution. Super-concentrated fiber either homemade or in the form of Metamucil should always be taken with lots of water.

Not to be outdone by *Prevention,* I will now reissue my favorite recipe for constipation that many of my constipated readers have learned to swear by! You will recall that the original trials of this laxative were done in my geriatric department with notable success. I've lovingly dubbed it my "gentle mover."

Here it is (revised a bit by a critical reader): Take a cup of dry senna leaves and add to two quarts of water. Bring to a boil and steep for about an hour. Then strain into an enamel pan and cook two pounds of prunes (figs or raisins are okay too) in the tea, adding more water if necessary. Store in the refrigerator in a glass gallon jar. Do not use a metal container. Dosage is the number of prunes needed to do the job; I would suggest two to three at bedtime for a start. It may be sufficient.

Patients often ask if it's okay to take the occasional enema if the going gets rough. The answer is yes, as long as it's occasional. Otherwise you may create a "lazy colon" and cause constipation! Use only clear water or saline enemas.

The term "constipation" in the old medical texts was also known as "costiveness," which is nowadays rarely used except in polite conversation. Under the heading "General Causes," Osler (1906) wrote, "Either a coarse diet (meaning fiber) which leaves too much residue, or a diet which leaves too little may be a cause of costiveness." (Obviously, Sir William's patient's with "too much residue" were not drinking enough water.)

Many of my older (now quite old) readers will remember the "autointoxication" craze of the midthirties. It all began as a theory championed by one of the foremost clinicians of the age, Sir William Arbuthnot Lane of England. He taught that retained feces in the colon not only caused constipation but allowed the release of toxins to spread "through the system" causing all sorts of dreadful maladies. This led to a generation of mothers believing that a daily bowel movement was an absolute "must" for the household, instigating a myth that staunchly persists to this day and is destined to continue.

I must end this erudite essay by recounting what the textbook of physiology of my medical student days had to say about a hapless patient with Hirshsprung disease, where the large bowel (colon) became tremendously dilated with stool "that had accumulated over a period from June 1st of one year to June 30th of the next."

Readers will be relieved to know that "on deliverance" the patient suffered no ill effects.

Now that *was* "costiveness"!

Heavy Run on Senna Leaves—Rochester (New York) Citizens Panic!

Dear Dr. MacInnis:

I read with interest your column on constipation, and your suggested cure—senna leaves and prunes. Everyone else in the city of Rochester read it, too, and there was a run on senna leaves!

I was under the impression that this was a "natural" way of curing a tendency to constipation. However, on the senna leaves box it states it is a laxative and could be habit forming.

Would you recommend this just as needed, or two prunes every night before retiring. Thank you.

Mrs. B., Webster, New York

Answer

Pharmaceutical companies are obliged to disclose all possible side effects, however remote, of their products. This serves to inform the patient and, I suppose, to protect the company in case of litigation.

The senna-prune compound you mention is indeed a "laxative" and like all laxatives tends to cause a degree of dependency after prolonged use. However, compared to other so-called irritant laxatives, its dependency quotient is low and should not cause concern when used with discretion. Should you use it only when needed or take two prunes before retiring every night? If your constipation is only occasional, then the senna-prune treatment should be taken only as needed. On the other hand, if your constipation is obstinate—the so-called obstipation—and does not respond to a mucilose (high fiber) regimen, then I would prescribe two or three of the senna-prunes at bedtime. This of course may be risking dependency over the long term, but it must be weighed against the almost certain risk with other harsher laxatives, or being hooked on daily irritant enemas.

Note: To you good citizens of Rochester: I apologize for being inadvertently responsible for that sudden senna stampede. But come to think of it, your health food stores will bless me!

And thank you for your letter, Mrs. B.

For Constipation: Lactulose *versus* Sorbitol

Dear Dr. MacInnis:

In your recent column on constipation you didn't mention anything about lactulose. In the chronic care hospital where I work as a nursing aid, lactulose is very high on our list as a safe, effective laxative. What is your opinion on this constipation treatment?

Miss M.N., Ontario

Answer

I, too, up to recently, worked in a geriatric hospital and I agree with you. Lactulose, a non-absorbable disaccharide (sugar), keeps the stool soft and bulky by increasing the osmotic pressure in the colon (large bowel). We found it safe, we found it effective, but we also found it very expensive, so much that we switched to another disaccharide called sorbitol, much cheaper, and in our opinion, just as effective as lactulose.

The cost to the pharmacist of a litre bottle of sorbitol is about $5 compared to between $30 and $50 for the same amount of lactulose (1989 costs).

In a recent study comparing the efficacy of the two laxatives and published in the *American Journal of Medicine* 89 (November 1990: 597–601), Lederle and co-workers concluded that sorbitol was not only cost effective compared to lactulose but was just as effective in their trial involving elderly men with chronic constipation.

I would suggest that you procure a reprint of that article from the medical library of your hospital.

Surgery in the Aged

About a year ago in these columns I printed a letter from a distraught lady whose father, age 82, was advised to have his gall bladder removed for recurrent cholecystitis. Her concern was that he couldn't stand the operation due to his great age. My answer was that he should go for it, pointing out that this was an elective (preplanned) operation, where the surgeon would provide adequate preoperative care, such as correction of electrolytes, pulmonary physiology, good nutrition, and proper counselling—all calculated to put his elderly patient into a proper frame of mind. I pointed out to his daughter that the mortality rate in an elective, well-planned operation at her father's age was about 5 percent, only slightly higher than an adult half his age (data from Mount Sinai [New York] Medical Center).

Where we find the dreadfully high surgical death rate in the elderly is in emergency operations, where the patient survival is limited due to pre-existing disease. At your father's age (82), there would be on the average at least five chronic conditions to contend with, all age related. Bronchopneumonia is one of the most common complications in elderly emergency surgery. Again, according to Mount Sinai records, a similar but emergency operation carried a mortality rate of 30 percent.

In this column of a year ago, I cited the difficulty in diagnosing an acute surgical abdomen in aged patients because they simply do not exhibit the traditional symptoms seen in younger adults. Take acute appendicitis for example. Mainly absent are the telltale signs—right-sided abdominal tenderness with rebound tenderness and a rigid belly. What the elderly patient may complain of is "just not feeling right" or he or she may not "look right" to the observer. Often the aged patient exhibits only mental confusion. Such abnormal presentations serve only to confuse the practitioner and thus delay the operation.

In an article in the *Annals of Surgery* 201: 695, a study is reported that revealed "that anywhere from 65 to 100 percent of diagnosed acute appendicitis in the 60 to 90 year age group ruptured before reaching the operating room." This is just one example of the cause of the extraordinary high operative death rate. Peritonitis from ruptured appendix is a serious complication at any age, but in the old it is always lethal carrying a mortality risk of 80 percent *versus* about 6 percent if the operation is done prior to rupture.

According to Dr. Clifton Sheets, assistant professor of emergency medicine, Wright State University School of Medicine, Dayton, Ohio, the most common surgical emergency in the aged patient is acute infection of the gall bladder (acute cholecystitis). Dr. Sheets points out that acute cholecystitis is often mistaken for lower lobe pneumonia, kidney infection, and even a heart attack (myocardial infarction). This, again, tends to delay the proper diagnosis, leading to higher operative mortality. "A very productive test, if immediately available, is ultrasound, and other tests always available are total bilirubin and liver enzyme tests," said Dr. Sheets.

So it is incumbent upon the medical practitioner when faced with a sudden change of behaviour in an elderly patient with minimal abdominal signs to think surgical. Again, according to Dr. Sheets, "Over one-third of aged people who come to the emergency department with abdominal complaints will require an immediate operation and 8 percent will die from the surgery. A correct diagnosis in the emergency room will reduce the death rate by half," Dr. Sheets stated.

How Safe Is an Anesthetic?

Dear Dr. MacInnis:

I am a woman, age 63, and in two weeks I'm due for major surgery. I would like to know just how safe is an anesthetic. Does the length of time in surgery play a key role in recovery? Is there much danger of an allergic reaction to either the anesthetic or painkilling drug? And, lastly, is it true that the most critical time is that following surgery when blood pressure may fall to a critical level?

Answer

You bring up points of great interest that are on the minds of everyone about to undergo an operation. And often the anesthesia is feared more than the surgery itself—the fear of the unknown.

Modern-day anesthesia, when administered by a skilled and experienced specialist, is eminently safe. Your vital signs —respiration, pulse, and blood pressure—are continually monitored and any possible deviation from normal is treated on the spot.

The length of time in surgery has some bearing on immediate recovery time, but not as much as you would think, again thanks to modern anesthesia, which maintains the patient's vital functions very near to, if not, normal for long periods of time. You will awaken as from a long night's sleep. Gone forever are the days of the monumental ether hangover, far worse than any surgery!

Is old age a risk? Not so much any more as long as the anesthetic is carefully selected and, of course, expertly administered.

Allergic reactions to the anesthetic or to drugs can occur but are exceedingly rare. Speed of action is the key to successful treatment and the operating room is the ideal place to handle the emergency. Is the period immediately following surgery critical? This is the time when monitoring of the vital signs is most important. You will not be wheeled out of the operating room until the anesthetist and staff are satisfied with your condition.

And then, off you go to the recovery room. Again, skilled staff take over till you awaken and slowly, ever so slowly, you open your eyes and look around. "No, this is not my bedroom," you say to yourself. And then it gradually dawns on you; it's not home, it's the hospital. The operation is over—and "look, I'm really alive and okay!"

Peptic Ulcer: Is It Caused by a Germ?

Dear Dr. MacInnis:

I am an active healthy 71-year-old male. However, I have the common nuisance problem of reoccurring duodenal ulcer. My recent recurrence has been healing with the Tagamet (histamine-blocking) therapy as have the previous two. The first ulcer occurred with a hemorrhage and under an excellent doctor's care was healed, prior to the Tagamet-type drugs appearing on the market.

My episodes have been in 1961, 1977, 1988, and 1992. My father and sister were also plagued with ulcer problems, so I assume mine was family related to a degree.

I would like your comments on the new treatment based on studies in England, and the U.S. that an organism called the Helicobacter pylori bacterium *could be the cause of ulcers in some cases. I understand that a combination of Pepto-Bismol, metronidazole, and the antibiotic amoxicillin for one or two weeks will kill the* H. pylori, *thus reducing the recurrence of ulcers in cases like mine drastically.*

Mr. G.J., New York State

Answer

For the benefit of readers who have not heard of the *Helicobacter pylori bacterium* as a possible factor in the genesis of peptic (stomach, duodenum, and esophagus) ulcers, here's a brief background.

For nearly a hundred years medical scientists have reported spiral shaped bacteria around inflammatory areas of the stomach (gastritis) and peptic ulcers. Nothing much was made of these germ colonies, as they were considered to be "normal flora" or inhabitants of the gastrointestinal tract. That is, until nine or ten years ago when investigators showed that under certain conditions, *H. pylori* might itself produce ulcers that respond slowly to conventional treatment and, at times, *cause recurrence.* (The most memorable of these early investigators was a team of Australian doctors who with incomparable zeal and dedication actually swallowed a hefty dose of *H. pylori* and, although healthy with no previous history of stomach trouble, all came down with peptic ulcers!)

More recently (November 16, 1991) Logan and colleagues writing in the *Lancet* 338:1249–52, reported that a one-week course of treatment consisting of bismuth (an antacid), amoxicillin (an antibiotic), and metronidazole (brand name Flagyl, an antifungal agent) "could eradicate *H. pylori* in a high percentage of cases." The cases that did not respond to the therapeutic regimen occurred almost always where cultures of the *H. pylori* were resistant to metronidazole. (This would indicate that there are various strains of *H. pylori,* some sensitive and some resistant to metronidazole.) The authors recommend that C and S (culture and sensitivity) tests be done on (endoscopically obtained) biopsy specimens from the ulcer to determine which patients would be likely to benefit from their one week "eradication package." Dr. Logan's findings were duplicated by a team of Texas researchers who published their findings in the May 1, 1992, issue of the *Annals of Internal Medicine.* From their study, it would seem that when *H. pylori* is present in an ulcer (over 75 percent of their cases), treatment with a routine quite similar to Logan's dramatically reduced their ulcer recurrence rate.

To determine, Mr. J., whether or not there's a *H. pylori* infection lurking around your recurring duodenal ulcer, you would need, first of all, a biopsy of the ulcer site to determine its presence and if present to find out if the bacterial strain is sensitive or resistant to metronidazole, as noted in the preceding paragraph. If resistant, then that's the end of the matter, for the one-week treatment package would most likely be useless. If the test shows that your strain of *H. pylori* is sensitive to metronidiazole, I would recommend the following one-week routine to eradicate your infection and (hopefully?) to prevent further recurrences: amoxicillin, 500 milligrams, three times daily; metronidazole (Flagyl), 250 milligrams, two tablets three times daily, along with Pepto-Bismol as prescribed.

Addendum: August 1993. Since I wrote the above column (in 1992) sufficient time has elapsed to determine just how effective this "triple therapy" (Pepto-Bismol, amoxicillin, and metronidazole) has been over the longer term. A number of studies have shown that it was successful in eradicating the *H. pylori* in 80 to 90 percent of cases when given for fourteen days. However, this was at the expense of quite bothersome side effects, such as nausea, vomiting, diarrhea, and abdominal pain, so bad that in many cases, patients gave up the treatment. It became clear that the ideal treatment would be a *single* antibiotic that was effective, had few side effects, and was not adversely affected by the stomach acids (as were most of the previously used antibiotics). The new generation antibiotic, clarithromycin, was recently found to meet the challenge—at least in a modest study—and may turn out to be the treatment of choice for recurrent peptic ulcer caused by the presence of *Helicobacter pylori*.

Piles Of Trouble

Dear Dr. MacInnis:

I am male, age 60, and suffer from one of mankind's most miserable maladies—piles. I went to a doctor about it and it must have been one of his quiet days, for he immediately recommended surgery (hemorrhoidectomy). He assured me that everything would be tolerable if not comfortable, but I didn't buy it as I remember what a friend went through for several weeks after the operation.

So that's why I'm writing to you with this question: Is there anything that can be done short of an operation and when is an operation definitely necessary?

Mr. D.L., Toronto, Ontario

Answer

It's impossible to offer you specific advice because you do not state the severity of your symptoms. Are they internal or external, are they painful, and if they bleed, how frequently?

As a general rule, a surgeon should not be consulted in the first instance. This could be left until later and only when conservative (non-surgical) measures fail.

Some non-surgical recommendations include: (1) frequent warm sitz baths, especially good for painful hemorrhoids; (2) avoiding sitting down for long periods of time (prolonged sitting in an office chair, an automobile, or at a long theatre performance causes congestion of the pelvic tissues and "inflates" hemorrhoids, which are basically anal and rectal varicose veins); (3) plenty of walking (walking tends to divert blood from the anal area thus "decongesting" hemorrhoids); and (4) avoidance of certain foods that in your experience aggravate the hemorrhoids.

Certain "preparations" are widely touted to "relieve" piles, and the Federal Drug Administration (FDA) warns that products or preparations claiming to "shrink" piles must also label that such products should not be used by people with diabetes or heart disease.

When the above-mentioned measures do not appreciably help, then you should seek surgical consultation. The surgeon may recommend simple injection of the hemorrhoids, laser treatment, or the standard cutting operation you have referred to. ("Banding" will be described in the next column.)

If you are still in doubt, then you should seek a second surgical opinion.

Banding Hemorrhoids

Dear Dr. MacInnis:

My doctor tells me that I have internal hemorrhoids, the kind that protrude whenever I strain at bowel movement. I've tried Preparation H and other ointments without benefit.

The reason I'm writing is that I saw a news item on TV announcing a "new treatment" for internal hemorrhoids called the "rubber band" treatment. Have you heard of this and, if so, is it a good treatment?

If you recommend it, I will ask my doctor to do it as an office procedure as I'm scared stiff of surgery.

Mr. L.T., age 70, Ontario

Answer

The rubber band treatment for protruding internal hemorrhoids is not new. I recall writing a column on it several years ago and recommending its use.

The procedure, done in the doctor's office, consists of tying a small rubber band around the hemorrhoid, causing it to drop off in a few days. Usually one hemorrhoid at a time is banded in a series of office visits.

Since I last wrote on the procedure, it has gained great popularity. At the May 1993 annual convention of the American Society of Colon and Rectal Surgeons (ASCRS), Dr. Robert Beart of Los Angeles reported on a comparative study of 177 patients who had single or multiple hemorrhoidal banding at the Mayo Clinic, Scottsdale, Arizona. Patients who had more than one hemorrhoid banded were more likely to report discomfort and pain than those who received only one banding per session (29 percent *vs.* 4.5 percent). Several other specialists reported similarly successful results. One in particular, Dr. Izhack Bayer of Israel, reported on the banding of 2,934 hemorrhoid patients over a period of twelve years. Here "treatment was successful without requiring sick leave in almost all cases," he said.

My advice: Go for it. As you can see, there are literally piles of evidence in its favor.

Crohn's Disease

Dear Dr. MacInnis:

My husband, age 53, has long-standing Crohn's disease with bouts of arthritis that is wearing him down. He has been on sulfasalazine for many years now and takes medicine for his arthritis as well. In spite of these treatments, he still complains of severe fatigue and bouts of abdominal pain with diarrhea and takes iron and BBB for his anemia.

My question: Is arthritis a complication of Crohn's or is it occurring separately? And does it turn into cancer?

Mrs. H.H., California

Answer

Crohn's disease is a type of inflammatory bowel disease that is often confused with ulcerative colitis. The most common symptoms are lower abdominal pain that may be mild or severe and at times requiring strong painkillers, even morphine. In addition, there is often a mild diarrhea. The diagnosis is made from history, X ray of large bowel, and visual examination of the large bowel with a flexible lighted tube called a colonoscope. Biopsy of the bowel wall can often provide a definitive diagnosis. Crohn's disease is sometimes associated with arthritis, probably because both are said to be caused by alteration in the immune system. The area where the small bowel joins the colon (ileo-colic) suffers the most from the slow but relentless chronic inflammation. The development of cancer in Crohn's disease is much less common than in ulcerative colitis.

Readers may procure more information on Crohn's disease by writing to Crohn's and Colitis Foundation, 444 Park Avenue South, New York, New York 10016.

I Had My Gall Bladder Out the New Way!

Dear Dr. MacInnis:

I read your column in today's Democrat & Chronicle *with interest as I had that new type of gall bladder operation a month ago that you described. I am 76 years old and had my operation at 1:00 P.M., and I went home the next morning about 9:00 A.M. The doctor said I could do anything I felt up to—climb stairs, walk, ride in a car, and eat anything. He said I perhaps shouldn't run out for a pepperoni or pizza right away but should go easy on them at first.*

My son had the regular operation (for gall bladder) a good many years ago and he had a very bad time. Nowadays, they do all the pre-op examinations before you go into the hospital, such as blood work, X rays, ECGs, etc. This also helps to lessen the stay in hospital. Incidentally, a woman in her 80s had this new type of operation the same day as I did, and she also went home the next day.

I had the X ray for gall stones about three weeks before the operation, and the stones showed up. I had been having gall bladder colic attacks for years, but not often. The most recent one was pretty bad, so my doctor told me not to wait, and I had it done.

I am sending you an article on this new type of gall bladder operation that my daughter copied for me. I hope you enjoy it.
Mrs. V.S., Canandaigua, New York

Answer

Most readers who read my two recent columns on the new type of surgical procedure for removal of the gall bladder will know what Mrs. S is talking about. You are the first of my readers to report on your experience, and it goes without saying it was a pleasant one.

For the benefit of readers who missed my columns on "laparoscopic cholecystectomy," as it is called, I will very briefly describe the procedure.

The term "laparoscopic" refers to an old procedure where a lighted tubular instrument called a "laparoscope" is inserted through the abdominal wall so that the operator can explore the abdominal organs both for diagnostic and curative purposes. (Gynecologists have been using "visualizing tubes" for female pelvic operations, such as tying Fallopian tubes, for over fifteen years, but it wasn't until 1987 that a French surgeon applied the technique for the removal of a gall bladder.) Laparoscopic cholecystectomy (removal of a gall bladder by means of a laparoscope) has definitely caught on and is rapidly becoming the procedure of choice for surgical removal of a gall bladder, with a few exceptions.

After the patient is anesthetized, the abdominal cavity is filled with carbon dioxide gas. This "balloons" the abdominal cavity, allowing the surgeon plenty of room to manipulate his or her dissecting and grasping instruments with ease. (A total of four tiny half-inch incisions are made through which a half-inch tube, or sheath, is pushed into the roomy abdominal space. The tubes serve as ports of entry for the laparoscope, and the necessary instruments for the operation. The outside (external) end of the laparoscope is connected to a video camera and cable that allows the contents of the abdominal cavity to be projected on two large television screens.)

The surgeon must relearn to operate looking at the screen, instead of the conventional direct method, something that seems awkward at first and takes time to get used to. The entire procedure takes about ninety minutes, slightly longer on the average than the "open" abdominal operation.

For the benefit of interested readers, the article that Mrs. B. sent to me appeared in the July 1991 issue of *Discover* magazine. Here, in the "Vital Signs" section, surgeon Sherwin B. Nuland writes a vivid and detailed recount of his experience in performing his first laparoscopic cholecystectomy.

Bad Time after Gall Bladder Operation

Dear Dr. MacInnis:

About ten years ago I had my gall bladder out for gall stones. My convalescence was four months, and I would not like such an ordeal again.

The reason I'm writing is that my wife, now 62, has been advised by two surgeons to have her gall bladder out. She has chronic cholecystitis (inflammation of the gall bladder) with three medium-size gall stones visible on X ray. With my bad experience still fresh in her memory, she is naturally apprehensive about surgery. My question: Is there any way other then surgery for treating gall stones?

Answer

First of all a comment on your bad experience from gall bladder surgery. In the majority of cases the conventional operation for gall bladder removal (cholecystectomy) is bothersome for the first few postoperative days followed by gradual recovery, allowing the patient to leave the hospital in about a week. Your case was the exception and, while quite unfortunate, should not influence your wife's decision to postpone surgery. In fact, for some unknown reason, women handle gall bladder surgery better on the average than men.

Over the years in these columns, I have reported on a number of non-surgical procedures for treating gall stones. The one that has commanded the most attention up to recently has been the fragmenting of the stones by extracorporeal (outside the body) generated electrical shock waves. This is a procedure widely used for the treatment of kidney stones and here it is quite effective. However, gall-stone fragmentation machines are not generally available, and even where they are, only a small proportion of gall stone patients are suitable candidates for this procedure.

The new procedure that's rapidly gaining ground involves the removal of the gall bladder through a laparoscope (an abdominally inserted lighted instrument) using laser technology. But for now the operation of choice for your wife is a cholecystectomy (surgical removal of gall bladder).

Laparoscopic Removal of Gall Bladder

The standard operation for removal of the gall bladder has been and still is through a large, right, upper abdominal incision under general anesthesia. Over the years we have become so inured to the relatively long hospital stay of one to several weeks and over a month of convalescence (minimum) before getting back to work that surgeons have taken these and other disadvantages for granted and have so advised their patients, that is, until recently.

In a previous column I responded to a reader who inquired about any possible options to the conventional gall bladder surgery. His wife was to have this operation and had some qualms about it. Although I had to advise the old standard operation, I had difficulty concealing my enthusiasm for a brand-new departure in gall bladder surgery. Due to space limitations I could only briefly describe the procedure but promised to explain it in more detail in a follow up column (and this is it).

The operation is performed through a lighted cylindrical instrument called a laparoscope, using laser technology for cauterization and coagulation. (The laparoscope has long been used in abdominal surgery for exploration of the abdominal contents to assist in diagnosis.) The procedure is called "laparoscopic laser cholecystectomy." Only three mini-incisions are used: One at the navel for the insertion of the laparoscope and two (one 5 millimeter and one 8 millimeter) incisions to insert the instrument (for the removal of the gall bladder under laparoscopic visualization). The detached gall bladder is pulled out through the navel incision. The laparoscope is connected to a video camera and cable. This allows the contents of the abdominal cavity (now greatly distended with carbon dioxide gas) to be easily visualized when projected into two large television screens. The surgeon must learn to operate "indirectly" while looking at the screen.

Writing in the medical journal *Surgical Endoscopy* 3 (1989): 131–33, Drs. E. J. Reddick and D. O. Olsen compared the results of laparoscopic laser cholecystectomy on 25 patients with that of twenty-five patients who underwent "open" abdominal gall bladder surgery but with a very small incision (3 to 4 centimeters, or 1½ inches).

Result: Average stay in hospital, 2.0 and 2.8 days respectively. Time till return to work: Average 6.4 days and 34 days respectively. (Source: *Internal Medicine Alert,* a semimonthly survey of current developments in internal medicine, November 15, 1990.)

Dr. Leon D. Goldman, assistant professor of surgery, Harvard Medical School and a consultant for *Internal Medicine Alert* commented (in part) as follows: "Laparoscopic cholecystectomy appears to be a major advance in the treatment of cholelithiasis [gall stones]. More and more patients are demanding this procedure, which has clear advantages in terms of length of hospital stay, reduced pain and discomfort, and earlier return to work. . . . In addition," said Dr. Goldman, "its availability may lead patients with cholelithiasis to seek earlier surgical consultation, thus preventing some of the complicated gall bladder disease that results from postponement of surgery."

This new procedure in gall bladder surgery calls for special training for abdominal surgeons. On this aspect Dr. Goldman comments: "First the technique requires special training and equipment. . . . Surgeons who perform this procedure need considerable time to master new skills. . . . The procedure is not appropriate for all patients. Those with a history of multiple surgical procedures who have adhesions are not well suited to laparoscopic cholecystectomy. In addition, patients in whom *common duct* stones are suspected or proven should probably have conventional surgery." Dr. Goldman quotes the American College of Surgeons and the Society for Surgery of the Alimentary Tract who suggest that "this procedure should be performed *only by surgeons who are prepared and competent to proceed with open (surgical) cholecystectomy.*" Despite these and other caveats, Dr. Goldman believes that "laparoscopic cholecystectomy is here to stay."

(I would like to acknowledge my indebtedness to *Internal Medicare Alert* and Dr. Goldman for the above quotations. *Internal Medicine Alert* is an educational publication designed to present scientific information and opinion to health professionals to stimulate thought and further investigation.)

Hirschsprung's Disease

Dear Dr. MacInnis:

What is Hirschsprung's disease? I don't have it, but I've heard that the child of a relative of mine was born with the condition. Any information would be appreciated.

Mr. M.J., New York

Answer

A more descriptive name for Hirschsprung's disease is congenital megacolon, which means "being born with a hugely distended large bowel." It occurs once in a thousand births, with boys more frequently affected. It is caused by the congenital absence of certain nerve cells in the wall of the colon whose function is to propel out fecal matter. Because of this colon paralysis and fecal stoppage, the large bowel becomes grossly distended and very evident on visual examination. Congenital megacolon usually becomes apparent in the first year of life. The usual constipation measures are not very effective and manual extraction of the impacted feces may have to be performed after oil retention enemas. The condition often seriously interferes with nutrition, causing retarded growth.

The acquired type of megacolon occurs usually in an emotionally disturbed child who refuses to follow the ritual of regular bowel movements. As in the congenital type, the rectum and colon is distended with accumulated feces. Here the treatment is basically psychiatric along with oil retention enemas and often manual extraction of feces.

Irritable Bowel Syndrome: Fact or Fancy?

Dear Dr. MacInnis:

My sister, age 40, has been diagnosed as having a spastic colon. The doctor at the clinic sent her to a specialist who made the diagnosis. Her main complaints were aches and crampy pains in the lower part of the abdomen with bouts of loose stools and sometimes just the opposite—periods of constipation. At first they thought it was bowel obstruction but after much testing and X rays, nothing showed up. He put her on 5 milligrams of Valium, which seemed to settle her a bit but she still has bouts of the old bowel trouble (now in its fifth year).

My question: What causes spastic colon? Will she ever get over it? Is there any better treatment for it?

Mrs. T.N., Edmonton, Alberta

Answer

Spastic colon can be considered a subset of the better known nervous gut condition called irritable bowel syndrome (IBS). People with IBS (and most are women) usually show a very rapid bowel movement transit time through the length of the small intestine and colon (large bowel). This may explain many of the symptoms, some that you have mentioned plus others, such as periodic bowel noises and an urgent desire to pass loose stools (often covered with mucus but seldom, if ever, blood). Another associated symptom and not uncommon is left shoulder pain that may radiate down the arm. This peculiar complaint is thought to be caused from intestinal gas trapped in the splenic flexure of the colon (where the transverse colon makes a 90-degree downward turn to become descending colon).

Patients with IBS are more often than not tense, anxious, and "nervous" people who tend to overreact to many of life's stresses. And it's the intestine that takes the brunt of this over-reaction. In describing the mechanism of IBS to my patients, I would like to remind how many of them reacted to the stress of a school examination with urinary urgency and diarrhea—and this they well remembered, for I can recall that many of these school-exam "overreactors" eventually "graduated" to the ranks of irritable bowel syndrome patients.

There are several other clinical conditions that more or less mimic IBS and must be ruled out. Most important is the one you mention—intestinal obstruction. Others like diverticulitis, ulcerative colitis, Crohn's disease, and lactase deficiency can, in most cases, be easily diagnosed. Since IBS cannot be detected by direct testing, like these others, the diagnosis is made largely by exclusion and by always remembering the associated "nervous" personality state.

The most important element of treatment is a thorough discussion with the patient of the fact that IBS appears to be an exaggerated intestinal reaction to emotional tension in a nervous person. This in itself tends to dispel the mystery of the condition and may go a long way in soothing the patient. But often the patient needs more than just reassurance, and sedation such as diazepam (Valium) is prescribed. If taken for long periods, sedatives like Valium can be addictive. (Most specialists recommend limiting such sedation to two or three weeks, or taking periodic drug "vacations" to minimize dependency.)

In cases of protracted diarrhea, "antimotility" medication like Lomotil can sometimes be useful. If constipation is bothersome, then a stool "bulker" like metamucil helps, especially if your diet is low in fiber.

There is nothing better for "calming the nerves" than a daily walking routine, so this type of exercise is highly recommended for IBS.

Irritable bowel syndrome is considered by many to be a "functional" rather than a truly organic condition that the doctor can determine by diagnostic tests. To others, it's the veritable "riddle within an enigma" leading to the extreme view that it is the typical example of a "non-disease," with a myriad of disconnected symptoms.

All of which in fine and dandy if you don't suffer from it!

A Case of Acute Appendicitis in an Aged Patient

Dear Dr. MacInnis:

I thought a long time before writing this letter. It's about my late husband, who was age 82 when his death occurred six months ago. He awakened one night in a confused state, and I called the doctor, who ordered an ambulance for the hospital. In the emergency they thought he was coming down with a stroke so he was admitted to the hospital for observation. His confusion and restlessness continued so he was given sedating drugs by needle, which made him even more confused. On the third day some doctor on the staff checked his abdomen, which was by this time very sore and tender. The diagnosis was acute appendicitis. At operation the appendix was ruptured and infection was spread all through his abdomen. He died three days later. I have often wondered if he would still be alive if the diagnosis was made earlier. Is it difficult to diagnose appendicitis in an aged person?
Mrs. J.H. (76), California

Answer

People often ask me, "How does geriatric medical practice differ from medical practice in general?" What's different is the older person's, particularly the "very old" person's, manifestation of disease. The old are generally more insensitive to pain than the young, as witness the so-called silent coronary and the relative absence of pain in an acute abdomen, like your husband's. Acute appendicitis, more often then not, goes undiagnosed until peritonitis sets in with its much more serious outlook. What the older patient often manifests instead of pain is delirium or confusion, with its disorganized thinking, that may be the cry not of a mental condition but of pain or infection or both.

In the *Annals of Surgery* 201: 695, a study reports "that anywhere from 65 to 100 percent of diagnosed acute appendicitis in the 60- to 90-year age group ruptured before reaching the operating theatre. Peritonitis (generalized abdominal infection) from a ruptured appendix is a serious complication at any age, but in the old it is most lethal, carrying a mortality risk of 80 percent *versus* about 6 percent if done before rupture.

Therefore, it behooves the medical practitioner to be most vigilant and have a strong index of suspicion when an aged patient suddenly becomes delirious, or "may not look right," or may say, "I just don't feel right."

He may be trying to tell us something!

"When in Doubt, Operate"

Dear Dr. MacInnis:

My husband (76) was operated on for suspected acute appendicitis. They found that the appendix was ruptured with infection all over the abdomen. He died three days later. The reason he wasn't operated on until two days after admission was because the doctors couldn't agree on the diagnosis. They said his symptoms weren't typical. With appendicitis so common, I always thought it was easy to diagnose. What went wrong here—or is it just hard to diagnose in old people?

Mrs. T.E., Ontario

Answer

As you correctly state, it's "just hard to diagnose in old people."

And this applies to any surgical condition in an elderly person—be it appendicitis, acute gall bladder infection, intestinal obstruction, or a strangulated hernia, to name a few. The lack of "typical" signs and symptoms often causes a delay in diagnosis that may result in sometimes fatal complications from peritonitis.

Some surgical specialists feel that aging in some way accelerates the infective process in appendicitis. One recent study revealed that "anywhere from 65 to 100 percent" of diagnosed acute appendicitis in the 65- to 90-year age group ruptured before the patient reached the operating room.

In many cases, abdominal pain, "rebound" tenderness, and rigidity—all telltale signs of appendicitis in younger folk—may be doubtful or absent in the elderly. And due to increasing longevity, there's been a seven-fold increase in "elderly" appendicitis in the past thirty years.

So it might be well to consider a new surgical maxim in the management of "suspected" appendicitis in the aged person: When in doubt, operate.

Delirium after Surgical Operation

Dear Dr. MacInnis:

My mother, age 77, who has what the doctor calls "early" Alzheimer's disease, recently underwent an abdominal operation. After coming out of the anesthetic she appeared very confused. The doctors called it "delirium," which seemed to lessen in a few weeks. Is this common following an operation?

Mrs. N.N., Manitoba

Answer

Delirium or acute confusional state frequently occurs in the elderly following an operation. It is particularly common if the patient is in early dementia like your mother. It is therefore a prudent practice in such cases to warn the relatives of this postoperative possibility before the patient goes to surgery.

Up until now it was thought by many doctors, including myself, that post-operative delirium was due to the anesthetic. But recent studies conducted at the University Hospital in London, Ontario, reveal that the type of surgery or the anesthetic played no part in he development of delirium. And neither did hospitalization itself have an important role.

What was important the researchers found, after analyzing 112 different factors that might predispose elderly patients to post-surgical delirium, was hearing impairment and the dose of narcotic medication given on the first post-operative day. Delirium associated with hearing impairment occurred within twenty-four hours after surgery while late onset delirium (occurring within one week post-surgical) was related to the narcotic dose.

Dr. Richard Knill, associate professor or anesthesiology at the University of Western Ontario, who presented a paper at the Canadian Anesthetist Society annual meeting in Ottawa, is quoted in Canada's *Medical Post:* "We think the relationship to hearing impairment in the early onset (within twenty-four hours) cases may reflect the practice in our institutions of removing hearing aids on the day of surgery and not giving them back until the next day .... Therefore those patients who are deaf have a type of sensory deprivation through the first postoperative night, which may precipitate their delirium," Dr. Knill said.

This is an exceedingly important observation that I'm sure will be heeded by all those entrusted with postoperative care of the elderly.

MedicAlert

One out of every three admissions to a hospital emergency department is an elderly patient. Emergency physicians tell us that their department, with its frenetic pace of organized confusion, is never the ideal place to calm a patient's anxiety. It can be specifically traumatic for the older person whose sometimes obscure medical history is often already complicated by confusion and disorientation.

With our ever-increasing geriatric population, the situation is bound to worsen. Ideally, emergency personnel should have access to a readily available and accurate medical history of older patients so they can provide quick and appropriate treatment and get them out of an uncomfortable environment.

Today I received a well-written and informative packet from the MedicAlert Foundation on this very subject. MedicAlert is celebrating its thirty-fifth anniversary by launching a nationwide program to help older people better protect themselves in medical emergencies.

In this column I will introduce MedicAlert to readers by presenting some important facts—the who, what, where, and why of this notable organization as related in its brochure.

1. What is MedicAlert? It is a nonprofit foundation dedicated to saving lives in accidents and medical emergencies. It is the most comprehensive medical identification system in the world.
2. Who needs MedicAlert? Any medical condition that places them at added risk such as hypertension, heart trouble, severe allergies, diabetes, asthma, and epilepsy to name a few of over 200 conditions.
3. Do physicians support MedicAlert? Over 95 percent of physicians acquainted with MedicAlert believe that it can speed treatment in an emergency and can save lives.
4. What can it do? It helps prevent tragic or even fatal mistakes from being made during emergency medical treatment. It speaks quickly for the patient unable to speak for himself due to illness or injury.
5. How does MedicAlert work? The MedicAlert emblem, which triggers the emergency medical data service, is custom engraved with the member's primary conditions,

identification number, and MedicAlert's twenty-four-hour emergency center's hot line phone number, emblem, bracelet, or neck chain.

6. The twenty-four-hour emergency line is accessible from anywhere in the world. The emergency number on Medic-Alert's emblem offers instant access to medical information, in addition to names of physicians and family members. In an emergency, MedicAlert supplies important lifesaving information to emergency care personnel. Your emergency hot line is guaranteed for your lifetime.

7. How much does MedicAlert protection cost? A one-time membership fee beginning at U.S.$30, including a stainless steel emblem, provides protection for a lifetime. Annually, you receive a wallet card copy of your computerized medical record with a reminder to keep your record up to date. You can update your record any time with a toll free phone call. In Canada write MedicAlert Foundation, Box 9800, Don Mills, Ontario M3C T29; phone 696-0267. Outside Toronto area phone toll-free 1-800-668-1507.

8. A universal symbol. The MedicAlert emblem bears the symbol of the medical profession and is recognized universally. The MedicAlert Foundation has affiliate organizations in twenty-two countries around the world.

9. How can I join MedicAlert? Write MedicAlert Foundation, 2323 Colorado Avenue, Turlock, California 95380. In U.S. call toll free 1-800-432-5378.

Chapter 11
Elder Sexuality

There is much more sexual activity and playfulness going on in the bedrooms of older men and women then the rest of the society seems to understand or perhaps is ready to believe.

Rev. Andrew Greeley, American R.C. priest, author, and sociologist

On the topic of sexuality, the Number One complaint of elderly males is impotence or the inability to successfully perform the sexual act. As you will read in one of the upcoming columns, the term "impotence" is gradually losing popularity because of its implication of *overall* inadequacy. I like the term "erection failure" because it immediately pinpoints both the problem and its anatomical locus. So as a pioneer of change, I'll try to use the term "erection failure" for "impotence" whenever possible or practical. It will be a slow start, but at least a start!

As you will see, some are successfully coming to terms with their sexuality, while others have already "given up"—victims of a societal verdict that sex in the elderly is at best somewhat comical or, at worst, unnatural. And unfortunately, that old saw, "What do you expect at *your* age," is still, in many doctors' offices, very much alive and well.

And how helpful are their adult children? From the letters I receive from them, not very much. For when the topic of Mom and Dad's sex life comes up, they transfigure into "instant puritans," which makes me wonder if they consider themselves the progeny of some modern style immaculate conception!

But out there in the very real world of the elderly (with over thirty million in the United States and three million in Canada) elder sexuality is still a very potent force—not without its problems—and many cry out for help. But I bring them good tidings for help is at hand.

If this chapter on elder sexuality seems to be male dominated, there's good reason. While men discuss their problems freely and often quite graphically, women are hesitant and when they do get up the courage to write, they often question their own perceived inadequacies when it's perfectly obvious where the blame lies. I hope that my columns on how aging affects the female sexual response—and the male's, too—will make informative reading for them.

Finally, a considerable part of this chapter is devoted to devices for treating "erection failure." Although for the most part these methods are "male operated," their success or failure rests on female acceptance or rejection. This is something the man must understand. He should never seek advice from a doctor or sex counsellor unless accompanied by his partner.

I'd Die Before I Ever Let Myself Get Old

Dear Dr. MacInnis:

In a column on elder sexuality you wrote long ago, you printed in sensuous poetry the thoughts of a woman, alone, ill, and close to death, who still felt the strong pull of love and sexuality and the memory of her experiences.

I've lost that poem. Could you share it again with your readers?

Mrs. L.B.

Answer

Over the years, many readers have asked for that intensely poignant poetry which I sent to them personally. This time I shall, indeed, share it with all. There's no need for further explanation. You've said it well. My only regret is that I cannot give credit to the unknown author.

Here it is again:

I'd die before I ever let myself get old,
I would always stay young,
I wanted then
The same as I want now
Everything!

To go everywhere in the world,
To be everybody in the world,
To slide under the ocean, climb over the moon,
Swing back and forth between them
Thumbing my nose.

You think I couldn't make you a good lover still?
You're crazy if you don't think so,
I could make you miserable with anyone else,
You would close your eyes with those tame little tootsies
And dream about me—plead for me!

Sexuality in the Elderly: Part 1

I frequently hear from men and women past middle age who feel they have problems with their sexuality, i.e., their negative response to sex. In most cases their problems are real; in some cases, however, their problems are more perceived than real. For instance a couple in their early 60s were convinced that since they indulged in sexual intercourse "only once a month" and were content with it, "there must be something wrong." When it was pointed out to them that whether it was once a night or once a year, it was normal when *both* partners were satisfied with the arrangement; they answered with thanks and relief!

In the interest of completeness, I must tell you that this couple rightly differentiated between "lovemaking," which in their case meant intimate affection—touching, kissing, caressing, and, fondling (sometimes culminating in ejaculation and orgasm)—and overt, preplanned coitus.

I can hear you thinking, "With all that lovemaking going on, that once a month sex was just the frosting on the cake!" And so it would seem. But there's an object lesson here that may be of help to a considerable number of impotent men who write about their inability to perform, leading to frustration for husband and wife. The lesson is this: There are alternatives to sexual intercourse and many wives would be forever thankful if husbands would "show a little tenderness now and then," as one wife put it.

So you husbands out there, get to it even though you can't have your cake and eat it, too. It might even help your "impotence"! The example I gave you was admittedly an ideal one and most likely a rare one. It was an easy "problem" to answer. All that couple needed was reassurance. What's not so easy to solve is the far more common situation where one partner (most often the husband) is the sexual athlete, demanding frequent (sometimes nightly) sex—his "normal"—with a harried spouse who seems perfectly content with her yearly "ritual." Here it's the wife who is worried that she's not "being fair" to her husband and perhaps secretly guilty about her inhibited desire. Here we're witnessing a sexual collision—intense sexuality *versus* inhibited desire—and the prognosis is not too good even with the best of sexual counselling, which should always be sought if at all possible in an effort to save this marriage by teaching the partners that "making sex" and "making love" should always be a part of their sexual interplay.

The question is often asked, "Is masturbation normal?" This query may be posed in either of two contexts. One, where the person, male or female, desires sex but for a number of reasons cannot procure a partner or, two, where mutual body pleasuring is an often necessary part of foreplay leading to intercourse. Medical myths like many "old wives' tales" die hard, but unless you are on a giant guilt trip about it, masturbation or "self-sex" is considered to be a normal part of sexuality and will not "make you blind," as the old family "doctor books" used to warn!

One of the amazing facts I've learned from correspondents over the years is the large number of couples (middle-aged and over) who have adjusted satisfactorily to the husband's impotence and are leading contented, happy lives (undoubtedly from indulging in the alternative intimacies referred to previously).

And another sexuality aphorism is worth noting. Couples who have enjoyed a strong, active, healthy sex life in their earlier years have a great tendency to continue the practice well into their later years, giving rise to a companion maxim: "If you always use it, you will never lose it"!

This column is meant to address sexuality in the elderly in a very general way. In the next column I'll be more specific with case histories of various problems and advice on their management.

Sexuality in the Elderly: Part 2

Dear Dr. MacInnis:

Is sexual functioning affected by aging? No matter what the experts say the old grey mare (or should I say the old grey stallion) is not what he used to be. I mean it's slower getting it up and when it's up it's never "very high"—to be frank with you.

I am happy to say, though, that we're both 72 years and enjoy what we think is a very gratifying sexual life. I make no bones about the "secret of our success." We have learned to respect and adapt to many aspects of a natural slowing down process and often "help nature along" when necessary. Perhaps some of your readers would like to know more about how aging can sometimes adversely affect the sex act but more often it can enhance it, thus making possible the "best years" of our adult life.

At least, that's the way we see it.

Mr. L.J., Vancouver, British Columbia

Answer

After reading your interesting letter (edited above), I'm convinced that *you* should write this column on sexuality in the elderly, not I!

Here are some physiological facts that you requested, Mr. "J." In males: slower erection time (your experience), diminished seminal fluid, more ejaculation control (Mr. J. has learned to prolong ejaculation even further by mental control), and briefer orgasm. There is quick loss of erection and several hours may elapse before re-erection. Mr. J. doesn't now turn over for a well-earned snooze. No, indeed, this is the time for post-coital pleasuring that can go "on and on," he says, "until pleasant natural sleeps wafts us on to dreamland." (This is perhaps a clue to Mr. J.'s reference to "the best years of our adult life.") Aging affects Mrs. J.'s sexual functioning to a lesser degree. Some elderly women feel no different than in earlier years. Mrs. J. experiences "increased desire" as with many women freed from the fears of pregnancy and a new intimacy with her husband in the "empty nest" with the children out and on their own. There is delayed vaginal lubrication in response to physical and emotional stimulation. The vaginal wall thins out, which can cause painful intercourse if not corrected. (Mrs. J. uses a vaginal lubricating cream.) She hasn't yet had to use estrogen but will if she has to. She is conscious of a "less intense" orgasm, but "it's still pretty good," she observes.

I believe that all elderly couples should be aware of these normal physiological slowdowns so that personal adjustments may be made.

Dear Dr. MacInnis:
After 42 years of happy married life, I find myself impotent. All the desire is there on both sides but there's practically no erection. It is causing unhappiness. She is wonderful about it all. The doctor says it is organic, that is, it's not "in the head" variety.
Mr. E.L., California

Answer

"Lovemaking alternatives" should, of course, be initiated, but I think serious consideration should also be given to using a device like ErecAid.

Dear Dr. MacInnis:
I am a woman 63 years old and in good health. I was never really interested in sex and, now, except for the occasional time,

I am totally uninterested. Is this normal? Is it hard on my husband?

Mrs. T.E., Kingston, Ontario

Answer

If there is little interest in sex early in life it's normal for it to go to pot in later years. Is it hard on the husband? If you're "two birds of a feather" in the sex department, there should be no problem. But if your husband hasn't yet put sex on the back burner, you both have a problem and I would advise you both to see a sex counsellor.

Dear Dr. MacInnis:

I am a healthy male, age 63, who is losing interest in sex. I can take it or leave it. I'm writing because it's causing problems with my wife, who is still quite interested.

Mr. M.R., Ottawa, Ontario

Answer

Apparently no impotence problem here—just loss of libido. He has an "interested" partner, but is she "interesting"? Is he just bored from years of sameness, or is it that his "blah" is of hormonal origin and just might respond to testosterone (sex shot)? Not too likely but it's worth a try. My guess is that it's an "all in the head" variety that will require intensive sex reeducation of both husband and wife for any measure of success.

A Penile Prosthesis

Dear Dr. MacInnis:

A doctor in the outpatient department of a large hospital in this city told me, after hearing my complaint, that I was impotent all right and that he couldn't do much about it, and dismissed me, saying, "And, anyway, what can you expect at your age." I'm a retired teacher, age 73.

Now, I've read all the columns you wrote on sex impotence in the older male and everything else on the subject I could get my hands on, and several things stand out: (1) impotence is very common in the elderly; (2) it's more liable to be caused by physical problems in the elderly than by mental (in your head) reasons; and this being so (3) my kind of impotence just might be treatable with a penile implant.

Here are two opposing views, with the patient often caught in the middle, fearing a marriage breakdown, particularly if his wife is quite a bit younger—as in our case.

I believe, however, since I'm fairly read up on the subject, that the implant route is the way to go. Of the two types available (semi-rigid rod and inflatable penile prothesis), I'm sold on the AMS (American Medical Systems) inflatable type and would like more information on it.

I may be in the "sexual wilderness," but I know I'm not alone.

No Name

Answer

No, you're not alone here, but you most certainly were in that large city hospital outpatient department. It's the worst possible place you could have picked for impotence advice, especially on a busy day!

But still, it may have paid off, for it's what sparked you to read and become knowledgeable. My advice to you now is to write or phone your local medical association for the names of doctors learned in this ever-growing area of medical practice. Only they can determine whether or not you meet the rigid physical and psychological criteria for the procedure.

Up to the mid 70s it was thought that 90 percent of chronic impotence was of the psychological or "in your head" variety. But thanks to a vast advance in diagnostic techniques, we now know that over 80 percent of all cases of chronic impotence are due to physical or "organic" causes.

Such cases include: (1) nerve and blood vessel damage from diabetes; (2) narrowing and hardening of the arteries due to aging (in this case the penile arteries), (3) chronic kidney failure,

(4) chronic alcoholism, (5) side effect of certain drugs (may be just temporary impotence here), (6) nerve damage from pelvic surgery, (7) injury to the spinal cord, pelvis, and genitals.

The common consequence of all these causes is penile nerve damage and/or reduction of blood flow to the penile arteries with resultant loss of erectile power.

Let me briefly describe in a general way the AMS inflatable penile prosthesis that has struck your fancy.

The device consists of three parts connected by tubing: a balloon-shaped reservoir, a pair of cylinders, and a pump with a release valve. The fluid-filled reservoir is placed under the abdominal muscles. The cylinders are inserted in the two chambers of the penis that normally fill with blood during an erection. The pump is placed in the scrotum. It's entirely within the body. The man looks and feels normal.

When the man wants an erection he squeezes the pump several times, thus transferring fluid from the reservoir to the penis cylinders. After intercourse he presses a small release valve on the pump and the fluid returns from the cylinders to the reservoir again. The penis then returns to its normal flaccid state.

For much more detailed information including the cost of various devices, write to American Medical Systems, P.O. Box 9, Minneapolis, Minnesota 55440.

The ErecAid Device for Impotence

I have received so many enquiries regarding the ErecAid system for impotence from male readers (and some females, too) that this column will again deal with it exclusively as it did a year ago. I will give you all the information available from the manufacturer that I have on hand and would beseech both the concerned and the curious *not* to write to me but to direct their questions to the Osbon Medical Systems in the U.S. or to its representatives in Canada whose toll free phone number will be given below.

ErecAid is the *non-surgical* treatment for impotence. It is an easy to use, natural-like method that imitates the natural process of erection more closely than any other technique by providing rigidity through vascular engorgement, resulting in tumescence of the entire penis. Once erection is achieved, engorgement can be maintained by slipping a small rubber ring around the base of the penis.

How it works: A vacuum source attached to a cylindrical chamber fitted airtight over the flaccid penis will cause a rapid influx of arterial blood into the corporal tissues of the penis when adequate negative pressure is utilized. Tumescence (engorgement) and rigidity are created, resulting in an erection maintained by the rubber ring.

Indications for ErecAid: (1) Psychogenic (in the head) impotence; and (2) organic impotence caused by diabetes, radical prostatectomy (often for cancer), spinal cord injury, vascular disease (causing reduced blood supply to penis), and multiple sclerosis. There are other causes for impotence, such as certain high blood pressure drugs and in some cases the etiology (cause) is unknown.

As to its effectiveness, a research study of more than 1,000 users indicates over 90 percent of them are satisfied with the results and would recommend it to others who are impotent.

Many would wonder if it is safe. Osbon states that there have been no reports of debilitating injuries (vascular or urethral damage) by more than 200,000 users of the ErecAid system since it was introduced in 1974.

Contraindications: Patients with bleeding disorders or on anticoagulant therapy (such as warfarin) should use cautiously, first maintaining erection for a short period of time, and then extending use for a longer period. Erection should be limited to no more than thirty minutes.

In a recent issue of the *Canadian Doctor* magazine, there is a report of a study from the Case Western Reserve University School of Medicine, Cleveland, Ohio, where twenty impotent men participated in "external vacuum therapy" trial where there was an overall effectiveness rate of 89 percent "in achieving erections of sufficient quality for intercourse." Their conclusion: External vacuum devices are "the least invasive, least expensive and safest of the current medical treatments for erectile dysfunction."

It is interesting that both the Osbon (ErecAid) company and the Western Reserve study report improvement in attaining *spontaneous* erections after using the vacuum for a period of time.

(In personal correspondence I was informed that the ErecAid system costs Can. $495, and that a doctor's prescription is required before they can send the device to a customer. This requirement applies as well to U.S. patients.)

I would strongly advise that you discuss this system with your doctor after you receive the information from Osbon Medical Systems.

Erection Failure

Dear Dr. MacInnis:

I am one of the many readers of your column and am writing for some advice on impotence.

Could you tell me if there's any treatment or medication for this condition? Are the symptoms permanent? I am in my early 60s and had a prostate operation in 1992.

Mr. E.L., Alberta

Answer

Impotence is by far the commonest complaint I receive from older men. Before answering your question I would like to comment on the term "impotence."

While everyone knows that it means the inability to perform sexually, it unfortunately carries the implication of general inadequacy to meet other challenges of life and is often devastating to a man's ego.

A better term and one that's catching on is "erection failure." This immediately localizes the problem anatomically, attributes it to a physical cause which it almost always is, and implies that there's a remedy, which is nearly always true.

Two decades ago, erection failure was considered to be 80 to 90 percent psychological or "all in your head"—difficult or impossible to treat, and when it was believed treatable, it often entailed time-consuming therapy from sexual counsellors (with a few acting the role of surrogates). Now experts believe that about 85 percent of impotence is organic and about 15 percent, psychological—a complete turnaround!

And times, too, have changed! Those of you who have followed my columns over the years have read about testosterone shots, "sex pills" like yohimbine, penile injections, "state of the art" implants (some requiring a journeyman's certificate to operate), and, more recently, simple, inexpensive, noninvasive vacuum devices that are rapidly gaining popularity in men of all ages.

Before commenting on these treatment options, a word on the often asked question, "What causes an erection?" and the more practical question, "What spoils it?" You may be sexually titillated "from here to eternity," but if you have little or no testosterone to kick in and direct the brain to engorge the penis, nothing happens. If your supply of testosterone is okay, full penile tumescence (engorgement) occurs and you're in business.

And what spoils it? Anything that interferes with testosterone production (e.g., removal of the testes for prostate cancer), anything that may injure the area nerves such as a prostate operation; or anything that reduces or prevents penile engorgement, such a artery disease from advanced diabetes or aging itself. And don't forget that certain medications you're on, like a high blood pressure drug or a tranquilizer, may be the culprit (as long as you're on them), and long-standing alcoholism may cause a permanent erection problem. Finally, there are "psychological" causes like fear of failure (as after a heart attack), waning interest in partner, overwork, and depression.

If examination reveals your testosterone level is truly low and you're otherwise physically fit with no sexual hang-ups, testosterone "shots" might be worth a trial, but don't count on it, for they don't always work. And there are drugs like papaverine (brand name Pavabid) and prostaglandin E1, when injected into the penis cause engorgement and rigidity. Although frequently successful, they are, in my opinion, somewhat masochistic and antierotic and only for the sexually intrepid. The yohimbine pills, from the bark of the South American yohimb tree and a well-known aphrodisiac, increases the blood supply to the penis and blocks its return. It is currently popular and often successful. But see a urologist to make sure you're a suitable candidate. My former enthusiasm for surgical implants has somewhat abated in favor of the ErecAid vacuum device that I have written about in detail on many occasions. I recommend the ErecAid device to you, Mr. L., and suggest that you contact the company for further information. The cost ranges from $400–450 (U.S.), and a doctor's prescription is required. Write to Osbon Medical Systems, P.O. Box 1478, Augusta, Georgia 30903 or phone toll free 1-800-438-8592. Canadians phone toll free 1-800-356-4676. Ask them about their two excellent booklets: (1) *Impotence: A Treatment Guide,* and (2) *Impotence: A Woman's Perspective.* Both are available for a minimal charge of $2 each for postage and handling.

More External Vacuum Devices for Impotence

Dear Dr. MacInnis:

Re your column on impotence and the ErecAid vacuum device. I was wondering if this remedy that you say costs around U.S. $500 could be purchased through the Manitoba Health plan. I am 64 years old and have "organic impotence" as the doctor puts it, and I have mislaid the Canadian toll-free number you gave. Thank you.

Mr. H.K., Winnipeg

Answer

The ErecAid vacuum device is made by Osbon Medical Systems of Augusta, Georgia, whose Canadian toll-free number is 1-800-356-4678.

Since writing that column, I have been advised of another similar vacuum device on the market. This is the Mentor Vacuum Constriction System (made in Santa Barbara, California), which can be purchased through its Canadian distributor, Canada Care Medical, Inc., One Raymond Street, Ottawa, Ontario K1R 1A2., telephone (613) 234-1222, FAX (613) 234-7806. The Mentor system requires your doctor's prescription.

I cannot tell you under what circumstances your provincial medical plan could assist, if at all. (In the States some private insurance and Medicare carriers may reimburse patients when the doctor's prescription points to impotence of an organic cause like yours.) I would suggest that you contact Canada Care Medical for further information.

The Mentor vacuum device sells for Canadian $535 (for the hand-operated version) and Canadian $625 (for the automatic type) with no GST or provincial tax. It is distributed at "no charge delivery" throughout Canada and offers a toll-free number service. They also provide video information and literature to both patients and doctors for use before the Mentor device is activated.

Dear Dr. MacInnis:
Re your column on "erection failure." If, as you say, only 15 percent is of the "all in your head" variety, what are the "not in your head" causes of impotence?

Mr. K.M., Avon, New York

Answer

A good stiff erection depends on a delicate balance between good blood supply to the penis and the ability for it to hold on to this blood for its adequate engorgement, intact nerve pathways to the blood vessels (of the penis), the right amount of male hormone (testosterone) secreted, and, of course, good motivation. Anything (or combination of things) that upsets, this balance may cause "erection failure" or impotence.

Here is a list of "NOT in your head" causes—better known as "organic" or "physical." Diabetes: Sixty percent of diabetic males may eventually become impotent. Disease of blood vessels nourishing the penis, pelvic surgery, or trauma (injury) to pelvic organs (prostate, bladder, and rectum); side effects of various medications (there are over two hundred drugs known to cause erection problems), e.g., high blood pressure and other heart drugs, major/minor tranquilizers and antidepressants; degenerative brain diseases such as Alzheimer's and Parkinson's; and chronic cerebrospinal disorders like multiple sclerosis that interrupt nerve pathways to the penis, may cause impotence. And subtance abuse is well up on the list. This would include excessive use of alcohol and tobacco (heavy cigarette smoking constricts blood vessels, and this includes the blood supply to the penis).

A Refrigerated Jock Strap

Dear Dr. MacInnis:
Did I hear the radio right about a new kind of jockstrap to increase male fertility? I'm a married man, age 45, but time is running out for both of us. . . .
Mr. H.J., California

Answer

Have you both been fully investigated at a reputable fertility clinic? If not, then please ask your doctor for a referral.

If your sperm on examination (microscopic) appears tired, weak, or both, then maybe you have overheated testicles. So say researchers at the New York University School of Medicine. They've come up with a testicular pouch filled with cold water and worn like a jock strap. It invigorates languid sperm, they tell us and to prove it, twenty-four out of sixty-eight infertile men were proud fathers within fourteen months.

Okay, but there's that immutable law of physics—that water eventually attains its surrounding temperature.

Unless, of course, this ingenious device boasts a hi-tech micro-cooling system.

The Long, Long Wait for Service

Dear Dr. MacInnis:

Your article on impotency was of considerable interest.

I recently went for an annual examination and complained of non-erection to my general practitioner. He referred me to a specialist, but I was rather taken aback when told there was no open date for six months. Have you any comments on this?

Incidentally, if the ErecAid system was prescribed, could I put the cost on my senior's prescription card?

My apologies for not signing this letter, but I don't want my name publicized.

(Letter dated May 14, 1990, with no address except "Ontario.")

Answer

You do not state what type of specialist you were referred to—a urologist, internist, or a physician specializing in sexual dysfunction. Regardless, my comment would be, "He/she is a very busy specialist and by the time you were seen, your impotence might very well have been past the point of no return." I feel that general practitioners who are unable to investigate impotence problems themselves should try to refer their patients to consultants with shorter waiting lists, no more than a couple of months at most.

In respect to the ErecAid system, I doubt that your Ontario Health Plan would pay for this (about $500). However, to be sure, you should check anyway.

Impotence: Is It My Age or the Water Pill?

Dear Dr. MacInnis:

I am a male, 78 years old, and have been taking a water pill called hydrochlorthiazide, 50 milligrams, every morning for several years because of high blood pressure. It has kept my blood pressure in check over the years and I am quite satisfied with that part of it. My problem is that over the past six months I believe I am slowly becoming impotent. I say this because I'm experiencing difficulty achieving an erection. I have spoken to my doctor about it and he suggested halving the dose. After one month I have noticed no difference. Do you think it is due to my age? I have received periodic medical checks over the years and my doctor tells me I am in good physical condition.

Mr. J.Y., Toronto, Ontario

Answer

It is a well-known fact that thiazide water pills can cause problems like yours in susceptible people. Several recent studies on water pills as a cause of sexual dysfunction have factored out age, diabetes, coronary heart disease, congestive heart failure, and kidney disease and concluded that the diuretic per se was several times more likely to produce impotence than a placebo (inert dummy pill).

The only information you provide is your age (78). This I believe may be an important, if not the principal, cause of your waning sexual dysfunction and not the water pill.

What about Yohimbine?

Dear Dr. MacInnis:

I am a 70-year-old male and beginning to experience what I think are the first signs of impotence. I guess I don't have to say much more; you know what I mean. I saw something in the paper about a drug called yohimbine. Do you know anything about it? I'm a bit reluctant to discuss this with my family doctor as he is my neighbor and friend. I would be pleased to hear from you.

Mr. J.L., Kelowna, British Columbia

Answer

Yohimbine is basically a heart drug made from the bark of an African tree. It has properties similar to rauwolfia, a high blood pressure drug. Yohimbine, probably because of its ability to dilate blood vessels, has been gaining popularity of late in treating some types of erectile problems leading to impotency. According to its distributor, Kramer Laboratories, Inc., of Miami, Florida, "it provides an extremely low cost, low risk therapy that will do the job for about one-third of men who see a specialist (urologist) for erection problems" (from an article in *Men's Confidential Newsletter,* September 1990).

Since it is available only by prescription, you will have to break the ice first of all by arranging, through your doctor friend, a consultation with a urologist.

Yohimbine is not recommended either as a heart drug or for impotence in elderly patients, (65 plus).

Note: Several months ago I recommended to a reader a book called *Impotence Options* "that has everything you need to know when things go bad down below." It is compiled by the editors of *Men's Confidential Newsletter* with up-to-date information on: Sex Counselling, Yohimbine, Vacuum Devices, Penile Injections, Implants, etc., etc. Price $9.95 plus $1.00 shipping and handling (in U.S. funds). Write to *Men's Confidential Newsletter,* 33 East Minor Street, Emmaus, Pennsylvania 18098 (4 to 6 weeks delivery).

Peyronie's Disease*

Dear Dr. MacInnis:

I am 60 years old and have Peyronie's disease. You will be surprised to know that despite my handicap I have fathered four children—all now grown up. I was always told by doctors that surgical treatment would probably make me impotent, and I didn't want that!

My question: Is there anything new for treating Peyronie's disease?

Mr. Y.F., Upstate New York

---

*Named after the French surgeon, Francois Gigot De La Peyronie, who first described the condtion in an article published in 1743 titled, "Some Obstacles Preventing the Normal Ejaculation of Semen."

Answer

You know about Peyronie's disease but a great many don't. It is a chronic disease of unknown origin characterized by a build-up of fibrous tissue in the shaft of the penis causing a curvature of the organ during erection. Some males are born with this curvature (known as Peyronie's curvature). You have the "curvature" and not the much rarer "disease," because with Peyronie's disease, the curvature is so extreme that sexual intercourse is impossible. (It resembles the more familiar affliction of the palms of the hands called Dupuytren's contracture where a build-up of fibrous tissue causes the fingers to permanently contract forming a partly or fully closed fist.)

In many cases (some authorities claim as high as 50 percent) the penile curvature disappears or diminishes to the extent that satisfactory, painless sexual intercourse is achieved.

There are several treatment options for Peyronie's disease. One is the conservative approach. Some urologists specializing in the area advise a course of vitamin E (said to be deficient in Peyronie's) and use this approach for at least a year. Before submitting to any surgical procedure for moderate to severe penile curvature causing erection and/or penetration problems, many patients have opted successfully for either a semi-rigid or inflatable penile prosthesis. This is the commonest and most popular remedy, because it usually achieves the prime objective—satisfactory sexual intercourse.

For cosmetic and reasons sometimes other than sexual, there's a simple and satisfactory surgical operation for moderate curvature (the Nesbitt procedure), and for severe curvature, an operation called "penile plication" has been developed in Germany that is said not to induce erectile failure (K. Erenbach, M.D., in *Journal of Urology*, November 1991).

Day Dreamer

Dear Dr. MacInnis:
I am a bachelor in my early 60s who spends a lot a time daydreaming about sex. Is this normal or should I have got it out of my system years ago? My general health is good.
Mr. L.Y., Toronto, Ontario

Answer

Normal, yet lamentable. The poet put it so well, "The saddest words of tongue or pen are these: 'It might have been.' "

According to psychologist Dr. Joyce Brothers in her book *What Every Woman Should Know about Men,* men under 40 think of sex six times every hour. When you hit the early 60s it's probably only once every hour or so.

I regret to inform you there's no statistics for bachelors, but I have a hunch their preoccupation with sex may exceed our national average.

Negative (Erotic) Ions Supercharge You!

Dear Dr. MacInnis:

I'm a bachelor in my late 50s living here in Ottawa where there are ladies galore. But I'm sorry to say I have had very little luck at the dating game.

This may seem like "last straw grasping," but is there anything to the idea that changes at atmospheric conditions affect a fellow's romantic urges, including the sex drive. I always feel better up in the Laurentian Hills.

Mr. M.A., Ottawa, Ontario

Answer

It's all got to do with ions (electrically charged particles) in the atmosphere, so say researchers on the subject.

When highly concentrated positive ions surround you, it makes you depressed, touchy, mean, and headachy, and your sex drive is well—blah! This can occur in low-lying areas of Ottawa or just before a thunderstorm.

But negative ions. They supercharge! You are romantic and devastatingly sexy.

Powerful concentrations of these erotic negative ions are found in high altitudes and in the vicinity of waterfalls—like Niagara—environmental scientists tell us.

So there just might be something ionic behind that old song about the two honeymooners who journeyed to Niagara and never saw the falls!

At your age (and attitude), Mr. A., Niagara's your final gamble and certainly worth a try.

Dear Dr. MacInnis:

What are pheromones? I hear they drive women positively wild. Where can I get some right away?

Mr. O.A. (80), British Columbia

Answer

This sounds like a rush order where time is of the essence! Pheromones are substances in body sweat that emit a fragrance that is sexually attractive to the smeller. Women seem to be more susceptible to its pungent aroma than men, authorities tell us.

Animal breeders, particularly pig farmers, have known this for years. A pheromone laced product sprayed in the pig pen will induce mating, so they say.

Human pheromones (in a man's after-shave lotion) were once marketed under the manly name of "Andron."

It is reported that a dentist (and Andron user) narrowly escaped assault from the dental chair when his 25-year-old female patient caught a whiff of the erotic scent.

"It was so sensual," she confided, "that I almost attacked him—and would you believe it, he was 71 years old"!

(Dentists, alas, can no longer buy Andron. I understand it's now off the market, presumably being too hot to handle!)

Chapter 12

Urinary Problems in the Elderly: Female Incontinence—Prostate Disorders

Male and female incontinence are exceedingly common problems besetting the elderly and many write in for advice. I have included in this chapter some of their more common complaints and hope that my suggestions will be helpful. I would strongly advise readers who find themselves with similar problems to seek counsel from their doctors.

What will become immediately apparent to the reader of this chapter is the abundance of repetitive subject matter. For this I make no apology, for two reasons. First, please remember that this chapter, and indeed this book, is an edited compilation of newspaper columns written over a period of twelve years. If you followed my columns over time, you would probably not notice the similarity of questions and answers, but compress them into the much smaller confines of a chapter and the repetition will become quite obvious—examples being my many references to the vagaries of incontinence, innovative versions of Kegel exercises, and various renditions of the enlarged prostate syndrome. My second reason for repetition is that it's good for memory. I am certain that after reading this chapter you will be well versed in what ails you in the urinary area or what might ail you in the future and in the various options for dealing with them.

There have been notable advances in several areas of urology that are noted here, again repetitiously! I am referring to the collagen injection treatment in selected cases of stress incontinence in women and post-operative prostatectomy incontinence in men. And heed well my reports on non-operative "prostate shrinkers," present and future. If my newspaper readers with prostate incontinence were polled today they most certainly would all opt for the non-surgical treatment, and who would blame them? I believe the time is not far off when they'll have the opportunity to choose from a wide variety of non-surgical options for benign prostate hypertrophy (BPH).

Meanwhile, the time honored TURP (transurethral resection of the prostate) continues to serve annually 40,000 Canadians and over 400,000 Americans with benign prostatic hypertrophy. But as I write this, news is out in the medical press that laser energy under the visual guidance of ultrasound is being used successfully through an ordinary cystoscope to not only destroy prostate tissue through coagulation but to cause, as well, a significant reduction in post-operative morbidity, e.g., from bleeding, electrolyte imbalance, and a hospitalization of one and a half days *versus* a two- to three-day hospital stay for the present TURP procedure. The laser technique, still undergoing Federal Drug Administration (FDA) evaluation, is not expected to completely supplant TURP (considered better in bladder neck hypertrophy) but will certainly, in time, whittle a huge dent in what has been for many years one of urology's most venerable institutions.

Recurrent Cystitis—The Female Scourge!

Dear Dr. MacInnis:

I have what my doctor calls "recurrent cystitis," which means that I get a troublesome bladder infection periodically that always clears up after sulfa treatment, stays OK for a while—several weeks to several months—and then flares up again when I get painful urination and frequency. On several occasions the infection went through to my kidneys, causing chills and fever until I got treated, this time with amoxycillin that seemed better than

*the sulfa, since the infection cleared up in a couple of days. But
again it came back—I mean the cystitis.*

*Why do I get it again and again? I usually take the medicine
for two to three weeks. Do you think this is long enough? I am a
married woman, 52, and feel well otherwise except for some hot
flushes that don't bother much.*

Mrs. M.H., Downsview, Ontario

Answer

I need not enumerate the symptoms of a recurrent urinary
tract infection, for you have done it for me, and masterfully at
that!

Many afflicted patients (mainly women) ask me, "What
causes it?" The culprit is nearly always a bacterium (germ)
called *Escherichia coli* (*E. coli*), a *normal* inhabitant of the colon
that when introduced into the urinary tract can cause an infection either in the urethra (rare), the bladder (common) or the
kidneys (not so common). And why does it infect women more
often than men? It's a question of anatomy. In the female there's
that close proximity between the anus and vagina and the much
shorter urethra compared to a man's (one inch to a man's four),
making it easier to introduce fecal matter into the urethra during defecation and particuarly so if tissue wiping is often or even
occasionally done from back to front. With those strikes against
her, plus the fact that women can't always void completely, her
bladder can become a stagnant cesspool of infection. And it
doesn't always stop there but can ascend right up the ureters
(urine tubes) to the kidneys, causing a pyelitis and occasionally
a system infection with chills, fever and vomiting. You know
what I mean; you had them both.

Other singularly female frailities rendering cystitis more
likely include a falling of the womb or bladder or both from
multiple birthing and the loss of estrogen hormone at menopause that makes the uretha less resistant to infection and the
vagina dry, sensitive and sore.

Lest my male readers feel they're being neglected, a common cause of bladder infection and shared by both sexes is the

indwelling catheter—almost routine after abdominal and pelvic surgery. And men, if or when your enlarged prostate gland encroaches on your urethra and prevents your bladder from emptying completely, your residual, stagnant urine becomes a powerful liquid compost for growing bacteria.

A urinary tract infection is diagnosed by demonstrating the bacteria in the urine under a microscope. Although not always done, a culture of the urine should be a part of the a regular urinalysis. This is particularly necessary in recurrent infection where it's important to determine what specific drug is the best for the infection. Remember, you should not "push fluids" before urinalysis, because it dilutes the urine, hindering diagnosis.

In office practice, we find that over 80 percent of urinary tract infections are caused by *E. coli* that is sensitive to practically all antibiotics as well as the sulfa drug you have been using. In the aged patient there's often a relative preponderance of resistant strains of other organisms, and here culture and sensitivity tests are a "must" to achieve any measure of success. In the case of a full-blown kidney infection that becomes generalized with fever, chills and vomiting, vigorous treatment in hospital may be necessary,

In your case, Mrs. H, it's quite possible that your treatment period may not have been long enough. Often six weeks or more are necessary. It's also possible that you are getting a *new* infection each time, and here is where low-dosage prophylactic (preventive) antibiotic treatment should be considered to prevent recurrences. Other preventive measures include proper toilet hygiene, pushing fluids, and always voiding after intercourse.

Stress Incontinence: It Happens When I Cough or Sneeze or Laugh

Dear Dr. MacInnis:

I am 58, female, and suffer from "stress incontinence." In plain English, I "leak" urine when I cough, sneeze, or even when I laugh. It's worse when my bladder is full. Physical exertion, such as jumping or lifting, can also cause it. Needless to say, this is a very embarrassing affliction and I have to be constantly on guard. But no matter how careful I am, accidents happen. I always wear a pad, which is helpful but not too reliable.

I am told by doctors that this condition is due to childbirth tears that were not properly managed. They all advise an operation. Is there anything short of an operation that you can suggest? What about physiotherapy and pelvic exercises?

Mrs. M.L.

Answer

Anything short of an operation? Very occasionally, a device called a pessary inserted vaginally will help hold up the sagging rectum and bladder and may reduce *mild* stress incontinence.

Pelvic floor or Kegel (named after the American gynecologist) exercises strengthen the structures supporting the bladder, rectum, uterus and vagina, which in turn may reduce or, in some cases, eliminate stress incontinence all together.

Here's how you get started: Sit on the toilet and begin to urinate. Then stop the flow and immediately restart. Do this as many times as you can so you can learn how to contract your pelvic floor muscles which is the whole point of the exercise. Then you can contract as often as you like where you like. Remember, you don't have to be voiding to perform the exercise.

You should set up a structured exercise program to ensure regularity, for that is the key to success. For example, before arising in the morning, contract a dozen times. Then every two hours during your working day do a dozen contractions, and get into the habit of always doing it when voiding. In fact, do it as often as you please—the more often, the better.

If you perform the exercise faithfully, regularly, and properly over a period of, say, five months, you should notice greatly improved pelvic muscle tone and, most likely, diminished stress incontinence. Once you have reached your peak of muscle tone, keep in shape by regular exercises—the Kegel kind, that is.

Another form of medical treatment that sometimes is helpful is vaginal female hormone cream or suppositories that serve to "normalize" the vaginal mucous membrane and strengthen the adjacent pelvic tissues.

Any one or combination of the abovementioned non-surgical measures is available to you from your doctor, along with clearing up of any urine infection that may be present. This may be all you need for reasonable control of your problem.

Even though you are reluctant to submit to surgery, I should, for the sake of completeness, advise readers that in the event non-surgical measures fail after a fair trial, there are a variety of excellent surgical procedures available to correct this distressing condition.

The Leaky Lady Syndrome

Dear Dr. MacInnis:

Your recent column on stress incontinence finally prompted me to write about a remedy my gynecologist has found for what some of us call the "leaky lady syndrome." It's a drug called Ditropan. The drug also helps to control the "undependable bowel syndrome" that seems to follow the "leaky lady" on occasion.

And sometimes during my ten years as a senior citizen I found that when I'm awakened morning after morning by leg cramps, an iron pill (one a day) for a few days stops the problem.

You probably know of all these remedies and more for the many ills of our creaking years, but I haven't seen any of them in your geriatric health column we all read.

Now if you could just come up with a remedy or a replacement for my "head stuffing" that's wearing out, I'd be eternally grateful.

This letter doesn't need an answer, thank you; just pass it on and check out my observations, and keep up your column we all find so useful.

Mrs. A.W.

Answer

Thank you, Mrs. W., for passing on to readers your new-found remedy for "stress" incontinence. I should point out, however, that oxybutynin chloride (brand name Ditropan) benefits mostly a particular type of incontinence, where there's an initial urgent desire to void. The secret of your success is that you may be the owner of the so called uninhibited neurogenic bladder, or something like it. The action of Ditropin is to relax the detrusor muscle that ejects urine from the bladder.

It was your good fortune to have had this special type of incontinence and being prescribed a remedy specific for the problem.

So congratulations to a very lucky leaky lady!

Replacing your head "stuffing"? Not a chance! Your very witty letter (that regrettably, I had to edit down) is clear indication you're still endowed with plenty of the "right stuff." My impression: You're a delight!

******

Still on the subject of female incontinence—there's a new urine collecting device for bedfast incontinent women that keeps the patient dry, thus preventing urine scalding, dermatitis, and often decubitus ulcers. It's analogous to the so-called condom catheter for men (where the urine drains into a collecting bag strapped to the inside of the leg). In women the "condom" part is held in place with adhesive that sticks to the *labia majora,* very much like an ileostomy appliance.

The new device recently described in the *Journal of Urology* was applied sixty-three times to seven bedridden incontinent women and remained in place for forty-eight hours. Result: Only 14 percent of the sixty-three applications had to be prematurely replaced due to "unacceptable urine leakage."

Caregivers at home or in hospital are well aware of infection complications from prolonged catheter drainage and know that absorbent diapering may cause skin breakdown.

The clinical trials on this device tool place at Veteran's Administration Medical Center, 3900 Loch Raven Boulevard, Baltimore, Maryland 21218.

Professional health care workers (doctors, nurses, and long-term care hospital administrators) should write to Dr. David Johnson at the above address.

(I am indebted to Canada's *Medical Post* [October 24, 1989] for its news item on this subject.)

Stress Incontinence: Is There a Remedy Short of Surgery?

Dear Dr. MacInnis:

I am a woman, age 55, who has a problem with what the doctor calls "stress incontinence." Anything that increases pressure in my abdomen, like straining at stool, lifting, coughing, or even hearty laughing will cause me to "leak" urine, sometimes only a few drops, other times a tablespoon or more, it all depends. The doctor has advised an operation to strengthen the muscles holding up the bladder and rectum that he said were stretched and weakened from having four big babies.

My question: Is there anything I can do in the way of exercise to strengthen these weak muscles or anything short of surgery? When I asked the doctor this question he said he didn't think so since my condition was quite advanced. I guess what I'm really asking for is a second opinion.

Mrs. J.C., Calgary, Alberta

Answer

I appreciate your consideration in realizing that I'm at a disadvantage in not knowing how severe was your childbirth damage. So my comments will have to be general and may not necessarily apply to you specifically.

In several previous columns I mentioned Kegel exercises that were devised many years ago by an American gynecologist for people suffering from varying degrees of incontinence and I am now going to purposely repeat myself. The basic reason behind these exercises is to strengthen the pelvic muscles that control the flow of urine. Dr. Kegel would advise you thus: Sit on the toilet and begin to urinate. Then abruptly *stop*. Immediately restart and *stop* again. Remember the *stop* contraction: You will be asked to perform this muscle contraction time after time and to do it in a structured and regular routine. For example, before you get up in the morning contract a dozen or more times. Every chance you get during your working day (say every two hours) do two dozen contractions and finally at night, after going to bed, contract a dozen times. The main things is to do it in a consistent way. If this exercise is practiced faithfully over period of five months or so, you may notice increased pelvic muscle tone and perhaps decreased stress incontinence. It's certainly worth a trial and costs nothing!

If stress incontinence appears after menopause a vaginal female hormone cream, such as Premarin, may be helpful and is something you should ask your doctor about. And while you're at it, ask about a pessary, a device inserted into the vagina to support weakened structures. It may be helpful in some cases. Several readers have asked about the value of collagen injections around the urethra. This is a rather new procedure (1990) for which there are good reports in selected cases of stress incontinence. Your doctor can tell you if it is available in your area.

Collagen Injections for Stress Incontinence

Dear Dr. MacInnis:

I read your column every week and have gained some useful information. Now I seek your help.

A friend and I had surgery for pelvic repair at different hospitals about five years ago. We are in our mid 70s and are experiencing increased problems (incontinence).

I need to get up at the same time every night. If I leave it too long I may not make it to the bathroom, which is next door to my bedroom. I practice the Kegel exercises you suggested. It works only after the overflow has slowed down. I only drink a half cup of tea without milk at supper time and a small cup of milk and crackers before going to bed. I should drink more water as I take bran and wheat germ on my morning cereal for constipation. I found that taking alfalfa tablets helps as well.

Is there anything that can be done to correct this (urinary incontinence)? I am going for a month's vacation next month and would be very grateful if you could get your answer in print as soon as possible.

Thank you.

Mrs. O.W.

Answer

You probably missed reading my column of a few months ago reporting on a new method of treating *selected cases* of stress incontinence. It involved the injection of collagen (one to three treatments) into the tissues lining the urethra and the neck of the bladder.

In that column (written in early 1992) I was unable to inform readers how generally available the procedure was in Canada, but since that time I have learned that it is being done at Sunnybrook Health Science Centre, Toronto; St. Paul's Hospital, Vancouver; and Victoria General, Halifax. (A lady has informed me that her 82-year-old mother recently [late 1992] received the collagen treatment at Sunnybrook Hospital, Toronto, which she reported successful at the time of writing. I would like to thank her for her thoughtful letter.)

It is far too early, I believe, to say that this represents a kind of breakthrough in treatment. At present, it should be considered as an interesting and promising treatment for *selected* types of incontinence.

You should discuss the matter with your family doctor who may be able to refer you to a medical center where the procedure is carried out. By the time this appears in print, other centers may be trying out the procedure. (U.S. readers please consult your urologist.)

In closing, let me quote from my original column on the collagen procedure: "Please remember the all-important qualifier, *selected*. Incontinent patients, young and old, who have accompanying 'falling' of the urethra or bladder will *not* benefit from collagen treatment. . . . It is only when the stress incontinence is due solely to urethral and bladder neck weakness should collagen treatment be considered, and this can only be determined by your urologist."

The U.S. Federal Drug Administration is currently evaluating the collagen procedure. Its Canadian counterpart, the Federal Health Protection Branch, has approved it specifically for female patients with stress incontinence and males with incontinence following a prostate operation.

And again, I urge you, do not make any personal decisions without consulting your physician or urologist.

Bashful Bladder Syndrome

Dear Dr. MacInnis:

I am one of those unfortunate people with the peculiar problem of not being able to urinate in a public washroom if there's someone present. It's not my prostate. It's just that I get embarrassed and tense up. So when I find myself in that predicament I have to wait till everyone leaves and, believe it, this hanging around a washroom can be embarrassing, too!

Is this just nerves? Can anything be done about it?

Mr. D.P., Merchantville, N.J.

Answer

My research on this subject reveals that you suffer from the "bashful bladder syndrome." But take heart. Let me proclaim to all victims the good news.

Psychologists at Georgetown University Medical School, Washington, D.C., have found that reciting your multiplication tables will relax the urine "nerve locks" and release the floodgates.

But a word of caution. I would strongly suggest that you recite quietly to yourself; otherwise your audible incantations might just have the opposite effect on your fellow participants!

Note: The multiplication table routine is only for seniors, now the sole repository of this historical mathematical intelligence. The younger afflicted male can only fiddle with his calculator.

What Is Benign Prostatic Hypertrophy (BPH)?

Dear Dr. MacInnis:

What is a BPH? It must have something to do about my prostate gland because that's what the doctor said after checking it. My symptoms are frequent urination during the day and getting up several times at night to urinate. If you were the doctor in my case, what would you advise? I am in good health otherwise.

Mr. N.M., Toronto, Ontario

Answer

BPH stands for "benign prostate hypertrophy," which means that you have an enlargement of your prostate gland which is benign (not malignant). "Normal" enlargement of the prostate gland usually begins in past midlife and can usually be detected by a simple rectal examination. If enlargement becomes excessive, the overgrown gland (situated at the neck of the bladder and straddling the urine tube) may gradually decrease urine flow, causing difficulty in starting urination, bothersome dribbling, and frequent voiding and getting up at night.

Long-standing BPH can sometimes lead to complete retention of urine. A common scenario is where after a night of beer drinking, a 70-year-old man is brought to the emergency department in severe pain from a distended bladder. As the bladder gradually filled up with urine, more and more pressure was exerted on the enlarged prostate at the bladder neck that eventually "blocked the gate." Here the urine must be drained with a catheter. Another common occurrence is where the already enlarged prostate becomes congested and swollen after prolonged sitting (several hours in a car, for example). Here the patient may be unable to start the urine flow. The usual remedy for this is to assume the upright position and walk around until the prostate congestion lessens to allow the urine to "pass the gate." The lesson to be learned here is that patients with BPH on a car trip should step out at least once an hour.

The advice I would give any patient with obstructive voiding symptoms caused by an enlarged prostate would probably be along this line: If you are unhappy with your complaints, such as frequent getting up at night (some patients don't seem to mind), dribbling, etc., then you should have something done about it. Another thing to remember is that symptoms tend to increase in severity over time.

Although there are advances being made in "shrinking the prostate" with certain drugs, these drugs are still in the experimental stage and although they seem to hold great promise, their use is still some years away. Another group of drugs, of which prazosin is the leader, can sometimes improve the obstructive complaints associated with enlarged prostate. It is sometimes used on poor surgical risks or for those who refuse TURP (transurethral resection of the prostate).

Either of two surgical procedures (prostatectomy) will relieve obstructive voiding from an enlarged prostate. The oldest procedure called "suprapubic prostatectomy," where the prostate gland is totally removed through an incision in the lower abdomen, is now rarely done except for a very enlarged gland. The commonest approach for removing the prostate is the TURP, where a lighted coagulating instrument is passed up the urethra (urine tube) to the bladder neck and bits and pieces of the prostate gland are whittled away to relieve the obstructive symptoms. Bear in mind that the TURP does not totally remove the gland, but enough to do the job, which doesn't usually have to be redone for five years or more.

Readers often ask how long they have to stay in hospital after TURP. The usual hospitalization is two to four days. For the total suprapubic operation the hospital stay is five to seven days.

Prostate Enlargement: The Time-Honored TURP

Dear Dr. MacInnis:

I am a male, 64 years old, and am told that I have enlargement of my prostate gland. The doctor says that my present symp-

toms of frequent urination, getting up at night, and slow stream
will undoubtedly get worse and will require an operation that
reams out the prostate gland, thus clearing the obstruction to
urine flow. To be honest with you I am scared stiff of surgery
and was wondering if there are other ways of lessening prostate
obstruction. I recall one of your columns where you discussed
"shrinking" the prostate with a drug treatment. Is this method
now generally used or it is just in the experimental stage? Any
other alternatives to surgery would be appreciated.

Mr. M.G.

Answer

Answering questions re enlarged prostate is one of my endless preoccupations! And for good reason. In the United States,
where statistics are available, 500,000 men underwent prostatic
surgery in 1989 for symptoms like yours. Nearly all of them had
their prostates reamed out by a procedure called "transurethral
resection of the prostate" or TURP for short. For TURP a lighted
cutting instrument is passed up the urethra (urine tube in the
penis) to the prostate gland where excess tissue is whittled away
to relieve the urine obstruction. The procedure is not minor surgery by any means, requiring either general or a type of spinal
(epidural) anesthesia.

Although TURP is a relatively safe procedure having stood
the test of time, there can at times be complications such as
bleeding from prostate tissue, and occasionally a degree of incontinence. Although postoperative erection failure is unusual,
there is always this possibility, especially if the patient's sexual
prowess was on the wane before the operation. Hospitalization
of four to five days is usually required with several weeks of
convalescence on the average.

The medical " shrinker" you refer to is called Proscar. And
you're right. It is still in the experimental stage and not available to your doctor. The future for Proscar looks bright because

302

it does not induce impotence like some of its predecessors. (See upcoming columns on Proscar.)

One of the latest non-surgical treatments of benign prostatic hypertrophy (BPH), or plain enlarged prostate, involved the insertions of a balloon-tipped catheter up the urethra (urine tube) into the prostate gland. Under fluoroscopic (X-ray) guidance, the balloon is inflated compressing the prostate outwardly towards its capsule and the obstruction is relieved. This procedure is now being tested in various university centers in the United States and Canada to determine how it compares with the venerable TURP operation, and so far reports show promise. Compared to TURP it is a "minor" procedure that can be performed on an outpatient basis requiring only local (topical) anesthesia for the insertion of the catheter into the urethra.

I would stress that transurethral balloon dilation of the prostate (TUDP) is still in its preliminary stage of development, and we will have to await more comparative trials before recommending it or advising the patient to await the outcome. Patient selection would appear to be very important. For instance, dilation of middle prostate enlargement was not nearly so successful as when the enlargement was present in either of the lateral lobes.

Currently, two large clinical trials of TUDP are in progress, one at the Veterans Administration Medical Center, Minneapolis, Minnesota, and the other at London's (England) Hammersmith Hospital. According to medical news reports, both groups are presently encountering conflicting results and only time will resolve the differences.

Prostate Enlargement: What to Watch For

Dear Dr. MacInnis:
My doctor tells me I have "benign prostatic hypertrophy." When I asked him to speak English, he translated it thus: "an enlarged prostate gland that is not cancerous."

At age 66, I have no urinary symptom—as yet. The doctor warned me that at some later date certain symptoms might arise. Could you give me some idea what symptoms in the course of time I could reasonably expect leading to a possible operation?
Thank you.

Mr. A.A., Calgary, Alberta

Answer

Your question is answered in a report of a research project from the University of North Carolina; Merck, Sharp & Dohme Research Labs., West Point, Pennsylvania; and the National Institute of Aging and published in *Prostate* 16 (1990): 25–261 (lead author, H. M. Arrighi, reported in *Year Book of Geriatrics and Gerontology,* 1991).

"Symptom questionnaires and physical examinations were administered to 1,057 men followed for thirty years. . . . The only symptoms that *positively* predicted subsequent prostatectomy for benign prostatic hypertrophy were a change in the size and force of the stream and a sensation of incomplete emptying."

According to this report, among men with these three risk factors—enlarged prostate, slowing of the urinary stream and a sensation of incomplete emptiness—37 percent eventually required operation, compared to only 8 percent in the remaining 945 men.

So you see, only time will determine whether or not you will need an operation and you now know what symptoms to watch for.

What Good Is the Prostate Gland and Where Is It?

Dear Dr. MacInnis:
Could you tell me exactly where the prostate gland is situated and what good does it do apart from enlarging and causing trouble in middle age!

I'm going on 55 and notice that I'm becoming a slow (urine) starter and when I get it going, I'm never quite sure if I'm really finished or not. And my stream that was once my pride and joy (I could overshoot a clothesline) now falls flat on my oxfords!

My doctor sent me to a urologist who recommends a reaming-out job. What are the options to an operation, if any? The specialist said there's now a pill available but I'm too far on for that. What did he mean?

Mr. E.T., New York

Answer

The prostate gland is the size of a large chestnut and weighs less than an ounce. It is situated at the base of the bladder and surrounds the urethra (urine tube) as it emerges from the bladder. Think of it as an undersized crab apple with a reamed out core through which the urethra passes.

Contrary to popular opinion, the prostate gland does serve the very useful function of providing a fluid vehicle for the sperm to travel to the outside during ejaculation. It also provides a nourishing medium for the sperm.

On the downside it has that pernicious tendency to enlarge in early middle age, thus constricting the urethra within the prostate (think of the crab apple core) giving rise to a number of urinary problems, some of which you mention. The culprit causing this hypertrophy (enlargement) is a hormone called di-hydrotestosterone that in most cases gets into high gear in past middle life and continues on to old age.

The operation your urologist recommended is called trans-urethral resection of the prostate (TURP), where a lighted cutting instrument is passed up the urethra, increasing the urine flow. It is still the "gold standard" of treatment and, as the urologist told you, is the most appropriate for your condition that would seem to be rather advanced. The pill that the specialist referred to is most likely a drug called finasteride (brand name Proscar) whose action is to prevent the production of that hormone I previously mentioned (dihydrotestosterone), thus "shrinking" the prostate. It takes about six months to determine its full effect. At present it works in over 30 percent of cases where the enlargement is not causing acute symptoms, as in your condition. When effective in relieving symptoms, it must be taken indefinitely, that is, for the rest of your life. The dose is one tablet (5 milligrams) once daily. There are other options (mainly devices still experimental) that I'll mention in an upcoming column.

Treatment of Benign Prostate Enlargement: Non-Surgical Options

Dear Dr. MacInnis:

I have some questions about the non-surgical treatment on enlargement of the prostate gland. One is Proscar and there may be others I cannot recall. And what about that method of "freezing" the prostate gland to make it shrink? As you may surmise, I'm opposed to surgical treatment.

As I do not have any problems, perhaps I can afford to wait until the surgical treatment of enlarged prostate, transurethral resection of the prostate (TURP), is no longer in fashion.

Am I expecting too much?

Mr. L.G., age 39, Florida

Answer

As I mentioned in a previous column, Proscar caused a shrinkage of the prostate gland by preventing the conversion of testosterone to dihydrotestosterone (the hormone that causes prostate enlargement in middle age and beyond). In contrast to TURP surgery that immediately relieves prostate pressure on the urethra (urine tube), Proscar may take up to six months or more to determine its maximum effectiveness. According to my latest information, Proscar can cause an appropriate mean decrease of 20 percent prostate volume in about 35 percent of patients, with an improvement in total as well as obstructive symptoms. According to the Merck product brochure, "The effects of Proscar are reversible if the treatment is stopped." Conversely, this means that if you find Proscar effective, you must continue the daily one pill (5 mg.) dosage indefinitely, i.e., the rest of your life.

The other drug you refer to is probably Minipress (a heart medication) that does not shrink the gland but is said to act on the urethral sphincter muscle to hold back the passage of urine in mild cases of incontinence.

You mention "freezing" of the prostate. This is medically called cryotherapy and has been much in the news lately. It is still in the experimental stage and I have no firm clinical news on it at present. An interesting device (on the other end of the temperature spectrum) is the Prostraton, a device that has a microwave antenna inside a urethral catheter that actually subjects the enlarged prostate to sufficient heat to cause shrinkage of the gland and alleviation of symptoms. It is quite popular in Holland. (In 1991 I heard from Prof. F. M. J. Debruyne, head of the Department of Urology at University Hospital, Nijmegen, The Netherlands, who reported a successful outcome in over 200 patients in his [Radboud] University Hospital. In June 1993, he reports that "almost 450 patients" have now received successful Prostraton treatment there and adds that "up to 17,000 patients have been treated worldwide".)

Another very interesting option, again undergoing clinical research, is prostatic ballooning, a procedure that dilates the urethra much in the same way as angioplasty opens up a coronary artery. It is often combined with the Prostraton method.

You ask the question whether or not the various non-surgical options—drugs or devices—may ultimately supersede the time-honored TURP (last year performed 5,000 times in my home province of British Columbia) and close to a half-million annually in the United States estimated to soon exceed $5 billion in costs per year and still soaring!

I believe the answer is yes, and a good analogy would be the ancient "ritual tonsillectomy" contrived to utterly devastate our school children's vacation break in the thirties, forties, and fifties. I can vividly recall being part of a nefarious surgical assembly line that wreaked havoc on the throats of innocents until an enlightened antibiotic age brought it to a merciful end!

The venerable TURP is still the "gold standard" of treatment, but I predict that by the turn of the century, non-surgical

307

options will have progressed to the point where surgery for enlarged prostate will go the way of the tonsillectomy and by the year 2010 the prostate resectoscope will be a museum piece just like me.

Zoladex for Prostate Cancer

Dear Dr. MacInnis:
Could you please give some information on Zoladex for the treatment of prostate cancer. My husband, age 76, has just been diagnosed as having this condition, and Zoladex was one of the treatment options offered. Thank you.
Mrs. M.M., Vancouver, British Columbia

Answer

Zoladex is a hormone that when injected under the skin once a month blocks the production of the male sex hormone, testosterone, which contributes to the development and spread of prostate cancer.

For many years, the standard treatment of cancer of the prostate has been surgical castration (removal of the testes). Zoladex has the same effect but without the severe psychological and physical side effects from that traumatic procedure.

Zoladex is contained in a depot about the size of a grain of rice and when injected under the skin, is slowly and constantly dissolved into the system over twenty-eight days. Then the depot injection is repeated indefinitely. It is establishing a good reputation and is probably the treatment of choice.

Update (March 1994): There's a recent report that the LH-RH group of drugs represented by Zoladex, when used continuously over long periods (two or more years), may cause prostate cancer to "adapt" and grow independently of testosterone. University of British Columbia researchers led by Dr. Martin Gleave of the Department of Surgery have begun testing a new intermittent drug schedule in laboratory animals of starting, stopping, then restarting such drugs at eight-month intervals in an attempt to prolong their effect. Dr. Gleave reports that preliminary reports are encouraging. (My thanks to Mark Nichols and *MacLean's Magazine*, March 21, 1994.)

What If the Cancer Spreads?

Dear Dr. MacInnis:

The doctor did a rectal examination and found my prostate gland to have a "hard area." A biopsy revealed cancer of the prostate well contained within the gland. Because of my age (78) the doctor at first decided to just watch it and do regular bone scans and blood tests but later changed his mind and sent me to a urologist, who removed my prostate just to be safe. That was a year ago and everything seems to be under control.

I was wondering what will be the procedure if the cancer should ever start to spread, say, to the bones?

Mr. A.B., Ottawa, Ontario

Answer

Since the spread of prostate cancer is aided and abetted by the male hormone, testosterone (secreted mainly in the testes), castration used to be the routine surgical procedure (along with female hormone injections). Although quite effective, castration is going out of favor because of its psychological implications. However, some urologists still practice the art and in deference to some patients' perceived "loss of manhood," provide them with two cosmetically acceptable plastic balls to fill the empty scrotum. Currently, the most popular male hormone blocker is an anti-testosterone drug called Zoladex contained in a depot the size of a grain of rice and injected under the skin every twenty-eight days and repeated indefinitely. It has recently been authorized for use in Canada and is available on prescription.

Collagen for Male Incontinence

About a month ago in this column I recommended and described a Kegel pelvic muscle exercise routine for incontinent

309

men who have undergone radical surgery for cancer of the prostate. It is reported that about a third of post-prostatectomy incontinence can be controlled by such pelvic exercises. For the remainder, the only hope was the surgical installation of an artificial sphincter in selected cases. That is, up until recently. There's now word out of the University of Arizona Health Sciences Center that urology researchers have come up with the novel approach of injecting Teflon (polytetrafluoroethylene) into the urethral sphincters. Although the immediate results were reported to be favourable, the beneficial effect soon began to wane in the majority of the injected patients. After seventeen months about 35 percent of the research patients reported that they were still better than before the injection procedure.

Readers may recall that I recently reported on the successful use of *contigen* (collagen) injection into the urethral sphincter in selected cases of female stress incontinence. This new approach, applicable to both sexes, may be heralding a sort of "breakthrough" for men who develop incontinence after a prostate cancer operation.

Kegel Exercises for Men

Dear Dr. MacInnis:

I have read where you advise Kegel exercises for women with incontinence. Why can't it apply to incontinent men as well? I have been having moderate incontinence ever since a prostate operation two years ago.

Mr. G.H., New Brunswick

Answer

Incontinent men should try Kegels. Here's the routine: You begin by starting and stopping your urine flow. Do this enough times so you can feel the muscles at work. Then you practice the contraction part alone, relaxing the pelvic muscles between each squeeze. The beauty of this routine is that you can practice without anyone being aware of it. Some urologists recommend twenty squeezes three or four times a day. I believe you should set up your own exercise routine and stick to it. You may notice a change for the better in three to four weeks and optimum urinary control in six weeks if it is going to work for you. Everyone should at least give it a **try**. You may be in that lucky 30 percent where it helps.

"Three-Dimensional Image" of Prostate

Dear Dr. MacInnis:

I know you write a lot about the prostate gland, and here's another question for you. I caught something on the radio news about a new method of viewing the prostate gland in three dimensions. Have you any information on this? I understand it will portray a much better view of the gland allowing doctors to detect cancer earlier than by present methods. Did I get this right?

Mr. M.N., Ontario

Answer

Yes indeed, the news is quite exciting and even more so to you, for it comes from your own home province!

Researchers from the John P. Robarts Institute in London, Ontario, have just recently announced their development of a new imaging system that will so vastly improve their ability to detect early prostate cancer that it could be 100 percent curable, they say.

Briefly stated, a series of computers are interfaced to an ultrasound system with special software. The resulting image of the prostate is three dimensional and can be "sliced" and viewed through any angle, much like a pathologist would examine slices of the actual prostate gland for cancer.

Early detection of prostate cancer before it breaks through the capsule and spreads to adjacent glands, bones, and other organs is particularly important in the "relatively young" man (fifty to seventy years) where surgery, radiation, or a combination of both modalities can virtually effect a complete cure. Up to now, our acumen for detecting early prostate cancer, while improved with the advent of the prostate specific antigen (PSA) blood test, still has its diagnostic limitations. This makes three-dimensional imaging a welcome addition to our armamentarium for treating prostate cancer when it's curable, i.e., *early*.

It is estimated that the early and accurate detection of potentially fatal prostate cancer could save the lives of 30,000 men annually in the United States and a proportionate number in Canada. (Three-dimensional imaging should be commercially available in 2–3 years.)

So What's Wrong with a Rectal?

Dear Dr. MacInnis:
What is wrong with the time-honored rectal examination to discover prostate cancer? I've been advised to have an ultrasound test by a doctor who says it is much better than the old fashioned finger test. And so is his fee—about $300 for the ultrasound versus $25 for the rectal (U.S. funds).

Mr. K.J., New York

Answer

There's nothing wrong with it. It's still the traditional diagnostic procedure for detecting abnormalities of the prostate gland, the most commom being enlargement (common past middle life and sometimes causing urine stoppage) and cancer, where the gland may not be enlarged but feels hard to the examining finger.

Proponents of ultrasound contend that it's far more sensitive and precise in detecting the early small cancerous nodule than is the examining finger. And early detection, they argue, means early treatment *before* the cancer spreads to the bones, where the outlook is poor indeed.

The urologists (urinary tract specialists), long the jealous wardens of the prostate, fiercely resent intrusion of radiologists on their sacred turf. They counterclaim that ultrasound, too, is

312

imprecise with its "blind spots" and "false positives." Even so, there are reports of some urologists beginning to use ultrasound on "suspicious" prostate glands.

What is needed here is a wise mediator with a license to marry the technical expertise of the radiologists with the treatment skill of the urologists. And all *three* would benefit—the urologist, radiologist, and, don't forget, the *patient!*

The Prostate Specific Antigen (PSA) Test

Dear Dr. MacInnis:

The PSA (prostate specific antigen) test measures the amount of antigen added to a blood sample to negate (I take it) certain antibodies present in prostate gland tissue. But what does this measure indicate? Is it a measure of susceptibility to prostate cancer or, if not, what does the test determine?

Is it possible that taking the drug Proscar might influence the level of the PSA test?

Mr. G.M., Ottawa, Ontario

Answer

The PSA test is not truly "prostate cancer specific" in the same way that, say, a positive pregnancy test is almost 100 percent correct. The PSA test merely assesses the risk of prostate cancer.

The PSA test can sometimes be positive when it shouldn't be—the so-called false positive—from simple enlargement of the prostate gland or from chronic prostatitis (infection). And yes, a prostate "shrinking" drug like Proscar is said to reduce the PSA level from the 4 nanograms per liter to sometimes as low as 2 per liter, which may lead in the future to "new normals" for patients taking prostate-shrinking medications.

Despite its limitations, the PSA test is the best we've got and should always be used as a screening agent. For instance, the PSA is better for detecting small cancers than the rectal examination, and these are the cancers that can be caught in the early state (while within the capsule) and cured by surgery or radiation, which can be lifesaving. This is particularly relevant in the relatively "young" patient of 50 to 60 years, where the malignancy may be more virulent than in advanced age.

Does this mean that the time-honored rectal exam is "over the hill"? By no means. The PSA test combined with a digital rectal examination (DRE) significantly increases the odds for detecting prostate cancer, keeping in mind their limitations. (Prostate ultrasound examination is fast becoming a very important diagnostic tool as well.)

Chapter 13
The Aging Senses: Disorders of Sight and Hearing in the Elderly

As we grow older we become more and more aware that our sharpness of vision is not what it used to be. Myopia or short-sightedness usually begins well before middle age when we notice we need longer arms to read the paper and as 60 hits, even our once perfect lens correction is getting a bit hazy reminding us that cataract time may be close at hand. These changes are normal visual events and are solely due to the gradual, insidious but always relentless aging of the eye, which prompted an authority to say that from the then available evidence of his time, if our lives could be extended to 130 years everyone would be blind!

Hearing impairment is said to be the second most common medical problem besetting the aged, being only exceeded by arthritis. This hearing loss associated with aging is called presbycusis. Several large studies have shown that this type of hearing loss can be detected in most people over 40 where it usually affects the higher frequencies. Like myopia, presbycusis creeps up on you, and a long time, even years, may elapse before you are convinced you're hard of hearing, often long after everyone else you know is sure of it.

Most readers write in about these common problems and in most cases they can be successfully treated with hearing aids that are becoming more and more miniaturized as well as more efficient. And the once formidable removal of "ripened" cataracts followed by the long convalescence and the fitting with "Coca-Cola bottle bottom" lenses have mercifully gone the way of the dodo, giving rise to the lens implant, a mere office procedure. No doubt about it, this is the golden decade of cataract surgery and the elderly are its prime candidates and fortunate beneficiaries.

Since the commonest things in life happen the commonest, the above-noted disorders are mainly featured. However, the two leading causes of blindness—glaucoma (past midlife) and macular degeneration (in the elderly)—are not forsaken nor is a column on low-vision services.

The chapter concludes with an in-depth study of the elderly driver, which I hope will postpone for a good time that unwelcome day when we all must "hang up the keys."

******

Macular Degeneration

Dear Dr. MacInnis:

What is "macular degeneration" and how does it affect sight? My husband, age 81, has had deteriorating vision for the past five years and gets little or no help from prescription glasses. The doctor says there's very little in the way of help. Any suggestions?

Mrs. T.H., Ottawa, Ontario

Answer

To answer your question, first a little eye anatomy. The macula is a small area located in the central part of the retina (behind the eye) that is necessary for the perception of clear central vision. By "clear central vision" I mean the ability to see objects straight ahead in fine crisp detail.

Macular degeneration is usually caused by a thinning or breakdown of the macula. The patient notices that straight ahead vision is becoming hazy and blurred when reading the words on a page. In addition, straight lines appear crooked or distorted. Side or peripheral vision is not affected.

Macular degeneration is the second leading case of blindness and occurs mainly in patients 65 and older. In many cases self-diagnosis is possible because the patient notices loss of central vision.

Some forms of macular degeneration can be helped by laser coagulation of bleeding retinal blood vessels. Where this therapy is unsuccessful, patients may derive useful vision from low-vision aids (hand magnifiers and special telescopic glasses etc.)

Low-Vision Services Offered

The following letter from the Canadian National Institute for the Blind (CNIB) refers to the availability of low-vision services offered by them for Ottawa and District.

Dear Dr. MacInnis:

I read your article on low vision for the elderly with great interest.

I have been working in the field of low vision for approximately six years and it has become apparent to me that the elderly experiencing vision loss need to have the necessary information and visual aids to continue living as independently as they wish.

I would like to inform you of all low-vision services available in Ottawa and valley towns.

The Ottawa General Hospital Eye Institute offers a low-vision clinic twice a month and referral is made through the patient's ophthalmologist. Visual aids are loaned through the CNIB and patients needing rehabilitation are referred to us. The CNIB (Ottawa office) provides low-vision clinics daily by appointment. We also offer a similar clinic in Cornwall twice a month and an optometrist adds his expertise to the multi-disciplinary team. At Pembroke, the CNIB is running one clinic a month out of a local ophthalmologist's office and all the usual services are available.

Individuals or family members wishing to obtain a list of low-vision services in Ottawa or the province of Ontario may contact Sandra Coady, RN, BA; CNIB, 320 McLeod St., Ottawa, Ontario, K2P 1A3. Phone: (613) 563-4021

Sandra Cady, R.N., B.A.

(Low-vision patients in other parts of Canada should contact the CNIB in their own province for information on their services provided.)

What is low vision? Here is the definition of low vision taken from the former Vision Canada Centre's booklet titled Focus on Sight Enhancement.

Question: What exactly is meant by the term "low vision"?

Answer: The low vision Association of Ontario describes persons with low vision as "all people *with* some vision where impairment of either central or peripheral vision seriously limits what they are able to do and where vision is not correctable with normal prescription lenses." In fact, "persons with visual abilities," says the booklet, "ranging from 30 percent to as low as 1 percent can be aided."

Free Radicals and Cataract Formation

We hear a lot nowadays about the role of "free radicals" in the causation of cancer, cardiovascular disorders, cataract formation, and a host of other chronic debilitating diseases and even aging itself.

Considered a rather wild and fanciful theory only a decade ago, the "free radical" hypothesis has finally come of age. This was the conclusion of an international conference on "antioxidant vitamins and beta-carotene in disease prevention" held in London, England (October 2 to 4, 1989). It was attended by six hundred delegates and scientists from around the world.

What are free radicals? They are atoms, ions, or molecules which contain one or more unpaired electrons. They are generally highly reactive and can become less reactive by taking an electron from or to another molecule. By electron transfers like these, free radicals create other free radicals, thus initiating chain reactions that can attack body tissues, damaging and eventually destroying them.

The body is continually generating billions of free radicals as a by-product of normal oxidation processes aided and abetted by environmental pollution from gamma radiation, cigarette smoke, and smog—to name a few. Free radical damage is so all pervading, scientists tell us, that it doesn't stop at the cell membrane but burrows into its nucleus, perhaps altering the genetic code and initiating predisposition to cancer and other chronic debilitating diseases.

How can we protect ourselves from the ravages of free radicals? Nature comes to the rescue by providing us with protective measures in the form of certain enzymes and especially the so-called antioxidant vitamins E and C and beta-carotene (the precursor of vitamin A).

At the International Antioxidant Conference, speaker after speaker from many parts of the world presented scientific papers suggesting that vitamins E, C, and beta-carotene may protect against heart disease, reduce the incidence of some cancers, and may help prevent the formation of cataracts.

I would like to briefly report on three scientific papers presented at this conference on the effect of antioxidants on the prevention of cataracts, said to occur in the U.S and Canada at the rate of half a million new cases a year in those past middle age.

Paper No. 1: Professor Paul Jacques and team at the Human Nutrition Research Centre on aging at Tufts University (Boston) presented evidence that cataracts are caused by the "oxidation of lens protein" (by free radicals) and that this oxidative process may be inhibited by the antioxidant vitamins E, C, and beta-carotene. Low levels of these vitamins in the blood "increase the risk for cataracts," Dr. Jacques said.

Paper No. 2: Prof. Shambhu Varma of the University of Maryland (College Park) observed that "a correlation exists between the incidence of cataracts in humans and exposure to sunlight. . . . Cataracts also develop in experimental animals and humans exposed to excessive oxygen concentration." He added that "high oxygen concentration enhances free radical production." Professor Varma believes that vitamin C as an antioxidant provides protection against cataract formation.

Paper No. 3: Dr James M. Robertson and colleagues from the University of Western Ontario (London) addressed the question of: "Cataract Prevention, Is there a Role for Vitamin Supplements?" Professor Robertson compared the self-reported consumption of supplementary vitamins over a five-year period with that of 175 cataract-free subjects. The study suggested that the cataract-free group consumed "significantly more vitamins C and E than the group with cataracts." His conclusion: "Increased vitamin use is associated with an apparent reduction in cataract risk of 50 to 70 percent."

Vitamins C, E and Beta-Carotene for Cataracts

Dear Dr. MacInnis:

Some time ago you wrote a column on the benefit of taking a combination of vitamin C, vitamin E, and beta-carotene to prevent cataracts. Could you give me some information on what vitamins C and E do? Does the combination with beta-carotene really prevent cataracts?

Mrs. E.J., Syracuse, New York

Answer

Your question was partly answered in the previous column.

What does each vitamin do? Let's start with vitamin C: briefly, vitamin C (ascorbic acid) has been found to increase resistance to infection and environmental pollutants. Its reported beneficial action against the common cold is hotly disputed by scientists with the "jury still out" on the matter. But even its most rabid opponents concede that vitamin C may help by drying up nasal secretions (due to its antihistamine effect).

Reports of its benefit in "preventing" cancer have been scientifically refuted. Despite this, there are always sporadic news flashes on its merit in this field. Just recently a report in the *Scottish Medical Journal* stated that low vitamin C levels found in elderly patients may be associated with *high* levels of LDL (Low Density Lipoprotein), the "bad" kind.

But its role as an antioxidant is what interests scientists working on cataract formation, and previously reported in these columns. It is postulated that free radicals cause deterioration and death of body organs (including lens damage and opacity) that in some way can be delayed or partly prevented by the use of antioxidants.

The above are some of the newer concepts attributed to vitamin C usage. But the only condition that we know for certain is due to low levels or absence of vitamin C in the human body is scurvy.

Vitamin E made the medical and lay news many years ago when the Shute brothers (both physicians) proclaimed to a sceptical world that vitamin E in the form of alpha-tocopherol could help prevent heart disease and other vascular disorders.

Although many doctors in my generation openly pooh-poohed the idea, it was well known that more than a few of them were "closet converts" who faithfully self-prescribed vitamin E "just in case"! But time, I believe, has vindicated the Drs. Shute, and Vitamin E is here to stay in its generally accepted role as an antioxidant or free radical fighter.

Beta-carotene (a precursor of vitamin A) is found in many yellow fruits and vegetables. It again has been credited as a cancer prevention by virtue of its antioxidant property. But it is in the field of cataract study that it is best known as a possible inhibitor of lens deterioration with formation of cataracts.

In my previous column on free radicals causing cataract formation, I cited the work of Prof. James Robertson and colleagues at the University of Western Ontario in London. His findings suggested that the cataract free group in his study used "significantly more vitamins C and E" than those in another group (same number) who had cataracts.

For the benefit of many readers who wrote in asking about dosage, I can tell them that the majority of Dr. Robertson's subjects on vitamins C and E took 300 to 600 milligrams of vitamin C daily and 400 international units (I.U.) daily of vitamin E (alpha-tocopherol).

Professor Robertson's results suggested that increased vitamin consumption was associated with an apparent reduction of cataract risk of 50 to 70 percent.

My Personal Cataract Experience

Dear Dr. MacInnis:

I read with interest your recent column on vitamins and cataracts.

I would appreciate receiving more detailed information from those cataract papers you referred to.

You may be interested in my personal cataract experience. About 1981 my ophthalmologist diagnosed the beginning of cataracts in both my eyes. About a year later I put myself on a vitamin/mineral program as follows:

Multiple B vitamins—1 daily

Vitamin C—600	*milligrams daily*	
Zinc—22	*"*	*"*
Selenium—100	*"*	*"*
Vitamin E—400 I.U.	*"*	*"*
Vitamin A—10,000 I.U.	*"*	*"*
Vitamin D—400 I.U.	*"*	*"*

As recently as June 1990, my ophthalmologist has recorded "essentially no change" in status of my cataracts. And I'm still wearing the same prescription in my glasses that was prescribed two years ago, which differed little from that of four years previously.

Also, my wife had a serious problem with carpal tunnel syndrome some seven to eight years ago. Since then, she has been able to keep it under control with a multiple B vitamin/zinc/vitamin C manufactured under the name of Z-Bec. I look forward to receiving further information.

W.J.P., Ph.D., Ottawa, Ontario

Answer

Your daily dosage of vitamins C and E is about identical to that used in the University of Western Ontario trials (under Professor Robertson). Here Dr. Robertson compared the self-reported consumption of supplementary vitamins over a five-year period by 175 cataract patients with that of 175 cataract-free subjects.

According to his report, "the findings suggested that the cataract-free group used significantly more vitamins C and E than the group with cataracts. . . . The majority of subjects," the report continued, "took supplements containing between 300 to 600 milligrams vitamin C and 400 I.U. of vitamin E." And "in contrast to the controls, cataract patients were only 30 percent as likely to have taken supplementary vitamin C and only 44 percent as likely to have taken supplementary vitamin E."

Professor Robertson summarized his findings by stating that his research "provides fair to good evidence for a causal association between supplementary vitamin C and E consumption and freedom from senile cataracts."

You appear, Dr. P., to have your cataracts under control so far with your program. I would be interested in your periodic progress reports.

"Wet" and "Dry" Eyes

Dear Dr. MacInnis:

I have excessive tearing in the right eye that's very bothersome. My doctor calls the condition "wet eye" and wants to refer me to an eye specialist for surgery. He described the operation but a lot of it escaped me. Could you explain it in plain English?

Incidentally, my next door neighbor has the opposite condition, called "dry eye." (We make a great pair!) What can I tell him about any possible surgery to cure him?

Mr. V.T. (age 76), California

Answer

Tears are composed of three substances produced by the eye: (1) the lacrimal gland situated in the upper outer part of the eyeball secretes watery tears; (2) tiny cells on the surface of the cornea called goblet cells produce a mucous material; and (3) the so-called meibomian glands situated in the lids secrete an oily substance. The excess tears normally drain into the nose. I say "normally" because in certain situations the tear duct becomes plugged—a cause of "wet eye." Sometimes merely dilating the tear duct with a probe-like instrument will clear the passage and allow the tears to drain into the nose. If the duct is damaged, then a surgical connection will have to be made.

Treatment for "dry eye" includes ointments and artificial tears but these remedies are rarely satisfactory. Sometimes, in extreme cases, surgery is beneficial.

What Causes Cataracts?

Dear Dr. MacInnis:
I am a woman 77 years with cataracts—worse in the right eye. Is aging the only cause of cataracts? Should I have a lens implant?

Mrs. H.F., British Columbia

Answer

Aging is the commonest cause of cataract—the so-called senile cataract—and is always present to some degree in most people over 70. A person can be born with cataracts, commonly known as a congenital cataract, which is usually present in both eyes. Most do not progress nor result in loss of vision. Trauma (from a blow on the eye) may cause the well-known traumatic cataract. Long-term use of certain psychiatric drugs (like phenothiazine) may cause deposits on the cornea and lens but, again, vision is not usually affected.

Yes, you should certainly have an intraocular lens implant, in my view, but the final decision is between you and your eye specialist.

Glaucoma

Dear Dr. MacInnis:
I am a woman, age 64, who has just been diagnosed as having glaucoma. This is how the diagnosis came about. I was in a car accident and didn't see the car that suddenly appeared and hit mine at the intersection. The eye specialist said that I was

losing my peripheral vision and that was why I missed seeing that car. I am now on treatment. Would you please give me as much information as you can on glaucoma, and I would appreciate knowing of any glaucoma organization in my state that I could contact. Thank you.

Mrs. J.M., Buffalo, New York

Answer

You are one of over 2,000,000 Americans and 134,000 Canadians with glaucoma, a serious eye condition mainly afflicting the elderly, which according to recent research is genetic in origin. It is estimated that about four out of every hundred seniors over the age of 65 have glaucoma, a figure that is certain to rise in line with our ever-increasing geriatric population. And its worst feature, next to possible eventual blindness, is that 50 percent have it and are not yet aware of it and may suffer irreparable damage to vision before the diagnosis is made.

What are the mechanics of glaucoma? There is a very gradual, insidious build-up of a liquid called aqueous humor in the eyeball. The aqueous humor is being continually produced within the eyeball, but normally the excess is drained through a channel (canal of Schlemm) out of the eye, thus keeping the pressure constant and normal. But in glaucoma this channel is blocked causing a rise of fluid pressure, resulting in damage to the blood vessels that nourish the retina and the optic nerve, the main nerve of the eye. Over time, then, vision is gradually lost, first from nerve and blood vessel damage occurring in the outer visual field that narrows progressively and in time causes tunnel vision. Field narrowing continues to total blindness. Briefly, then, that is the natural progression of (untreated) glaucoma.

The popular notion that chronic glaucoma always causes pain and redness and blurred vision and "halos" around street lights is incorrect, except in the case of *acute* closed-angle glaucoma that occurs in about 20 percent of cases and is an emergency condition that requires immediate treatment to prevent blindness occurring in as little as twenty-four hours. This sudden onset of symptoms brings the *acute* glaucoma patient to the doctor immediately. But 80 percent of glaucoma is of the *chronic* wide-angle type and creeps up on you slowly and insidiously, often over months or years, and, as aforementioned, one can have a far-advanced case without being aware of it and where, as in your experience, Mrs. M., an automobile accident brings the matter to light.

It becomes apparent, then, that in chronic glaucoma, *early* diagnosis is of paramount importance so that the benefit of early treatment can be given to the greatest possible number of people. This can only be achieved by a routine eye examination for glaucoma once a year and more often for those at risk—diabetics and those with a family history of glaucoma.

The main object of treatment is to lessen pressure within the eyeball by reducing the production of fluid (aqueous humor) and/or improving its drainage. This can be achieved in the majority of cases by the use of eye drops given three or four times a day. (For those who are unable to self-administer eye drops, there is a sustained release pellet available that is inserted under the eyelid and releases the drug constantly for a week at a time. (It is more expensive than the regular eye drops.)

Ten percent of chronic wide-angle glaucoma do not respond to conventional eye drop treatment, and laser beams must be used to reduce eyeball pressure by reopening drainage of the pent-up aqueous humor. If this fails, surgery to build a new drainage system is the last resort.

For further information on glaucoma, Americans should write to the National Society for the Prevention of Blindness, 79 Madison Avenue, New York, New York 10016. Canadians should contact their provincial branch of the Canadian National Institute for the Blind (CNIB). The phone number can be found in your phone book.

Tears from Winter Cold

Dear Dr. MacInnis:

My parents (father, age 80, and mother, 75) both complain of an excess of tears. The problem is intensified by the winter cold

*when they can have tears streaming down their cheeks if they go
outside.*

*Their doctor prescribed "artificial tears" for them, which
seems to be for "dry eye." They were puzzled by this but tried it
anyway, only to find out that it didn't work.*

*Another doctor probed the tear ducts on my mother's eyes,
but that didn't help either.*

*Have you any advice for their problems? They are otherwise
in very good health.*

Mrs. A.B., Ottawa, Ontario

Answer

Excessive tearing in the aging eye is commonly due to recurrent infection of a tear sac with accompanying conjunctivitis
(infection) of the same eye, with the inability of the natural
drainage system of the eye to the nose to handle the excess
amount of tears.

Tear sac infection with conjunctivitis can be successfully
treated with an appropriate antibiotic after a culture and sensitivity test of the eye secretion is done. Sometimes a tear duct
becomes obstructed, which can be relieved by passing a probe
through the duct.

You will note that tear duct/sac infection, with its often
attendant tearing, commonly involves only *one* eye. It is rare
for excessive tearing from infection to occur in *both* eyes of one
person at the same time and unheard-of to occur in two people
at any one time, unless the cause is environmental, e.g., cold
air initiating an irritant reaction in both your parents' eyes
when they venture outside.

But whatever the cause, the main problem would seem to
be inadequacy of the natural drainage system to dispose of excess tears from the eyes to the nose.

I would suggest that your parents consult with an eye surgeon to determine whether or not a by-pass operation (establishing an artificial connection between the tear sac and nasal cavity) would be a practical measure. It is probably not, unless the
tearing is absolutely incapacitating.

Avoiding exposure to the cold winter air would seem to be the better option in my view.

Can Eyes Wear Out?

Dear Dr. MacInnis:
Is there such a thing as the eyes wearing out from too much use. And another question: Do "aging" eyes need more light than "young" eyes?
Mr. M.N., Rochester, New York

Answer

The idea of eyesight "wearing out" from too much reading, for example, is a popular myth that I would like to put to rest forever.

There is no need whatsoever of "saving" your eyesight so the eyes will last longer.

Older people need more light than younger folks. Experts tell us that a 50-year-old eye needs about twice as much light as a 20-year-old eye, and a 90-year-old eye needs more than three times as much light as a 20-year-old eye. There are a few rare exceptions to these general rules, so we must always remain aware of special individual lighting requirements (source: *Geriatric Care*, vol. 14, no. 7).

Tear of the Retina

Dear Dr. MacInnis:
I read about retinal tear in your column in our local paper. I have the floating spots and a curtain sweeping across my field of vision.
I saw two eye specialists and all they said was, "I sure hope it clears up."
I am very interested in the laser treatment you mentioned. Please send me an address or phone number of any doctor who does this laser treatment on retinal tears.
Mr. N.J.

Answer

My advice to you, Mr. J., is to see an eye specialist again and this time ask the question, "Do I have a retinal tear or not?" If your symptoms are caused from a tear, the best treatment is by laser and is performed by most eye surgeons.

If, on the other hand, your symptoms are *not* caused by a tear, the usual cause, at least of floaters, is the deposition of debris from an aging retina. In this case there is no specific treatment but sometimes the spots "dry up" and disappear. And then sometimes they recur.

So the all-important thing is to find out whether there is a tear in the retina or not, and any eye specialist can tell you.

Laser Repair of Retinal Tear

Dear Dr. MacInnis:

My husband has just recently been diagnosed as having a retinal tear. His main problem was seeing flashing lights. The eye specialist has strongly advised him to have it repaired with laser so as to prevent retinal detachment at a later date. Although the doctor explained how a retinal tear takes place, we didn't understand it very well and wonder if you could repeat it in layman's language. My husband is 60 years old.

Mrs. M.H., Mississauga, Ontario

Answer

The retina is an extremely thin layer of brain tissue that lines the back of the eye. Visual images are recorded on the retina much like what happens to a film in your camera. There, images are transmitted to the brain, which interprets what you're seeing.

In front of the retina in the eyeball there's a gelatinous material called the *vitreous*. At birth the vitreous is firm and adheres to the retina. As we get older it tends to become like molasses or syrup and collapses away from the retina in certain areas; in doing so, it can cause a retinal rip or tear. If the retinal tear is not repaired the syrupy vitreous may seep through the tear "bubbling" the retina of the inner wall of the eyeball. If you've ever seen new wall paper bubbling on a wall, you get the picture. This is the commonest cause of retinal detachment. Trauma from an injurious blow is another cause.

You mention only one symptom of retinal tear—seeing flashing lights. Two other common symptoms are seeing floating spots and something like a curtain sweeping across the field of vision. Any reader with one or more of these symptoms should see a doctor.

Laser is now the standard treatment for retinal tears. The process has been picturesquely described as "spot welding."

I would advise you to have the tear "welded" as soon as possible. The success rate is reported to be approximately 90 percent.

Retinal Detachment

Dear Dr. MacInnis:

My husband, age 70, recently experienced vision problems such as flashing lights and the appearance of floating objects in the right eye.

The doctor referred him to an eye specialist who discovered what he described as a small tear in the retina. He treated the tear with a laser beam that he said would prevent what he called retinal detachment, which I gather is much more serious than a retinal tear.

Would you kindly explain what retinal detachment is and what causes it?

Mrs. F.R.

Answer

Your husband has shown excellent judgment in procuring medical aid quickly, because otherwise it would have likely gone on to retinal detachment with all its serious consequences including total blindness.

Before discussing your question, I would like to say something about some structures of the eye as they relate to retinal detachment.

First, about the retina itself. It is a thin transparent membrane covering the back wall of your eyeball. Just behind the retina is a layer of little blood vessels that nourish the eye so that it can perform its visual functions. When the retina separates from this layer, called the choroid, you have retinal detachment.

Another term you need to know is the "vitreous"—a transparent jelly-like "humor" that fills the back of your eyeball and adjoins the retina. Tearing of the retina allows vitreous fluid to leak under it, tending to lift it off the blood vessel layer previously referred to.

Retinal tearing often leading to detachment commonly occurs in the elderly. It is said that aging softens the vitreous humor causing it to shrink and in the process tugs on the retina producing a hole or a tear. (When retinal tearing or detachment occurs in the young it is invariably caused by eye trauma.)

A retinal tear must be attended to at once, and the most common and beneficial procedure is to seal it by laser beam. This is commonly done in the eye specialist's office. If there are several holes or tears or if retinal detachment is occurring, the patient must be hospitalized where the retina can be reattached.

Outlook: The speed in attaining quick surgical attention may make the difference between sight or blindness in the affected eye. In general, the surgical success rate is 85 to 90 percent if the central part of the retina (macula) is not affected. Even when the macula is detached, surgery can sometimes result in useful central vision.

Detached retina most often occurs in near-sighted people, males, and Caucasians for reasons not understood. About one in every 10,000 people in the industrialized world suffers retinal detachment.

Let me repeat the symptoms of retinal tearing: Flashes of light, sparks, or stars, and seeing floating objects (floaters). When detachment occurs you may notice a shadow or curtain on your line of vision in the affected eye.

When any of these symptoms occur, consult your doctor at once.

No More Horrible "Coke-Bottle Bottoms"

Dear Dr. MacInnis:

I have been told that I need a cataract operation. I understand that thick cataract glasses are no longer needed if a lens implant is done. What about ordinary glasses for reading or distance? Will they be necessary after a lens implant?

Mrs. L.K., age 61, Calgary, Alberta

Answer

In most cases yes, but having to wear bifocal glasses is a small price to pay compared to the old horrible "Coke-bottle bottoms," with all their problems.

You will be pleased to know that the Gimbel Eye Clinic in your city (Calgary) is now pioneering the use of this new *multifocal intraocular* lens in Canada. This will allow patients fitted with the new lens to switch from close to long distance, as with bifocal glasses.

According to Dr. Howard Gimbel, this new lens "has real potential and I am convinced it is the way of the future. It is probably the biggest breakthrough since the development of the artificial lens implant itself," he said.

Lens Implantation in the "Old Old"

A column on lens implantation after cataract surgery in the "old old" sparked a very positive response. Most correspondents were considerably senior to the 75-year-old who wondered if he was "too old" for implantation of a plastic lens.

Here's a letter that should dispel any doubt about having the procedure done:

Dear Dr. MacInnis:

In answer to that 75-year-old gentleman's enquiry, I would like to say that I am an 81-year-old lady who had a cataract operation with an implanted lens last year that was very successful. This year I had the other eye done successfully. The operation is so simple that I wouldn't hesitate to have it done if I had a third eye!

Mrs. L.S.

Blepharitis

Dear Dr. MacInnis:

My father, age 78, has crusting of his eyelids and eyelashes. Sometimes there's irritation and itching as well. What is this condition and do you have any suggestions re treatment?

Mr. A.B., Toronto, Ontario

Answer

From your description of your father's eyelids, it is most likely that he has a condition called "blepharitis," a very common eye infection in the elderly. The disorder affects the function of the meibomian (oil) glands of the eyelid. It is thought to be due to a staphylococcus infection. Pus from the infection causes matting of the eyelashes and crusting along the lid border.

Warm compresses twice a day or more loosen the crusting and can be made more effective by the use of a clean, warm, moistened washcloth wrapped over the patient's index finger. In this way the washcloth is used to rub vigorously to remove the crusts and stimulate the oil glands. An antibiotic ointment should be applied to the eyelid margin once or twice a day after the eyelid "scrub" previously mentioned.

Ectropion and Entropion

Dear Dr. MacInnis:

My lower eyelid is turned in almost completely. The eye lashes rub against the eyeball causing irritation, redness, and tears. Is there any remedy for it?

Mr. E.L. (78)

Answer

In medical language you have an "entropion." It is caused by excessive loss of fatty tissue in the eye socket resulting in a backward displacement of the eye and a rolling backward of the lower eyelid. The treatment is a simple operation that is completely satisfactory.

There is another condition just the opposite to your case, where the lower eyelid rolls *out*, which I believe is the commoner. It is called an "ectropion." When the roll-out is excessive, it can be quite disfiguring with a rim of red membrane emerging in place of the lower eyelid. Again, the treatment is a simple operation and what a satisfying one it is!

The commonest cause of excessive production of tears affecting one eye only is obstruction of the tear duct, usually the result of repeated infection. This tear duct runs from the inner corner of the eye to the nose, draining off the excess tears produced in the eye. If this obstruction cannot be relieved by passing a probe down the tear duct, there is a satisfactory operation for it.

Floaters

Dear Dr. MacInnis:

For some time I've been winking at a spot floating in my left eye. Lately, the spot has grown legs and become a darting water strider.

How do I live with this without taking residence in a swamp?

Mr. A.B., Michigan

Answer

You have a so-called floater in your vitreous humor (a gelatinous substance filling the front of the eyeball behind the lens). You can "see" all sorts of little creatures such as flies, bugs, and exotic marine life (like your water strider). It most commonly occurs in the aging eye and usually represents tiny particles of detached tissue from the vitreous gel. The motion of the eye causes exits and entrances with ballet-like grace of your favorite flora and fauna.

Such theatre becomes in time, boring, distracting, and often exceedingly annoying, and it appears that you see it this way. Nothing much in the way of treatment is available, I'm sorry to say.

Although most floaters are benign and don't affect vision, a sudden appearance of "specks" could be heralding a slow hemorrhage in the retina from diabetes or from a tear in the retina leading to detachment. Both require immediate treatment by an eye specialist.

Bifocal Contact Lenses

Dear Dr. MacInnis:

I am a male, 45 years old, and have been wearing contact lenses for about ten years. As I was having trouble reading, I tried out my wife's reading glasses and noticed marked improvement. My question: Do I have to get reading glasses to wear over my contacts or are there bifocal contact lens available? About five years ago an optometrist told me about the possibility of bifocal contacts "some time in the future" but not then. What's the situation now?

Mr. T.G., Mississauga, Ontario

Answer

Over the past five years great strides have been made in the development of bifocal and even trifocal contact lenses. Practically all of the "big names" in contact lens marketing (Bausch

& Lomb, Allergan, Pilkington) and a host of smaller companies are preparing for the huge demand for multifocal contacts when the "baby boomer" generation turns presbyopic at around 45 like yourself. (Presbyopia is where the aging lens loses its elasticity in which near objects are seen less distinctly than those at a distance.)

Most contact lens users got them for myopia, or near-sightedness. But again, in the course of time, near vision also becomes blurred when presbyopia develops.

The American Academy of Ophthalmologists predict that 40 percent of people with presbyopia will need bifocal correction. As there are an estimated 45 million people in North America with presbyopia—a figure that will double in the next decade, there will be an ever-increasing demand for bifocal contacts.

I would suggest that you consult an ophthalmologist or optometrist to give you up-to-date information on the subject.

Excimer Laser Treatment for Myopia

Dear Dr. MacInnis:

I read recently an article about the laser treatment for near-sightedness. It appeared to be a very successful method to treat this condition and at 45 years of age I am looking forward to having it done. As you live near Calgary where the operation is now being performed, I was wondering if you could tell me more about it. Thank you.

Mr. M.L., Toronto, Ontario

Answer

Dr. Howard Gimbel, head of the Gimbel Eye Clinic in Calgary, Alberta, has to date (March 1991) performed eighty-one operations using excimer laser therapy and reports that the results have "exceeded all expectations." It is considered by some eye specialists to be one of the biggest breakthroughs in the history of eye therapy since the intervention of corrective lenses. It has been used in Europe and the U.S. for the past three years.

The U.S. FDA has approved of its use, but Canada's Health Protection Branch hasn't, at the time of writing, given it the green light. Despite this, Dr. Gimbel carries on.

The excimer laser technique involves the use of a mix of argon and fluoride gas in a mirrored tube which produces a beam of "cold" ultraviolet light that, in effect, sculpts the cornea to correct myopia (near sightedness). (In myopia, which usually occurs in the mid-40s, the eyeball becomes elongated so that the rays of light from an object converge in *front* of the retina, producing a fuzzy image.) The laser beam flattens the cornea, causing light rays from objects to properly converge at the retina producing a sharp image. (The same effect is obtained by a myopic patient with corrective glasses.)

It is important to stress that the excimer laser beam does not produce heat like ordinary laser beams and, therefore, doesn't burn the cornea or deeper tissues. It is said that its emitted energy sculpts the cornea not from searing the tissues but by breaking down their molecular bonding.

Some "veteran" readers may recall I wrote a column about six years ago on "radial keratotomy," a procedure originating in the then Soviet Union where a similar "fore-shortening" of the eyeball was effected by making a tiny radial incision around the circumference of the cornea resulting in shrinking of the cornea when the scars healed. It looks like laser therapy will in time totally supplant the "cutting"operation because "it is safer and more predictable," according to Dr. Gimbel. Nevertheless, there are still outspoken critics of the procedure.

Arcus Senilis

Dear Dr. MacInnis:

A few months ago you wrote in your column about a "white ring" around the iris of the eyes. I believe you said it correlated with certain medical conditions and generally was a natural consequence of aging. Quite recently my sister spotted a white ring around my mother's irises and asked me if I had any idea what they meant. I then recalled you had written about it but for the life of me I couldn't remember the name of the condition. I would be pleased to hear from you as I'd like to know if there's any cause for concern.

Mrs. T.E., California

Answer

You are describing an exceedingly common condition called "arcus senilis" or more literally "senile ring." Here's what Dr. Isadore Rossman says about it in his *Clinical Geriatrics,* Second Edition (Philadelphia, PA: Lippincott, 1979, reprinted by permission). "It is common among the elderly . . . due to deposition of droplets of fatty substances in a ringlike fashion around the margin of the cornea. . . . In some instances it completely encircles the cornea; in others, it is present above, below or both. It is initially greyish, gradually getting heavier, whiter and occasionally yellowish as the person grows older. Attempts have been made to correlate arcus senilis with arteriosclerosis [hardening of the arteries] or increased blood cholesterol. A combined study of internists and eye specialists seems to indicate a relationship between the degree and severity of arcus senilis and retinal arteriosclerosis but no significant relationship to other indices of aging."

Arcus senilis has been with us for a long time. Sir William Osler remarked in his 1906 *Practice of Medicine,* "Fatty arcus senilis is of *no moment* in the diagnosis of fatty heart"!

To which your faithful scribe affirms "Amen."

The Older Driver

Whether we sense it or not, driving ability begins to deteriorate ever so subtly in the 50s but it's usually not till 65 that we're bothered more and more with headlight glare that didn't seem so bad before. Furthermore, the glare effect may persist longer than usual, making night driving so uncomfortable that we try to avoid it whenever possible.

Night driving presents other hazards for the older (and not so older) driver. Consider that it takes a 52-year-old driver about one second longer to switch from the roadway to the instrument panel. There is also a narrowing of side vision, requiring us to look further and further over our shoulder. This all adds up to keep our eyes more and more off the road.

A study of older (65 plus) night drivers revealed that they had to drive one-third to one-quarter closer to a series of test signs at night than drivers under 25 in order to read them properly. Daytime driving may also have its problems, such as difficulty in picking out a relevant directional sign amidst a clutter of other signs. This, of course, worsens at night.

Aging also affects decision-making abilities. Have you noticed that you are taking longer to make the appropriate response particularly when you are in unfamiliar territory?

Looks bad, doesn't it? But read on.

An automobile safety study, providing information on the driving problems, was developed in 1988 by the American Medical Association and General Motors Environmental Activities staff. Here are some questions and answers from the study:

Q. Can people expect to have more (car) crashes after middle age?

A. No. Research indicates that we adapt quite well to the gradual changes that take place in vision, hearing, reactions, and decision-making capabilities. In fact, drivers over 65 have fewer crashes as a group than do drivers of any age group.

Q. Do the crashes of older drivers differ from those of other drivers?

A. Definitely. A person over 65 is more apt to be in a crash where he or she: (1) failed to yield the right of way, (2) changed lanes without checking to see if another vehicle was coming alongside, or (3) ignored a traffic light. Also, drivers over 65 are involved in almost twice as many left-turn accidents as younger drivers, although it's not generally understood why.

Q. At what age should a person quit driving?

A. There is no specific age at which a person can be considered too old to drive, as long as he or she remains healthy, and if the declines that takes place in the senses and other capabilities are normal. There is no basis on which to say that anyone should be refused a driver's license simply because of age.

Q. Are we, as older people, more at risk in crashes?

A. Yes. People over 65 are about five times more at risk than a 19 year old involved in the same crash.

Q. What kind of car should older drivers buy?

A. The older driver should attack less significance to the car's exterior appearance and pay more attention to the interior, especially the instrument panel. As people age, they may prefer speedometers, gauges, and legends that are simple and *bold*. They may select certain colors for sharper definition of symbols within easy reach. (A personal beef of which I have complained, in vain, is the turning directional light that's invisible in bright sunlight and which cannot be heard over the fan and radio.)

Q. Do you have any tips for older drivers?

A. Do not become complacent about driving because it has become a routine based on forty or fifty years of driving experience. Be sensitive to quick changes in traffic movement or the possibility of an unexpected stop sign or traffic signal. And don't become distracted by other passengers (including back-seat drivers). Select roads or streets where the pace of traffic does not make more demands than you can adequately meet. At night, stay on well-lit streets where possible. Keep mentally and physically fit.

Q. What about driving only at certain times?

A. Many elderly people have the option of selecting the time they drive. For instance, they may choose to avoid night driving whenever possible as well as fast paced traffic hours. They are also cautious if driving at dawn or dusk. They avoid driving after drinking alcohol or taking a sedative or when overly tired.

In conclusion, please contact your local automobile association, many of whom conduct regular refresher courses for the older driver.

(My thanks to the American Medical Association and General Motors Environmental Activities Staff.)

Tinnitus

Dear Dr. MacInnis:

I am a man 72 years old bothered with continuous ringing in the ears. This started with a buzzing sound about five years ago and has never left except to change into ringing. I have talked to a number of people my age who suffer from the same problem, some mild, some worse than mine. My hearing is somewhat impaired but still reasonably good. My doctor says it goes with old age and there's nothing much to do about it. I'm not looking for a miracle cure but there must be something in medical science that's helpful.

Mr. J.G., Saint John, New Brunswick

Answer

The annoying condition you describe is called "tinnitus" (from the Latin *tinnire,* which means to "ring like a bell"). Although ringing and buzzing are the commonest sounds heard in one or usually both ears or only in the head (less common), sufferers may complain of clicking like the sound of a cricket in both ears. One of my patients had a sensation of "high seas breaking on a reef." Yes, your doctor is right in stating that it is age related (40 or more). It may get worse over the next ten years and then may seem to improve (probably because the victim gets used to it). "Aging" tinnitus is caused by damage (over time) to microscopic hairs on the surface of the auditory (hearing) cells in the inner ear. These tiny, sensitive hairs move in response to sound waves transmitted to the inner ear by the ear drum. When damage occurs, the hairs become irritated and move wildly in all directions causing random impulses that your brain interprets as bizarre sounds (in your case, buzzing and ringing).

Management: First, the elderly tinnitus patient should get a medical checkup and audiometric (hearing) test. (Tinnitus is

85 percent associated with hearing loss.) You may be referred to an audiologist (hearing specialist) who may prescribe a device worn like a hearing aid that produces a static-like radio sound that may "mask" the more disagreeable sound of tinnitus. It's worth a try.

Hearing Getting Poor

Dear Dr. MacInnis:

I believe my hearing is getting poor. If I don't set the TV myself, it's never loud enough for me. I am at my hearing worst in a crowded room where everyone's talking. Things like that. My age is 71. Should I get my hearing tested? And how?

Mr. Y.L., Ontario

Answer

You can always have your hearing tested by an audiologist. I suggest that you contact one in the department of audiology in any large hospital where you will get an unbiased consultation.

(You will find below a quick simple screening test for hearing loss devised by the American Academy of Otolaryngology that offers guidance depending on your score.)

A Quick Screening Test for Hearing

Do feel you're becoming hard of hearing? Here's a quick screening test put out by the American Academy of Otolaryngology (specialty of ear, nose and throat). It takes about five minutes to answer the questions and should indicate whether or not you should see an ear, nose, and throat specialist for more detailed examination and advice. Here's the test:

Answer each question with the most appropriate of the following responses: Almost always; half the time; occasionally; never.

1. I have trouble hearing over the telephone.

2. I have trouble following conversation when two or more people are talking at the same time.
3. People tell me I always have the TV on too loud.
4. I have to strain to understand conversation.
5. I sometimes don't hear sounds like the phone or doorbell.
6. I have trouble hearing at a noisy party.
7. I get confused as to where sounds come from.
8. I misunderstand some words in a sentence and need to ask people to repeat themselves.
9. I especially have trouble understanding the speech of women and children.
10. I have worked in noisy environments such as assembly lines, jackhammers, jet engines, etc.
11. Many people I talk to seem to mumble or don't speak clearly.
12. People get annoyed because I misunderstand what they say.
13. I misunderstand what others are saying and make inappropriate responses.
14. I avoid social activities because I cannot hear well and fear that I might reply improperly.

To be answered by a family member or friend:
15. Do you think this person has a hearing loss?

How to score: Count three points for every "almost always," two points for every "half the time," one for each "occasionally," and zero for every "never."
How to interpret:

0 to 5—Your hearing is probably fine. No further tests needed.
6 to 9—Seeing an ear specialist is suggested.
10 and above—Seeing an ear specialist is *strongly* recommended.

Please note: The above is only a screening test to determine the advisability of seeing your doctor or an ear specialist. It should *not* be construed as a definitive test in itself. (My thanks to the American Academy of Otolaryngology.)

I'm Losing My Sense of Taste

Dear Dr. MacInnis:

I am a farmer, age 62, in good health, so why should I write to you? I believe I'm losing my sense of taste for sweets and to some extent, salty foods. Is there any reason for this apart from the fact that I'm getting on in years? Can anything be done about it?

Mr. L.T., Ontario

Answer

The ability to taste and smell food declines in later life, often compounded by certain diseases and medications. Some diseases that may adversely affect taste and smell are flu, liver disease, kidney failure, nervous diseases such as Parkinson's disease, diabetes, and cancer. And drugs like anticoagulants (blood thinners), diuretics (water pills), antihistamines, muscle relaxants, and antibiotics can also interfere with smelling and tasting.

Some interesting research in taste and smell is being carried out at Duke University, Durham, North Carolina, by Dr. Susan Schiffman, who has discovered that sodium transport plays an important role in the perception of taste in both humans and rats. She placed the diuretic drug *amiloride* (brand name Moduretic) on the tongues of human volunteers and then tested their ability to taste a variety of flavors. (Amiloride prevents the transport of sodium ions that carry taste sensations to the taste buds.) Dr. Schiffman found that this did not affect the ability to detect bitter or sour flavors but salty and sweet taste sensations were definately impaired. This seems to indicate that sodium ion depletion may have some relation to your taste problem possibly leading to a practical solution some time in the future.

While you're waiting for something better, Mr. T, Dr. Schiffman suggests several things to enhance food flavor: Take alternate bites of different foods (when several bites of the *same* food are taken the first bite gives the stronger flavor); "And chew your bites thoroughly," advises Dr. Schiffman, "because chewing breaks down food, allowing more food molecules to interact with your taste buds."

I've Lost My Sense of Taste

Dear Dr. MacInnis:

What can you do for an old guy like me (age 81) who has lost his sense of taste. Everything tastes the same—flat, even vinegar! My sense of smell is not like it used to be either. What causes it?

Mr. J.L., Mississauga, Ontario

Answer

I regret I cannot be of much help other than suggest that you try to make your food servings as attractive as possible.

Your loss of taste sensation is due mainly to your diminished sense of smell. Readers will recall how a plugged nose (from a cold) can affect the taste of food and usually the first sign of a head cold clearing is when your taste comes back.

The taste buds in the tongue decrease from an average of 248 in children to 88 in persons 74 to 85 years of age. Taste buds help you to recognize strong sensations of taste, such as sweet and sour. But to discern subtle flavors it takes a good sense of smell as well.

In a recent study, age was correlated with the ability to identify by smell four common odorous substances (coffee, oil of almonds, peppermint and coal tar).

Age	Percent of Subjects Who Smelled Nothing
20 to 39	0
40 to 59	0
60 to 69	8
70 to 79	10
Over 80	29*

(Although it was not stated, I presume that the percentage of *taste* loss in the same subjects would be similar if not greater.)

*From M. P. Anand, "Accidents in the Home," in W. F. Anderson and B. Isaacs, eds., *Current Achievements in Geriatrics* (London: Cassel, 1964), p. 239.

Chapter 14
Cancer in the Elderly

A reader recently asked me two questions about cancer. His first question was, "Does cancer run in families?" Question number two was, "Is cancer more common in old people?" and he went on to say that "in the past year, three of my friends here in the senior lodge have passed away, all with cancer of the rectum."

The hereditary nature of many types of cancers has long been observed. In certain families, for example, mothers, daughters, and granddaughters have shown susceptibility to breast cancer, while other family generations succumb to cancer of the gastrointestinal tract, particularly of the stomach, colon, and rectum.

We, as medical students many years ago, were taught that for cancer to develop, two prerequisites were necessary: (1) a genetic background or susceptibility (which is not constant for every kind of cancer), and (2) an inciting or causal factor or group of factors that triggers the development of cancer in *susceptible organ tissue*. In many cases it may take many years—even a lifetime of these inciting factors, such as environmental trauma—to produce the necessary mutation or change in an originally normal cell to produce a cancerous cell. And this could explain why most cancers are most prevalent in the elderly, who have over the last century been experiencing an ever-increasing life expectancy.

Examples of the rapid escalation of certain cancers with aging would include cancer of the large bowel, breast, lung, skin, and prostate gland. Some authorities have ascribed this aging-cancer correlation to a gradual dysfunction of the aging immune system, but a better explanation might be the aforementioned time factor necessary to complete the mutation (change) process from a normal cell to a malignant one.

It's a giant leap from these scientifically valid observations of yester-year to the Nobel Prize–winning medical research of 1989. But that's what medical scientists Harold Varmus and Michael Ponds of the University of California have now determined—that the origins of all human cancers are carried within the gene like a signature or logo, and that these cancer genes are nothing more than mutated or altered normal genes that in time, given the necessary prodding by cancer-causing agents, will ultimately express themselves as clinical cancers.

Genetic scientists tell us that of the 100,000 or so genes making up the human genome (our genetic map), probably no more than 300 are the so-called cancer causing genes. This is heartening because molecular biologists, thanks to the landmark findings of Ponds, Varmus, and co-workers, can now concentrate on a relatively small area of cancer cell research, such as normal to cancer cell mutation and, better still, know they are finally in the right field.

And what are these cancer-causing factors that trigger cell mutation? We've been hearing about them for years; the admonitions are familiar—e.g., avoid smoking, excessive alcohol, and the midday sun! The question is: Will we be better listeners now that the scientific basis of much we have known before has been firmly established?

I believe we will. And to those of you getting up in years, it's still not too late to change your lifestyle a bit. Some of these 300 cancer genes so frantically trying to mutate further may be stopped in their tracks!

And you may still enjoy a healthy old age.

Why Is Lung Cancer So Deadly?

Dear Dr. MacInnis:

Why is lung cancer so deadly? My father died from it last year and chemotherapy, which is usually fairly successful in most other cancers, did no good at all. Surgery and radiation weren't tried, but I'm told that they are not all that good either.

Mrs. K. T., Toronto, Ontario

Answer

The mortality (death) rate from primary cancer of the lung has changed little over the past half-century. In Canada, over 15,000 deaths occur every year, and in the industrialized world it accounts for 30 percent of all deaths from cancer.

A research team from Queen's Cancer Research Laboratories (Queen's University, Kingston, Ontario) made an important discovery late last year that may serve to answer the oft-repeated question: Why is lung cancer so resistant to chemotherapy?

The Queen's researchers, headed by Drs. Susan Cole and Roger Deeley, discovered that lung cancer cells possess certain genes that produce a protein rendering these cells resistant to cancer drugs. Their findings were reported in the December 1992 issue of *Science.*

It will take from five to ten years, the researchers say, before we will see the development of a new generation of strong drugs capable of penetrating this protein armor around lung cancer cells and treating the patient more effectively.

The yew-based anticancer drug, taxol (see below), is showing very significant activity against advanced non-small-cell lung cancer (NSCLC). According to Dr. Alex Chang, a cancer specialist at Genessee Hospital, Rochester, New York, NSCLC accounts for about 75 percent of lung cancers (it is highly malignant, drug resistant, and spreads rapidly).

Taxol for Ovarian Cancer

Dear Dr. MacInnis:

About a year ago you had a small item in your column about a treatment for ovarian cancer using a product made from the bark of the yew tree. Now I have heard that my sister, age 48, has cancer of the ovary and I want to send her some information on it. Do you have any up-to-date information on this treatment? I hear it is a very serious kind of cancer and difficult to treat.

Mrs. C.L., California

Answer

The drug you refer to is taxol, which you correctly state is processed from the bark of the yew tree, mainly found in the ancient forests of Washington, California, Oregon, and British Columbia, where it is known as the Pacific or western yew. It is a hardwood tree that can grow to a height of fifty feet or more and is widely used in furniture making.

Taxol is still undergoing clinical trials and about a thousand cancer patients are receiving it on an experimental basis. It has shown to reduce by up to 30 percent advanced malignant ovarian tumors, which have always responded poorly to conventional methods of treatment—e.g., chemotherapy, radiation, or surgery. The drug is being developed by the National Cancer Institute (NCI) and the Bristol-Myers Squibb Drug Company, which has official access to the bark in U.S. national forests. The NCI is now expanding the experimental use of taxol for women with breast cancer.

Currently, the processing of yew bark into taxol is severely limited by a shortage of the bark brought on, environmentalists claim, by poor cooperation of the logging industry with the U.S. Forest Service's regulations for bark conservation. It takes 27 kilograms of bark, equivalent to three very old trees, to process enough taxol to treat an ovarian cancer patient for a year.

Because yew bark is the only approved source of taxol, this constitutes a great incentive for researchers to attempt to develop the drug synthetically.

According to the American Cancer Society, ovarian cancer will each year cause the death of 12,500 women in the U.S. (over 1,000 in Canada) and 45,000 from breast cancer (about 5,000 in Canada).

Lung Cancer in Women

Dear Dr. MacInnis:

I got the surprise of my life when I read that lung cancer in women now causes more deaths than cancer of the breast. When I told my wife (age 60 and a two-pack cigarette smoker) she laughed at it, arguing that I'm hearing rumours again and that "everybody" knows that cancer of the breast is the number-one woman killer. I'm sure I read it somewhere but have no proof. Maybe if she reads it in your column she will believe me. I hope I'm right.

Mr. C. E., Avon, New York

Answer

You are indeed right. Just recently (1993) the Center for Disease Control (CDC) in Atlanta stated that "lung cancer *already* has passed breast cancer as the most common cause of cancer death among women." This statement is based on U.S. statistics, but I'm sure the trend is becoming evident in other parts of the world as well.

It is true that more men die of lung cancer than women—about 74 deaths per 100,000 for males in 1986 compared to 27 deaths per 100,000 for women. But consider this: From 1976 to 1986 the death rate for women jumped 44 percent while the rate for men was up only 7 percent.

According to the CDC report, male smoking "has been on the decline since the early 1950s but female smoking peaked later—in the 1960s."

There has been a decrease in smoking among women—from 32 percent in 1965 to 27 percent in 1987. "But that isn't nearly as sharp as the drop in smoking by men—from 50 percent to 32 percent," says the CDC. The result: "The death rate from lung cancer among women continues to climb and will do so until the turn of the century." This is because "peaks in cigarette smoking appear (statistically) to be followed by a peak in lung cancer deaths about thirty-five years later," said the CDC report.

351

Addendum, 1993: A University of Toronto study reveals that women who smoke cigarettes put themselves at about three times the risk of developing lung cancer than men who smoke cigarettes.

Brain Tumor

Dear Dr. MacInnis:

My mother died at 61 from brain tumors (metastases) that spread from breast cancer. During her last month of life she became quite unaware of everything and didn't recognize Dad or any of the children. The doctor said she was suffering from dementia—something I thought could only happen in Alzheimer's disease. They decided to treat the brain tumors with radiation, but she passed away before anything was done. We have wondered if radiation given earlier might have helped this dementia and prolonged her life. I would appreciate your opinion.

Mrs. K.L., Ottawa, Ontario

Answer

In my own hospital department of 212 beds we admit over a hundred patients in far advanced dementia—the majority with Alzheimer's disease and a lesser number with dementia associated with disorders of brain circulation. Only rarely do we see patients in dementia as a result of a primary brain tumor or a secondary one, as in your mother's case. This is because such patients usually remain in the neurological department of the general hospital where the diagnosis was made.

Would your mother have benefited from brain radiotherapy? I regret to say I don't believe so even if given earlier. And whole brain radiotherapy can often itself cause a devastating dementia if the patient survives long enough to develop it.

The long-term consequences of brain radiation are seldom observed because of the patient's usually short life expectancy. But in certain cases, where the patient lives longer than usual, various degrees of dementia, from mild to extreme, have been observed. There is a recent report out of Memorial Sloane Kettering Cancer Center citing twelve patients who developed progressive dementia, ataxia (muscular imbalance), and urinary incontinence within five to thirty-six months of radiation. (None of the radiated patients had tumors when these neurological signs and symptoms appeared.) The authors of the report advise smaller daily fractions of radiotherapy in brain tumor patients with a better than usual outlook so as to delay the onset of possible dementia *(Neurology* 39, [1989]: 789–96).

Letter To Bill

Dear Dr. MacInnis:

My husband, age 51, is a two-pack-a-day cigarette smoker. When I tell him repeatedly that he is flirting with lung cancer, it falls on deaf ears. I'm at the point of giving up, but before I do, I wonder if you can provide me with some cold, hard facts that might impress if not scare him into quitting cigarettes? Perhaps it would be more effective if you wrote to Bill himself. He has promised to read your answer.

Mrs. T.F.

Dear Bill:

In the early 1900s lung cancer was a rarity, with undertakers of this condition about as busy as Maytag servicemen! But over the last fifty years with the tremendous increase in cigarette smoking, lung cancer now accounts for 70 deaths per 100,000 men every year in the United States. Due to an overall decrease in cigarette smoking, the death rate as depicted on a graph is now in a plateau and there is a good possibility that a gradual decline will follow.

But women have not stopped smoking to any extent. In fact, more young girls are starting to smoke than ever before. This is why lung cancer deaths in women have recently exceeded breast cancer as the leading cause of cancer deaths in women.

And a few more statistics to ponder. While non-smokers are at very low risk of developing lung cancer, a one-pack-a-day cigarette smoker runs thirty times the risk of a non-smoker. You, Bill, a two-packer, have sixty times the risk of a non-smoker. Add to this the fact that your wife as a *passive* inhaler of cigarette smoke runs two to three times the risk of developing lung cancer than if she lived in a cigarette-smoke–free environment.

The question is frequently asked, "Does quitting the weed reduce the risk of coming down with lung cancer?" The answer is yes, although it may take about ten years' abstinence before your lungs are as free of risk as that of a non-smoker. While it's true that quitting early in life provides better protection than if you stop later, your relative youth (51) will reap the profits in your 60s, where the incidence of lung cancer is high.

I do not have the time nor the space here to submit proof of the correlation between lung cancer and cigarette smoking except for one very telling case study: Ninety-three percent of the 807 patients with lung cancer seen at one U.S. institution between 1980 and 1985 were cigarette smokers.

And on a national scale, according to the *Scientific American Textbook of Medicine,* "Lung cancer is responsible for more deaths among men and, as of 1985, among women than any other type of cancer in the United States"—and the same would apply to Canada. You take it from here, Bill.

Beta-Carotene

Two readers have written in requesting information on the beneficial effect of beta-carotene on helping to prevent lung cancer in smokers. Both are admittedly "confirmed diehards who just can't stop"!

I have finally been able to procure the information they want. I apologize to these readers for the long delay.

Most people don't know (except the two readers) that beta-carotene is a safe nontoxic form of vitamin A and that, along with other carotenes, has been associated with a protective effect against cancer, especially lung cancer.

And my two readers know something else that most people don't know. It's that smokers as a group could possibly obtain benefits by increasing their intake of fruits and vegetables containing carotenes. According to my sources there is consistent evidence that a high dietary intake of carotenoids and a higher blood plasma level of beta-carotene is associated with a *decreased* risk of lung cancer in smokers.

In a study conducted at the Western Electric Company in Chicago, over 2,000 males were asked about their food-consumption habits, once at the beginning of the study and a second time, one year later.

It was discovered that there was a seven-fold difference in the risk of lung cancer between groups of subjects with the lowest and highest levels of beta-carotene intake. When subjects who had smoked for thirty years were evaluated separately, the risk of lung cancer was almost eight times greater in the men who had low intakes of carotenes.

Another study conducted on 1,271 residents of Massachusetts showed that after controlling for smoking and age, subjects with the highest consumption of fruits and vegetables containing beta-carotene had a risk of death from cancer 30 percent lower than subjects with the lowest intake of carotene-containing green and yellow vegetables.

The largest study of all is now being carried out in Finland on healthy smokers. This study involves 29,000 Finnish male smokers age 60 to 69, who are taking 20 milligrams of beta-carotene daily. The trials will run till 1993.

While the results of this research are eagerly awaited, beta-carotene continues to make a name for itself in the scientific community as a powerful antioxidant vitamin. It acts as a "scavenger" of free radicals—dangerous compounds formed spontaneously through oxidation in the body at all times. (It is speculated that free radical damage to body tissues may play a part in initiating cancer.)

Beta-carotene is associated with a lowered risk of cancer in the epithelial (lining) cells of the esophagus, stomach, colon, rectum, and cervix. It has also been shown to reverse certain pre-cancerous lesions.

Where is beta-carotene found? In bright orange and dark green leafy vegetables such as carrots, squash, pumpkin, spinach, kale, and broccoli, and fruits, such as melons and papaya.

What most people don't know (maybe not even my two correspondents) is that cooked vegetables deliver more beta-carotene than the raw variety. For example, one-half cup of cooked carrots offers more beta-carotene than two or three raw carrot sticks. (It is a well-known fact that cooking lowers the vitamin content of most foodstuffs.)

According to Health and Welfare Canada, consumers should be eating at least five servings of fruits and vegetables daily.

(I am indebted to the "Media Backgrounder" compiled by Lederle Consumer Health Products and distributed by Barry Ashpole Associates of Toronto for most of the information on beta-carotene contained herein.)

Am I Too Old to Give Up Smoking?

Dear Dr. MacInnis

My husband, age 52, has been a two-pack-a-day cigarette smoker for almost forty years. As he puts it, the only positive things about his addiction is that he has never in his long smoking career exceeded two packs and that he has really tried several times and "partly succeeded," when he quit for six months. He has agreed to give it another try if he can find a suitable program for a heavy smoker getting to middle age.

We would both like to know if quitting smoking at this late age would have beneficial effects on the heart and lungs.

Mrs. T.Y., California

Answer

I'll answer your last question first. No less an authority than Dr. Tom Glynn, research director of the National Cancer Institute's smoking, tobacco, and cancer program, tells us that quitting smoking between the ages of 40 and 55 can add, on the average, five years to your life. And these could well be the best years of your life.

Authorities, too, are convinced that quitting the weed even in later years will lessen the risk of coronary heart disease and major or fatal heart attacks. And the risk of stroke, that ruthless disabler and killer of past middle life, can be reduced on the average by 50 percent. Add to this a decreased risk for cancer of the lungs and bronchitis and emphysema, and you have ample reason to quit smoking at your husband's age—or at any age for that matter.

You ask for a good quit-smoking program tailored for "middle age." The National Cancer Institute finances a do-it-yourself quit smoking program for smokers over 50. It is called "Clear Horizons" and consists of a helpful serialized reading course. It is free.

For more information on the "Clear Horizons" program please write to Clear Horizons, Fox Chase Cancer Center, Dept. NC., 7701 Burholme Avenue, Philadelphia, Pennsylvania 19111. Allow six weeks for delivery.

Granddaughters, Cigarette Smoking Gives You a Prune Face!

We all know that cigarette smoking over time causes lung cancer. There's also a relationship between smoking and emphysema and numerous studies attest to its relation to heart disease and leukemia. Over the past decade, I've written many columns on the hazards of smoking, but I fear to little avail, for more young people than ever (particularly girls) are beginning smokers, and lung cancer has recently superseded cancer of the breast as the number-one cancer killer in women.

What I want to report on this week is one more study with a new twist, in that it proves that cigarette smoking, independent of other factors such as age, sex, and sun exposure, is a direct cause of premature facial wrinkling and increased with pack years of smoking. Add to this years of excessive sun and you have concocted all the ingredients of the well-known "California prune syndrome."

357

The authors of this superbly conducted study from the University of Utah Health Sciences Center have reprints available for professional workers and they may be obtained by writing to the head researcher, Donald P. Cadence, M.D., Division of Dermatology, Room 4B454, University of Utah Health Sciences Center, 50 North Medical Drive, Salt Lake City, Utah 84132.

Their article, published in the May 15, 1991, issue of the *Annals of Internal Medicine,* merits an accompanying editorial that addresses a conviction that our anti-smoking fire-and-brimstone scenario is just not getting across to a young smoking public who seem to be more influenced on how they look *now* than by the more remote possibility of death from cancer. "To sell the idea of smoking cessation to patients," said the editorial, "we need to speak *their* language, not *our* language and we need to speak to their concerns, not to our own. . . . A brief survey of the magazine advertisements in the grocery store should provide enough evidence to convince any doctor that many people are very concerned about the possibility that their skin may be a little too oily, may be a little too dry, or may be getting a little bit wrinkled."

Yes indeed, death warnings on cigarette packs are getting us nowhere with the youngsters. So what to do?

Appeal to their vanity, not their pathology.

It will sure get to the girls! And boys, too, are more terrified of their wall-to-wall acne than of lung cancer any day!

Is Breast Cancer Hereditary?

Dear Dr. MacInnis:

My mother developed cancer of the breast and died from it five years after her operation (radical mastectomy) followed by radiotherapy.

Her mother, she told me, also had breast cancer, and I know that one of her sisters also came down with it.

My question: Is breast cancer hereditary?

Mrs. J.H. (52), Toronto, Ontario

Answer

Cancer of the breast is considered by experts in the field to be hereditary in 5 to 10 percent of cases. From your family history there is a higher-than-normal risk factor present. Other factors increasing the risk are a large number (larger than yours) of relatives with breast cancer, when breast cancer occurrs at a relatively early age, when both breasts are affected, and a history of occurrence in male relatives. Genetic research has revealed that a gene (p 53) considered to be a cancer suppressant is absent in patients with hereditary breast cancer. Furthermore, a cancer-causing gene has been found to be present in high-risk patients.

For the 90 percent that is not hereditary, it is thought that genetic damage may also play a part, but here it occurs after birth, causing "mutation" in breast cells that may lead to breast cancer that is not transmitted to offspring.

The "Pill" and Breast Cancer

Estrogen replacement therapy (ERT) and breast cancer: Can taking the "pill" cause breast cancer in later life? Does estrogen hormone replacement for menopause increase the risk of breast cancer? Over the past twelve months in these columns I've written more often on this subject than on any other topic.

This is because it has lately become so controversial.

Last year, based on evidence of Wingo and colleagues (*Journal of the American Medical Association* 257, [1987]), I reported "no definite link" between estrogen replacement therapy (for menopause) over a twenty-year observation period.

In a subsequent column I quoted from a study published in the *American Journal of Epidemiology,* where researchers at the Boston University School of Medicine found that women who had used oral contraceptives had, on average, twice the risk for breast cancer than those who had never used them and four times the risk after ten years of use.

Then there was the study by the Royal College of General Practitioners (Great Britain) involving 46,000 women that reported "a threefold risk" for breast cancer in women aged 30 to 34 who had used oral contraceptives for two to seven years.

But a Federal Drug Administration (FDA) Advisory Committee found so many inconsistencies in the two last-mentioned studies that this drug-regulating body decided not to act decisively on the matter and recommended that further studies be carried out.

I mentioned in that column, "We are probably back to square one again," with very little to do but wait for an upcoming big study, this time conducted by the National Cancer Institute and being completed in 1995 where 1,000 women with breast cancer and 1,000 without will be followed to see if estrogen played a part or not. "This could provide more definite data," NCI scientists said.

But yet another study has hit the medical headlines and is all the more serious because it tends to incriminate as well the hormone progestin, very frequently given with estrogen in menopause replacement therapy to help prevent cancer of the lining of the uterus (a long-known side effect of estrogen).

The study by Swedish and U.S. researchers and published in the *New England Journal of Medicine* (first week of September 1989) showed that women who took a combination of estrogen and progestin for more than six years were "4.4 times more likely than others never taking it to develop cancer of the breast."

The number of Swedish women in the study was large—23,244 of them age 35 or older, all who received various kinds of estrogen replacement therapy over a period of six years. The researchers compared the incidence of new cases of breast cancer in this group to a similar group from the same geographical area who never received estrogen replacement treatment.

Their findings: The women who received estrogen replacement therapy were on the average 10 percent more likely to get breast cancer. The longer they were on estrogen, the greater was the risk. For example. after nine years of estrogen the cancer risk increased to 70 percent.

Some cancer specialists view the findings as "important but preliminary and must be confirmed by further studies." At present they do not recommend any change in prescribing habits, preferring to weigh any suspected cancer risk against "proven benefits," such as protection against heart disease and stroke.

And here the controversy stands to await still "another study." My advice is that you always discuss ERT with your gynecologist.

Breast Cancer Statistics

Dear Dr. MacInnis:

Is it true that one woman in ten will get breast cancer? If true, is that the average over a lifetime or does the figure apply to a certain susceptible age group? Are young women of childbearing age at more risk than, say, a woman of my age, 51? I'm confused.

L.G., Kelowna, British Columbia

Answer

This oft-quoted one-in-ten statistic is extremely misleading. What it actually represents is the *accumulated* risk over a woman's life expectancy (now about 80 years).

Now, to answer your question, your risk of cancer increases with age. For example, from birth to 24 a woman's cancer risk is one in 40,000. By your age (51) your risk is about one in ninety. And this risk continues to increase the longer you live until it reaches one in ten at around the age of 80. In other words, you'd have to reach 80 before your statistical risk would be 10 percent.

Properly used, these statistics should dispel another popular myth—that the risk of getting breast cancer somehow lessens at 50.

As you see, it just ain't so.

Breast Cancer in Men

Dear Dr. MacInnis:

My brother, age 67, who resides in the States, has been diagnosed as having cancer of the breast. I was very surprised to hear this as it never occurred to me that it could happen in men. I asked our family doctor about it and he told me that he had read about it but had not actually seen one either in his training or practice.

Could you please briefly comment on its incidence, treatment, and general outlook compared to women. I thank you for this.

Mr. J.M., Canada

Answer

Carcinoma (cancer) of the male breast is relatively uncommon. The *Annals of Internal Medicine* in its November 1992 issue, reports American Cancer Society estimates that, in 1992, "1,000 new cases of breast cancer in men will be diagnosed in the United States, compared with 180,000 cases in women and that about 300 men will die of the disease."

The basic local treatment is modified radical mastectomy (removal of breast and armpit glands, with sparing of muscles). Radiotherapy may be a part of this procedure. If the armpit glands are positive for cancer, combination chemotherapy along with tamoxifen is administered. If the cancer has spread to bones or distal organs, additive hormone therapy, e.g., tamoxifen, has proven beneficial in producing partial remissions. Please bear in mind that these are only general statements. Your brother's treatment would depend on the stage of his disease, i.e., whether or not the cancer is localized or has spread and how far it has spread, as in the case of a woman. These factors also dictate the prognosis (outcome) that again is generally similar to that of breast cancer in women.

Breast cancer in men represents less than 1 percent of all male malignancies.

Cancer of the Colon and Rectum

Except for cancer of the prostate in men, cancer of the colon and rectum is the most common malignancy in old age, with about 90 percent of such cancers found in people over 50 years. The risk for colo-rectal (colon and rectum) cancer begins around 40 and doubles with each successive decade and reaches its highest incidence at age 80. Long-term survival depends on at what stage the cancer is detected, with a 90 percent five-year survival rate for *very early, in situ* (localized, non-spreading) cancer, to less than a 50 percent five-year survival for cancer that has spread to adjacent lymph nodes. It strikes about 150,000 persons annually and causes about 60,000 deaths in the United States. (In Canada, the figure is approximately 6,000.) Men and women are equally at risk.

Polyps (benign intestinal growths) are precursors to colo-rectal cancer, and their detection and removal are sure ways of stopping a possible cancer right on the spot. This is done with the colonoscope. Colonoscopy, the most sensitive and specific screening method, is usually performed on an outpatient basis. Using this long, flexible, lighted, tubular instrument, doctors visually examine the full lining of the colon and rectum and may remove polyps as they are discovered.

Although one in every twenty-five people develops colo-rectal cancer in their lifetime, it is important to know that this rate is increased threefold in those with a first-degree relative affected with colo-rectal cancer. About a quarter of those with colo-rectal cancer have been found to have at least one affected first-degree relative. (First-degree relatives include a person's parents, brothers, sisters, and children.)

In the April 1992 issue of *Diseases of the Colon and Rectum,* Dr. Malcolm Stuart of Sydney, Australia, reported on a study conducted at Saint Vincent's Hospital (Sydney)) where colonoscopies were performed on 600 patients with a family history of bowel cancer from 1982 to 1990. Results: Polyps or cancer were detected in 45 percent. But in patients with *more than one* first-degree relative, polyps or cancer was discovered in 67 percent.

Dr. Stuart recommends repeating the colonoscopy every four years if the initial examination is clear, unless two first-degree relatives are affected, when it should be done every two years.

Addendum, July 1993: Researchers at Johns Hopkins University have located the gene site for hereditary colon cancer on chromosome 2. This may lead in about two years to a genetic test that will detect those at risk. Only one out of seven colon cancer patients have the inherited type, the remainder being the so-called sporadic kind. However, Mayo Clinic scientists believe that sporadic colon cancer may also be genetically determined with an overall common gene operating in both types. It should be stressed that only the *site* of this gene has been discovered, and *not* the gene itself, but the researchers feel that they will be able to identify it in a year to two.

A Family History of Colo-Rectal Cancer

Dear Dr. MacInnis:

I have a family history of colo-rectal cancer. My uncle died with it thirty years ago. As I recall (with the help of my brother), some of his symptoms were loss of appetite and weight, anemia, bloody stools, and bouts of pain in the abdomen. In the hospital, they did X rays (barium enemas) and made the diagnosis. The doctors told him that the cancer had spread. There was very little they could do for him.

As for myself, I don't have any complaints except some constipation over a period of several months (which is somewhat unusual for me). My question: Should I see a doctor about this?

Mr. B. (55), California

Answer

I received your letter while I was compiling the above column on colo-rectal cancer. You should heed well the advice given in that column, for it applies particularly to those with a family history of colo-rectal cancer like yourself. See your doctor immediately.

Cancer of the Rectum

Dear Dr. MacInnis:
What are some of the important early symptoms of cancer of the rectum?

Mr. F.M., age 73, Calgary, Alberta

Answer

The Canadian Cancer Society in its booklet "Facts on Colorectal Cancer" lists four symptoms that might indicate the presence of cancer but emphasizes that such symptoms are "much more likely to be due to some non-cancerous condition which can be relatively easily corrected." With that caveat, here they are:

1. Change in bowel habit, such as increasing constipation or alternating constipation and diarrhea lasting over two weeks.
2. The presence of bright or dark red blood in the stool. (If no blood is seen on examination the doctor may do a chemical test for occult or "hidden" blood.)
3. Crampy abdominal pain and swelling of the abdomen. These symptoms appear only after changes in bowel habit have occurred.
4. A persistent desire to move the bowels associated with little passage of stools and little relief of desire.

If you have one or more of these symptoms you should see your doctor who will take your history (including family history) and perform a physical examination including a rectal where the rectum is explored by the examiner's finger.

This preliminary examination is usually followed by further tests, such as a barium enema (X ray) or sigmoidoscopy, where a flexible tube bearing a light is passed into the rectum to its junction with the large bowel (sigmoid) and the interior area visualized. Sometimes a flexible, lighted instrument, called a colonoscope, is used for visual exploration of the higher large bowel. If suspicious lesions are seen a biopsy is taken for micro-scopic tissue examination.

For further information on colo-rectal cancer contact your local unit of the Canadian Cancer Society and ask for the booklet.

U.S. readers, contact your nearest American Cancer Society branch.

Will High-Roughage Diet Prevent Colon Cancer?

Dear Dr. MacInnis:

Is it true that a high-roughage diet will prevent cancer of the colon(large bowel)? There was a report on the radio to that effect.

I am 58 years (male) and had a successful operation for cancer of the colon ten years ago. If this preventive measure is true, then I feel it would be prudent for me to begin a high-fiber diet—just in case. Would you please give me some guidance as to the proper foods to take.

Mr. H.F.

Answer

A high-fiber or roughage diet will not *prevent* cancer of the colon but the risk can be reduced "dramatically and fairly quickly" by adopting a high-fiber diet. Such is the recent declaration of the National Cancer Institute. According to Dr. Jane Henney, a deputy director, the average person consumes from 10 to 20 grams of fiber a day. This should be doubled to about 35 grams daily, said Dr. Henney. And fat intake should be reduced to 30 percent from the present 40 percent of total calories eaten.

It is relatively easy to meet the optimum daily fiber requirements of 35 grams. The cancer Institute tells you how by simply adding three high-fiber foods every day. An example would be a bowl of whole-fiber cereal with a sliced banana or berries to make up two high fiber foods. To this add a bowl of pea or bean soup, a vegetable salad, and a slice of coarse bread—and there you have it.

As for reducing fat in your diet, the Institute advises to cut down on foodstuffs containing the highest amount of fat. In ascending order these are: ground meats, hot dogs and luncheon meats, full-fat dairy products, cookies and other pastries, ice cream and frozen desserts, salty snacks such as potato chips and nuts, fried chicken and fish, and gravy and meat sauces. But cheer up! They're *not* forbidden. Just cut down.

Many years ago, Dr. Denis Burkitt, a British doctor practicing in Uganda, East Africa, noted the relative absence of large bowel disorders, such as diverticulitis and cancer in his patients—all of whom ingested a very large daily amount of roughage in the form of fruits and vegetables. Similarly, the cancer institute has studied groups of people in America who have a low incidence of large bowel cancer such as the Mormons and the Seventh-Day Adventists. All of these people consume a high fiber diet.

And then there's the oft-quoted observation of the 13 percent decrease of breast cancer deaths in wartime England and Wales, when the consumption of cereals, fruits, and vegetables was very high and dietary fat very low.

It is estimated that these dietary changes could in fifteen years, prevent 29,000 deaths from colon cancer in the United States every year. And there's evidence that the same measure could reduce the breast cancer deaths by about 30 percent, but may take a little longer than in the case of colon cancer to achieve it, said Dr. Henney.

Despite the fact that you are free clinically of cancer of the colon, you should still, I believe, adopt the prudent course to help prevent a possible recurrence.

Marked Drop in Stomach Cancer

Dear Dr. MacInnis:

I read recently that cancer of the stomach is not nearly as prevalent in the United States as it used to be. If this is so, what appears to be the reason?

Mr. K.M., California

Answer

What you read is right and no one knows exactly why. In the 1930s stomach cancer was the most frequent cause of cancer death in the United States. Since that time the death rate has dramatically dropped from 25 per 100,000 to a present-day 6 per 100,000.

One engaging theory for this drop is that with the advent of almost universal home and industrial refrigeration sixty years ago, there has been a marked reduction in the consumption of pickled and smoked food products, thought to be a cause of stomach cancer. Another factor could be the much easier availability of fresh and frozen fruits and vegetables in our diet.

(Though Japan has the highest rate of stomach cancer in the world, the children of Japanese immigrants to the United States enjoy the low American rate, which again suggests a nutritional cause.)

Cancer of the Pancreas

Dear Dr. MacInnis:
My husband, age 63, has just been diagnosed as having cancer of the pancreas. He has lost considerable weight, as his appetite is poor. The doctors have given a very poor outlook for this condition and tell me it is too late for surgery. Is there any other type of treatment that might help him? I have just about given up.

Mrs. D.R., Ontario

Answer

It is not easy for me to affirm what your doctors have told you, but since you are well aware of the outcome, you have made it less difficult for me and for this I thank you.

For the information of other readers, I can state that cancer of the pancreas has the lowest survival rate of all cancers. There is no treatment other than surgery, and that must be performed very early for any measure of success. The procedure involves total resection of the pancreas (Whipple operation). Again, in the early case, chemotherapy and radiation may improve survival.

According to specialists in the field, the only advance in the management of this dreadful cancer is early diagnosis—mainly by ultrasound that allows earlier treatment with a better prognosis.

Don't Give Up on Cancer of the Pancreas

Dear Dr. MacInnis:

I have just read your reply to the lady whose husband was diagnosed as having cancer of the pancreas.

I would like to comment that while all your medical pronouncements are true, there is still hope. A person can never just give up. There is still living to do; one takes only a brief time to die.

I, myself, have been diagnosed as having a malignant brain tumor and am under "palliative care." But I will not just give up. Just because a team of medical doctors say your time has come does not necessarily make it true. No one should play God.

You must have hope and a belief in yourself. You have to work to stimulate your immune system. You can conquer cancer and I am going to do so.

There is a book out called The Cancer Conqueror *by Greg Anderson, and it is a wonderful book for people like myself and the lady who wrote you that letter.*

I just wanted to write and comment on your reply and I thank you for listening.

I don't want my name, address, or anything pertaining to my identity revealed as this is at present a very close family secret.

Answer

I am sure readers who have cancer or other serious problems will be inspired by your letter.

The Cancer Conqueror that I recommended some time ago to a reader received a tremendous tribute from Abigail Van Buren in her "Dear Abby" column.

I am pleased to report that it is now published in paperback and is available in most bookstores in Canada and the United States.

Duragesic for Cancer Pain

In the last few years I've written about the transdermal (skin patch) delivery of various medications. Two come to mind: a nitroglycerine skin patch for angina and a scopolamine patch for motion sickness. The value of transdermal delivery is that it predictably and systematically secretes its medication over a specified period, minimizing to some extent its "peaks and valleys" of effectiveness. Minimized, too, are the drugs' side effects, and being non-invasive, they are readily accepted by all patients.

Today, I was introduced to another transdermal product, Duragesic, recently approved by Health and Welfare, Canada's Health Protection Branch (equivalent to the U.S. Federal Drug Administration), which is the first cancer pain medication in a transdermal patch. This new treatment system developed by Janssen Pharmaceuticals offers continuous relief for seventy-two hours with fewer side effects and a higher safety profile than traditional medications. It is specifically designed for stable cancer patients with moderate to severe chronic pain.

It is estimated that between 20 and 50 percent of cancer patients have pain severe enough to justify using opioids (e.g., morphine), yet *up to 25 percent will die without adequate pain relief.* For those whose pain is severe and long term, Duragesic is particularly applicable.

"Almost seven million patient days of clinical experience in the U.S. confirm the value of Duragesic for treating the chronic, excruciating pain of cancer," says Dr. Mary Simmonds, assistant professor of medicine at the Pennsylvania State University College of Medicine. "The combination of a convenient, safe administration method and a proven, effective medication make Duragesic ideal for use with patients requiring long-term potent opioids for relief."

In an article published in *Clinical Pharmacy,* vol. 11 (January 1992) the authors concluded that Duragesic "may be particularly appropriate for outpatients or institutionalized individuals with relatively constant chronic pain who are medically stable and require opioid analgesics (pain killers) but who are unable to ingest oral (by mouth) drugs because of vomiting."

Duragesic is not a new drug. Its generic name, fentanyl, is a potent synthetic narcotic analgesic with pharmacological effects similar to morphine or Demerol and has been around since the early 60s.

The side effects associated with Duragesic include transient and mild skin reactions to the patch; other adverse events common to other narcotic analgesics (constipation, sedation, confusion) are reported as being mild. Specific advantages of Duragesic include convenience and prolonged efficiency leading to an improved quality of life, noninvasive administration (i.e., no needles), the absence of stomach side effects, and its overall safety.

And again quoting Dr. Simmonds: "Duragesic satisfies the need for more effective yet convenient and uncomplicated pain management. It also overcomes caregiver concerns about medicinal misuse, reducing the costs associated with health care, and maintaining patient independence."

Of interest to doctors and other caregivers, the Duragesic transdermal patch is available in four strengths: delivering 25, 50, 75, or 100 micrograms per hour depending on the severity of the pain (a microgram is 1 millionth of a gram).

What are some important spin-offs from Duragesic therapy for intractable cancer pain? Remember the 25 percent of cancer patients who will die without adequate pain relief? It will provide for their comfort and that in itself would make it all worthwhile. Equally important is that in cancer patients where intractable chronic pain is the predominant symptom, most of them can now, thanks to Duragesic, be adequately managed at home.

Malignant Melanoma

Dear Dr. MacInnis:

My husband, age 55, noticed a growing dark-colored mole on his neck that the doctor diagnosed as a malignant melanoma. He was referred right away to a surgeon who cut out the mole with a wide incision. Fortunately, the cancer had not spread and two years have passed without any further problem. I understand that malignant melanoma is a very serious type of skin cancer. Could you please tell me more about it, including what causes it? Also, does it run in families? My husband's brother had a malignant melanoma. It was also cut out but last year it recurred and the doctor says that it has spread to nearby nodes. He is now on chemotherapy and doing well so far. What is immunotherapy?

Mr. O.A., Edmonton, Alberta

Answer

To say that malignant melanoma is "serious" is putting it mildly!

But let me put it in proper context. Although malignant melanoma is 100 percent fatal if allowed to spread, it's 100 percent curable if caught in time and cut out. Microscopic examination of the excised mole and surrounding tissue will determine whether or not the cut-out is successful. (If a melanoma is diagnosed and found to be less than 1/32 of an inch deep, it can usually be completely cured by cutting it out. If it is deeper, there's a good chance that it has spread and is then highly lethal.) If everyone handled suspicious moles like your husband and brother-in-law, there would be few deadly melanomas.

But in the real world where people just put it off until too late, they become some of the estimated 7,000 malignant melanoma deaths a year in the U.S. (with a proportionate 700 to 800 in Canada).

What should arouse your suspicion about a skin mole? The U.S. Skin Cancer Foundation has published a booklet called "The ABCDs of Moles and Melanomas" that I am reprinting in part to help you decide. I would strongly suggest that, if after studying your ABCDs, you have even the slightest doubt, then see your doctor. Here they are:

A— is for A-symmetry (out of symmetry). A normal mole is round. An early melanoma loses its roundness and symmetry.

B— is for Border. A normal mole has a regular border. A melanoma, in contrast, has an uneven border.

C— is for Color. Moles normally are nearly always brown. A melanoma can exhibit a variety of colors, tan, brown, black, white, and even red. All combinations of colors can be present *in any one melanoma*.

D— stands for Diameter. Moles are usually less than a quarter inch in diameter. Melanomas are wider.

Melanomas are quite rare in black- and brown-skinned people because of a protective substance in their skin called "eumelanin." Fair-skinned persons have a much less protective skin substance called "phaeomelanin." It's the fair-skinned victim of a blistering sunburn who runs the risk of developing a melanoma later on in life.

Melanoma is not only the most curable of cancers, if discovered in time, but it's also the most preventable of cancers. Remember, use sun screen liberally and avoid like the plague that midday sun!

You ask if melanoma runs in families and what is the cause.

Yes, there are high-risk families, and these constitute about 10 percent of the 30,000 new cases of melanoma each year and rising yearly (the remaining new cases are the so-called nongenetic sporadic cases).

In the past five years, cancer scientists have been studying the genetic or hereditary aspects of these "melanoma families" and just recently they have "tracked down" a gene to chromosome 1 that makes family members highly susceptible to developing malignant melanoma. They have not yet identified the gene.

For advanced melanoma, immunotherapy in the form of lymphokine-activated killer (LAK) plus interleukin 2 or high-dose interleukin 2 alone is sometimes used with marked tumor regression reported in some cases. But there can be toxicity as a side effect from either form of treatment.

Chapter 15

Osteoporosis, Menopause, and Post-Menopausal Disorders

Over the years, I've written many times on osteoporosis. In almost every column the question of dietary and supplemental calcium came up and as a dutiful scribe, I reported faithfully the prescribing trends of the day.

But now, in retrospect, I feel I should have discerned as long as five years ago that the heady hype in calcium supplement advertising was clearly getting out of hand. Yes, there were some muted protests from the medical profession, but when you compare their meagre publicity resources with Madison Avenue multimillions, there was a resounding "no contest."

In a column a few months ago, I did report that there was increasing doubt being expressed in scientific circles about the value of calcium supplements alone in the prevention of post-menopausal osteoporosis. The consensus: "It has not been scientifically proven."

So kudos to the Osteoporosis Society of Canada for its steadfast reluctance to officially endorse in principle the concept of calcium supplementation per se in the prevention and treatment of osteoporosis. Rather, it has always referred the prescribing of calcium (with or without estrogens) to the discretion of the doctor.

The society's stance on calcium supplements has again received support from a study by Riis and associates published in the *New England Journal of Medicine* 316 (1987):173–77.

They studied the effect of calcium supplements to prevent bone loss in forty-three women in their early post-menopausal period. They received *one* of three treatment regimens: estrogen, 3 milligrams (by needle) daily; calcium tablets, 2,000 milligrams daily, and a placebo (a dummy inert pill). To determine the effect of each treatment, measurements of the spine, forearm, and total mineral content were made.

Results: Those taking the placebo showed progressive loss of mineral content in all three measurements. Those receiving estrogen (progestin added) after the second year evidenced no bone loss. Those on calcium alone showed approximately the same mineral loss at those on placebo.

Conclusion: Dietary calcium supplementation in the dosage used cannot retard early post-menopausal bone loss and is not an alternative to estrogen/progestin therapy.

Estrogen replacement therapy for post-menopausal osteoporosis has not been devoid of controversy. Despite its well-documented benefit, there was always the lingering feeling on the part of the patient, and her doctor, too, that its long-term use might be associated with an increased risk of breast cancer. This doubt is expressed frequently in this chapter, and I am glad to discern a strong desire in the literature to dispense both estrogen and progestin in the very minimal effective dosage. Perhaps some day soon, synthetic parathyroid hormone (reported in this chapter) will be the definitive answer. The remainder of the chapter is taken up with menopausal and post-menopausal problems, which I hope will be informative and even comforting to the patient.

Osteoporosis: What Is It?

Dear Dr. MacInnis:

My mother, age 62, stumbled and broke her hip. X rays showed a condition called osteoporosis that the doctor said caused the hip bone to break. Is osteoporosis common and is there any way to prevent it?

Mrs. T. Y., New York

Answer

Your mother is one of the 300,000 American woman who last year suffered a fractured hip from osteoporosis. Of this number about 30,000 died within three months from complications, making it the twelfth leading cause of death. An estimated five million women in the United States are affected by osteoporosis.

It is unfortunate that the diagnosis of osteoporosis is nearly always made (by X ray) after a fracture has occurred, or when an X ray has been taken for some unrelated condition. No wonder it's called the "silent thief."

Osteoporosis means loss of bone density due mainly to loss of calcium in the bones. In your mother's case the loss of calcium in her bones is most likely related to insufficient calcium in her diet along with a loss of female sex hormone that naturally occurs at the menopause. Osteoporosis reaches its peak about ten years after the change of life. Males, too, can develop osteoporosis as a result of loss of male sex hormone.

In the 60- to 75-year range, women with osteoporosis outnumber men two to one, but in the very old (85 plus) there is no sex difference.

With the loss of minerals (mainly calcium) from the bones, they become brittle and break easily from a trivial cause. When it affects the vertebrae (spinal column bones), there is a forward bowing of the upper spine resulting, in severe cases, in a hunchback appearance. This is frequently seen in elderly women of slight build—the so-called "dowager's hump." Here the vertebrae literally collapse due to loss of bone substance.

The prolonged muscular inactivity of bedridden patients leads to calcium loss and osteoporosis. A bone in a plaster cast for an extended period of time shows a degree of it as well, as the bones of astronauts after a period of weightlessness in space.

Conversely, muscular exercise builds not only muscle but the involved bone as well. This is one of the basics in preventing osteoporosis.

Finally, osteoporosis may be a preventable condition. Dr. Robert Lindsay, director of the Regional Bone Center at the Helen Hayes Hospital in New York, said recently that if we did these three things we could reduce osteoporosis by 75 percent: (1) increased calcium in the diet (two or more grams daily), (2) maintained a regular vigorous exercise program, and (3) determined bone density at menopause and took estrogen if indicated.

The Pain of Osteoporosis: What Causes It?

Dear Dr. MacInnis:

I am a woman in my late sixties in good health except for osteoporosis that is not too well controlled with both female hormone and a high-calcium diet, 500 milligrams of calcium carbonate, plus a daily exercise program. My problem is a curvature of the spine that causes a continuous gnawing pain in the back where the hump is. The doctor says there is no fracture.

What causes pain in osteoporosis?

Mrs. L.

Answer

The cause of pain in your case is most likely the "squashing" of several vertebrae on one another on the front of your bent spine. This is not exactly a fracture as we know it, but can be just as painful. As the long bones thin out, they become susceptible to regular fractures such as of the hip bone and wrist, the commonest fracture sites in osteoporosis.

Your present plight, Mrs. L., indicates that despite the completeness of your treatment program (except for a rather low-calcium supplement intake), you are still suffering the ravages of osteoporosis, a condition that afflicts one in every four women over the age of 50. Males, too are not immune. It can hit them a decade or two later.

It's becoming increasingly apparent that calcium, although playing an indispensable role in the "mineralization" of bone, has been oversold both in the lay and medical media by the current hype, not on dietary calcium, but on the so-called calcium supplements. Some say that the benefit of calcium supplements in preventing calcium loss in bone has never been scientifically proven. Others declare that estrogen (female hormone) is the all-important ingredient in management. All agree that prevention, starting about the age of 45, would be the "ultimate cure," ideally forestalling osteoporosis in later years. The trouble is that nobody knows what constitutes "ideal prevention." And although estrogen and adequate dietary calcium might seem a good prevention package, there's always the lingering controversy over long-term estrogen usage.

But there may be good news ahead. Researchers at the University of Toronto and Canada's National Research Council—Drs. Cherk, Tam, and Wing, have produced a new synthetic parathyroid hormone from the human parathyroid gland (using DNA technology) that has shown great promise in stimulating bone formation in laboratory animals.

Parathryoid hormone "parathormone," derived from the parathyroids (four small nodules embedded in the thyroid gland) has long been known as an important controller of calcium levels in the body. It has been successful in treating human osteoporosis, but high cost prohibits its general use.

The newly cloned parathyroid hormone (at time of writing still without a name) can be cheaply mass produced. And if it's as beneficial in human osteoporosis as in animal studies, this might be the ideal prevention package—adequate dietary calcium and a safe inexpensive hormone. All of which provides little comfort to you, Mrs. L., with your intractable pain from osteoporosis.

I would recommend that you discuss with your physician the question of using etidronate (discussed in the next column). An alternative would be Calcimar (calcitonin-salmon, USV Laboratories), but it suffers the drawback of daily needle administration and close medical supervision.

For further information on osteoporosis write to Osteoporosis Society of Canada, Suite 601, 76 St. Clair Avenue, Toronto, Ontario M4V 1N2.

Etidronate for Severe Osteoporosis

Dear Dr. MacInnis:

I'm told I have two compression fractures of my spine as well as osteoporosis. I am a male in my late sixties.

Would you please comment on these two conditions, such as the prognosis of each. I am quite interested in knowing whether I must simply learn to cope with this pain or if there's some

*medication that would help, or if it would be wise to consider
some type of operation. At present I am taking extra strength
Tylenol along with Advil. Thanking you in advance.*

Mr. G. L. D., Rochester, New York

Answer

I presume that your two vertebral fractures are due to your
osteoporosis, which must be quite severe.

In my opinion there's nothing in the way of surgery to fix
the compression fractures. What you need now is preventive
treatment for your osteoporosis to eliminate or at least limit the
occurrence of further fractures.

For this I would recommend a drug called Didronal, which
has been for some years quite effective for a bone disorder known
as Paget's disease of bone. More recently it has been found very
beneficial for increasing the bone density in severe osteoporosis,
according to an article in the *New England Journal of Medicine*
322 (1990):1265–1271. Here it was reported that over a two-year
period of taking Didronal (generic name, etidronate), the rate
of new vertebral fractures in post-menopausal osteoporosis was
reduced by 50 percent.

These results were confirmed in an even more recent study
published in the *New England Journal of Medicine* 323 (1990):
73–79.

Etidronate (Didronal) is available on prescription in the
U.S. I suggest that you discuss this recommendation with your
physician.

Provera to Help Prevent Uterine Cancer

Dear Dr. MacInnis:

*I am confused about the drug Provera. We are three friends
who go to different doctors and we've all been on Premarin (conju-
gated estrogen) for post-menopausal problems for the past fifteen
years. Let's call ourselves A, B, and C.*

A has one ovary removed due to cysts. She takes Premarin for twenty-one days and stops for seven days. During the last nine days of Premarin, her doctor prescribed Provera (5 milligrams per day). She is 68.

B is also 68. During the last eleven days of the Premarin treatment, she took ½ tablet (2 ½ milligrams) of Provera, but very heavy bleeding occurred and her doctor took her off the Provera.

C is 63 and had a complete hysterectomy (total uterus and ovaries removed) at age 50. During the last seven days of the Premarin, she takes two tablets (10 milligrams) of Provera.

In a previous column on estrogen replacement therapy, you said that Provera was given to keep the lining of the uterus "healthy" so as to prevent cancer of that organ.

My question: Why would the heaviest dosage be prescribed for C when she didn't have a uterus?

Mrs. B. J.

Answer

Provera is the brand name for methyl progesterone acetate, or progestagen. According to the *1993 Compendium of Pharmaceuticals and Specialties* (our "Blue Book"), the action of Provera is to inhibit gonadotropin production, which in turn prevents ovulation.

Indications: "For dysfunctional uterine bleeding due to hormonal imbalance. As adjunctive and/or palliative treatment of endometrial (uterine lining) cancer. As adjunctive and/or palliative treatment of hormonally dependent, recurrent breast cancer in post-menopausal women."

As you mentioned, I reported that there is indeed a link between estrogen replacement therapy and endometrial (uterine lining) cancer, and Provera is commonly employed here as a cancer-preventive agent.

But to be effective, Provera requires the presence of a uterus to work on. It would appear that if your story is correct, Mrs. C is receiving treatment for a nonexistent one!

Should I Have My Womb Out?

Dear Dr. MacInnis:

I hope you can help me with my problem as you have helped others. Here are the details.

I am a woman in my early fifties who has had three children. A Pap test done last year was "suspicious." This was followed by biopsy of the cervix, which was normal. No cancer.

The doctor then advised me to have a hysterectomy, which I am not thrilled about. She said I have a strong chance of getting cancer, and this despite the fact that I've never had a positive Pap in the past—only "suspicious," requiring repeats.

Now, my question: Can one have cancer of the womb with a Pap test okay? And should I have my womb out?

Mrs. L. W.

Answer

A positive or negative Pap test has only to do with the state of affairs on the surface of the cervix. Yours was "suspicious." You then had a cone biopsy of the cervix and it was negative for cancer. It can therefore be assumed that you do not have cancer of the cervix.

Yes, you can develop cancer of the womb independently of the cervix. But you have given me no evidence that you have cancer of the womb or a "strong chance" of getting it.

But perhaps the doctor knows something I don't. Should you have a hysterectomy? As a medical columnist, my professional advice is only appropriate as general advice. I never specifically "diagnose" or "treat" from long distance.

And my general advice to anyone in your predicament is this: Always get a second opinion from a specialist gynecologist.

Is There Life after Menopause?

Dear Dr. MacInnis:

Do women really ever get over the menopause or is it just relative, with some faring better than others? I'm five years into it, and although I've learned to live with the hot flashes, sex is becoming an ordeal for me, being very painful indeed. I have used various types of vaginal creams, some containing hormones, but they have been of little help. If it wasn't for a kind and understanding husband, our marriage would have been on the rocks years ago. We are trying to make the best of it, hoping that there is life after menopause. Any suggestions in the meantime?

Mrs. X (49)

Answer

If what you say is correct, you are receiving some pretty awful medical advice, if indeed any guidance at all. It seems incredible that here you are, teetering on the brink of a broken marriage with help no further away then your nearest caring physician or gynecologist.

I am referring of course to estrogen replacement therapy (ERT) that makes up for the female hormone lost at menopause. Loss of this hormone (17 beta-estradiol) mainly accounts for the telltale "change of life" signs and symptoms of hot flashes and flushes, night sweats, vaginal dryness causing painful sex, and a host of emotional disturbances. It is estimated that 75 percent of menopausal women suffer from one or more of these problems.

Results of a recent poll of 500 menopausal women on ERT indicate that estrogen plays a significant role in controlling symptoms and enhancing a woman's self-image and outlook on life. Approximately 90 percent cited estrogen as improving their hot flashes. About half the respondents said that once on ERT they felt "more healthy" than before, while more than half again perceived that their bodies functioned better overall since taking treatment, and this included sexual function.

According to Dr. Lila Nachtigall, professor, Department of Obstetrics and Gynecology at the New York University Medical Center, the above-mentioned poll data confirm on a broad scale some of her own findings from twenty years of clinical research and practice. Says Dr. Nachtigall, "For the menopausal woman who suffers symptoms, estrogen can make the difference between a healthy productive life and one marred by continuing discomfort and resulting fatigue."

"Menopause is a sexual turning point for most women," according to Dr. Philip Sarrel, associate professor of psychiatry at Yale University School of Medicine, and adds that "a woman's intimate relationship may be suffering, and in some cases a woman may not fully realize that the sexual problems impacting negatively on her sexuality are menopause related."

And to again quote Dr. Nachtigall, "ERT can definitely enhance sexuality for many menopausal women and they should know that help is available."

The newest and probably the most dependable delivery system of ERT is the Estraderm patch containing estradiol (the same kind of hormone produced by the woman's own ovaries). Worn on the abdomen, the patch delivers estradiol directly to the bloodstream. In this way it has the advantage over oral (by mouth) administration in by-passing the liver, thus permitting an extremely small dose to be consistently delivered to target organs. The patch is applied twice weekly.

Note: ERT may not be appropriate for some women. Therefore you should always consult your physician for personal advice.

Hot Flushes and Flashes: Are They the Same?

Dear Dr. MacInnis:
Is the term "change of life" the same as "menopause," and what does the term "climacteric" mean? And finally, are they "hot flushes" or "hot flashes"?

Mrs. K. N. (51)

Answer

The term "change of life" was probably more meaningful to your grandmother than to you. At the turn of the century the average life expectancy of a woman in this country was about 50 years. A woman's "change of life" or "menopause" took place at about 46 and more properly signalled the "end" rather than the "change" of life. But nowadays it's different. Your average life expectancy, Mrs. N., is a whopping 78! This means that you can live one-third of your life after menopause, sometimes referred to as "the best years." It marks the end of reproduction only, in contrast to animals where the end of reproduction signals the end of life.

The "climacteric" is that period of time leading to the menopause and here's where the flashes and flushes may sometimes give you a bad time. Three-quarters of women in the climacteric experience the well-known hot "flash" or "flush." The hot "flash" is a feeling of heat, while the hot "flush" is where the skin turns red and becomes visible.

He's Going through the Viropause

Dear Dr. MacInnis:

My wife, aged 56, is going through the menopause with all the usual symptoms—night sweats, hot flashes, and periods of depression. She is taking hormone pills and is feeling better.

But that's not why I'm writing. I, at age 63, have had the same symptoms going on two years and am beginning to wonder if the menopause is catching! "Male menopause" is not a very manly diagnosis, so I am reluctant to see a doctor in case he applies that label. Here's a brief outline of my various problems: marked tiredness not helped by adequate rest and sleeping. I get periods of depression or perhaps "blueness" that I think is more persistent than my wife's kind. And would you believe it, I get night sweats just as she does; in fact, worse than hers (because she's on treatment), and sex is now pretty well on the back burner—and it's my fault.

Now tell me straight, doctor, do I have it—I mean the menopause? I hope you can come up with a better name for it. Is there as good a treatment for men as you have for women, and is it common amongst men? I would certainly be relieved to know that it was and could probably live through it, but I tell you, it's rough!

Thank you.

Mr. M. N., Quebec

Answer

I believe you're in the so-called male menopause, but forget I ever mentioned it for I have the "manly" diagnosis you desire that should make you feel better already! Experts call it the "viropause" (from the Latin *vir*, meaning "man," "man of courage," "hero," and the like). It's relatively common and is said to have a wider age range of onset than in females, anywhere between 45 and 80. But some doctors are still wary.

The rationale of testosterone replacement therapy is similar to estrogen replacement in females and both are predicated on a low level of male or female hormone. Frequently the viropause may occur without a low level of testosterone and has been puzzling to doctors. But now a British clinical endocrinologist, Dr. Malcolm Carruthers, believes this seeming paradox can be explained by his theory of testosterone resistance, which, in effect, suggests that the body can increasingly resist the action of testosterone as in some cases of late-onset diabetes, where there is resistance to insulin. Dr. Carruthers has treated these testosterone-resistant cases with larger than usual doses of male hormone with notable success. However, his work has not been accepted yet by fellow clinicians, who are bothered by the possible effects from this larger than normal testosterone dosage given to the 400 test viropause patients he's been observing over the past four years. (I will keep readers informed of new developments in this exciting study.)

What would I recommend in your case, Mr. N.? I suggest that you see an endocrinologist (gland specialist) who could confirm or negate the diagnosis of viropause, both on clinical and laboratory grounds, and then you leave it to his/her good judgment to initiate treatment or not.

Relative Cost of Calcium Supplements

Dear Dr. MacInnis:

In your column about calcium absorption in the stomach you said that calcium carbonate is the most widely used calcium supplement. *You didn't mention anything about the cost. There are so many different calcium products in the market, every one a different price for the same amount, that I'm utterly confused. For instance, calcium carbonate is around eight cents a tablet, while calcium gluconate costs only three cents. Would you please untangle this mess? And what about dolomite and bone meal?*

Mrs. M. E., Toronton, Ontario

Answer

You're right, it looks like a mess and unless you read the labels carefully, it *is* a mess. What matters is the weight of elemental or pure calcium in each tablet. A calcium gluconate tablet weighing 650 milligrams contains only 60 milligrams of pure calcium—9 percent—(the rest is pure filler). A calcium carbonate tablet weighing 1,500 milligrams contains 600 milligrams of pure calcium (40 percent).

According to your pricing, eight cents buys 600 milligrams of pure calcium in a calcium carbonate tablet.

For a post-menopausal woman like yourself, the recommended daily intake is about 1,500 milligrams (of pure calcium).

Now supposing you get 1000 milligrams of pure calcium daily in your diet (two cups of skim milk have 600 milligrams, one cup of plain yogurt has 400 milligrams). That leaves 500 milligrams daily from a calcium supplement, which is roughly one calcium carbonate tablet costing eight cents or eight calcium gluconate tablets costing twenty-four cents. Calcium gluconate, then, is about three times more expensive than calcium carbonate.

Dolomite and bone meal? Both are high in calcium—22 percent and 31 percent respectively, but may be contaminated with potentially toxic metals like lead.

The Osteoporosis Society of Canada provides all the information you need on dietary and supplemental calcium. Write to them at 76 St. Clair Avenue, Toronto, Ontario M4V 1N2.

And there is an excellent booklet put out by the Dairy Bureau of Canada titled *Calcium, Your Mini Source Book*. Address: 20 Holly Street, Toronto, Ontario M4S 3B1.

Note: As this column was written several years ago, prices given are now only relative.

Calcium Carbonate Supplement for Osteoporosis

Dear Dr. MacInnis:

You write a lot about osteoporosis and one time you said that calcium pills are not nearly as well absorbed into the system as natural calcium in foodstuffs. Why is that? I take two calcium carbonate pills daily as a supplement.

Mrs. L. P. (60)

Answer

Calcium carbonate is the commonest form of calcium supplement prescribed for osteoporosis. If given on an empty stomach it requires the presence of stomach acids to be absorbed.

As you get older, the ability of your stomach to manufacture these acids is impaired. So if there's little or no acid present in your stomach, there's little or no absorption of calcium carbonate when taken on an empty stomach.

But don't despair. I bring you glad tidings. The *New England Journal of Medicine* has recently reported that calcium carbonate pills taken with food resulted in "completely normal absorption" even in the absence of stomach acids.

Rx: Take your calcium pill twice a day *during* a meal.

Chapter 16
Diabetes in the Elderly

The diagnosis of diabetes mellitus in the elderly differs from that in younger people mainly because their glucose tolerance decreases as old age progresses to about 75 to 80 years, where it remains static.

Medical management of the elderly diabetic also differs in that their manifestations are often chronic *complications* of diabetes rather than the acute metabolic changes seen in the younger adult versions of the disease.

It would be difficult to compile this chapter without injecting a personal opinion that pertains particularly to the aged patient receiving insulin. I learned long ago that it could be in the patient's best interest if (in the fortunately rare occasion) I "threw away the book," for any attempt at rigid scientific control was nearly always doomed to failure, leaving only a distraught, uncooperative, and generally sicker patient on my hands. I feel that one should operate with a realistic leeway, where the best gauge of success is the patient's clinical appearance and quality of living rather than foolish, futile attempts to adhere to strict laboratory "standards of excellence" and fail miserably.

The incidence of diabetes in the elderly is high. If we extrapolate the figures of the National Health and Nutritional Examination Survey, it suggests that when undiagnosed cases are included, between 15 and 20 percent of all people in the 65 to 74 age group are diabetic (*Diabetes* 10, [1967]: p. 126–534).

Finally the chapter concludes with the announcement of a dramatic breakthrough in the treatment of insulin dependent diabetes, an event exceeded only by the discovery of insulin itself.

Diabetes Catechism

I receive many letters from readers in the 65- to 75-year age group who tell me they have diabetes. Some are on "tablets." One is on insulin but the majority, by far, say that they have a "touch of diabetes" and are "just watching" their diets.

All showed great interest in their diabetes and for the most part were fairly well read on the subject. There were, of course, misconceptions and occasionally expressed total myths!

The most concerned, and rightly so, were true diabetics who were well versed in the care of the feet, such as avoiding poor fitting shoes and, whether or not they realized it, were practicing good preventive medicine in their efforts to stave off chronic foot infection and gangrene. Two concerned elderly diabetics had eye problems, one with cataracts and the other with poor circulation in the retina (back of eye).

While it's true that diabetes in the elderly is often "overdiagnosed" it is nevertheless important that it be "picked up" in its early stage. This allows the doctor to give advice on the control and prevention of circulation problems in the legs, eyes, and kidneys. And why is diabetes in the elderly "overdiagnosed"? Mainly because a blood sugar reading that may be diagnostic of diabetes in a young adult is not necessarily so in an oldster. In other words, a "diabetic" reading in, say, a 30 year old may be perfectly normal in a 70 year old.

And then there are differences in the manifestations of diabetic symptoms, e.g., frequent urination, excessive thirst, loss of weight, and tiredness. The elderly diabetic may have none of the symptoms. The diabetes may have been discovered accidentally in the course of a medical workup for something else, which usually turns out to be a complication of diabetes such as cataracts, boils and carbuncles, recurrent fungus infections, and perhaps the most common complication—rectal and/or vaginal itching.

Although much commoner in the elderly, diabetes is generally less severe and, in the majority of cases, managed successfully by diet, weight control, and programmed exercises. Oral (by mouth) tablets are used occasionally in selected cases and insulin rarely, certainly in the "old old" (over 80).

Here is a sampling of the most frequently asked questions about diabetes in the elderly, to which I append a brief answer—brief, not by design, but because of space limitations. For more detailed comment please consult your family physician.

Here is your "Diabetes Catechism." Paste it on your fridge door.

Q. Is diabetes more common in the elderly than in the young?

A. Yes. For example, about 5 percent of 75 year olds are truly diabetic (0.25 percent of the population). This does not take into account yet undiagnosed diabetes. (See following columns.)

Q. Can you have diabetes and not know it?

A. Yes, this is true for all ages but more so for the elderly. As aforementioned, the elderly tend to present the *complications* of diabetes.

Q. Does diabetes run in families?

A. Yes, a familial tendency is seen in the so-called "non-insulin dependent diabetes mellitus (NIDDM), the kind most frequently found in the elderly.

Q. Does age affect glucose tolerance?

A. Yes, glucose "tolerance" is reduced in the elderly.

Q. What is the formal fasting blood sugar in a 70 year old?

A. Quite a bit higher than the "normal" for a young person. For instance, a blood sugar of 130 milligrams per deciliter (7.2 m/l) would be diagnostic of diabetes in a 30 year old. In a 70 year old with this reading, I wouldn't be so concerned. It very well could be "normal for age."

Q. When would you be quite concerned?

A. When it's over 140 (7.7) certainly.

Q. Then what would you do?

A. If there was sugar in the urine as well, I would make a diagnosis of diabetes then and there. If there was no sugar in the urine and the blood sugar was 140 (7.7) or more I would order a two-hour glucose tolerance test.

Q. Then what?

A. If your two-hour blood sugar is found to be one and a half times your age plus 100, I would consider you have diabetes. At age 70 that would be a two-hour level of 205 (11.3). This is a pretty reliable "rule of thumb."

To sum up: The diagnosis of diabetes mellitus in the elderly is not easy because of: (1) different blood sugar "normals" for the aged and the young, (2) absent or different manifestation of symptoms in the elderly, and (3) lack of strict diagnostic criteria to guide the doctor in diagnosis. (Note: American blood sugar reading is followed by its Canadian equivalent [in parentheses]. To convert American to Canadian, multiply by conversion factor 0.0551. [American is in milligrams per deciliter (mg/dl); Canadian is in minimols per liter (mmol/L).])

NIDDM versus IDDM

Dear Dr. MacInnis:

My father, age 81, has had diabetes for about ten years. He is on twenty units of NPH Insulin daily and according to his doctor is well controlled. I know several old people my father's age who have diabetes and all are on pills. My question is this: Why is my father on insulin when the others are all getting along okay on pills?

Mrs. L. B.

Answer

I cannot comment on your father's case specifically, as it's not my policy to "personalize" treatment by mail.

But you've given me the opportunity to answer, in a general way, a very valid question.

About 90 percent of all older diabetics are non–insulin dependent. This means they do have insulin-producing cells in their pancreas. But these specialized cells are "lazy" and require the stimulation of diabetes tablets to produce their natural body insulin. This non-insulin diabetes mellitus (NIDDM) used to be called Type 2 or "maturity onset diabetes" because it begins in adult life. The most serious acute complication of NIDDM, hyper-osmolar coma (HC) is uncommon and managed in the same manner as the so-called diabetic coma encountered in insulin dependent diabetes mellitus (IDDM).

The other 10 percent of elderly diabetics have an absolute deficiency of body insulin due to a lack of beta cells. They have what is now called insulin-dependent diabetes mellitus (IDDM). It used to be called Type 1 or "juvenile onset diabetes" because it usually begins in childhood. Here, diabetes tablets are of no use and the body's insulin deficiency must be replenished with insulin by needle. (Insulin cannot be taken by mouth because it is destroyed by small intestine juices.) There are at least a half-dozen brand names of diabetes tablets—the so-called sulfonylurea group of beta cell stimulators, all differing in the speed and duration of the sulfonylurea action on beta cells to produce natural body insulin. Some, like Tolbutamide, are short acting and need more than one tablet daily. Diabenese, on the other hand, is long acting and only one tablet daily is usually needed. Only your physician can decide what kind of diabetes tablet is the most appropriate. Cost, too, is a factor.

Your question, Mrs. B., regarding the indications for insulin treatment in an elderly patient with diabetes, can now be answered. Generally speaking, the patient must be switched to insulin when he or she responds poorly to tablets and a dietary regimen. There may be acid bodies (acetone) in the urine as well as sugar and the fasting blood sugar may be well over 250 milligrams per deciliter (14 m/l) most of the time. I would presume that your father's diabetes would present some or all of these features. A rule of thumb is that if insulin requirements are above twenty-five units a day, the chance of a successful switch to tablets is remote.

Please check with your nearest Canadian Diabetic Association branch for information on all aspects of diabetes. American readers please write to the American Diabetes Association. (The local branch address and phone number is in your phone book.)

Note to Mr. T. L., Fort Myers, Florida: "Peripheral neuropathy" means nerve problems in upper and/or lower limbs caused (in your case) by diabetes. Common symptoms in the legs are pain, tingling, and burning sensations. But the commonest complaint I get from readers—burning soles—is usually not due to diabetes at all. This "burning" sensation arises from damaged nerve endings in the sole of the aging foot arising from loss over time of its natural protective pad of elastic tissue. These damaged or irritated nerves transmit bizarre messages to the brain and are wrongly interpreted there as "burning" soles, even though the sole may be cool to touch. It's always at its worst at night in bed. Here's a case of your nerves really playing tricks on you! Treatment is unsatisfactory. An antihistamine at bedtime may be helpful because of its sedative property (see "diabetic neuropathy" in an upcoming column).

A Chronic Diabetic Infection of the Foot

Dear Dr. MacInnis:

Have you any advice to offer my husband with a chronic foot infection from long-standing diabetes? It started out about six months ago with an infection around the nail of the left big toe. The infection gradually spread to the foot and a chronic ulcer developed, which has not been helped by antibiotics. Sometimes it seems to improve but it always breaks down again. The foot is so painful that he cannot bear weight and has to get around with crutches. He takes forty units of NPH Insulin and twenty of Toronto daily. He is 48 years old.

Mrs. T. J., Toronto, Ontario

Answer

What you have described is one of the serious complications of diabetes mellitus. This chronic diabetic foot infection is exceedingly difficult to treat even with expensive intravenous antibiotic therapy. Diabetes causes accelerated vascular deficiency with diminished blood supply to the tissues of the feet. This may proceed to gangrene of the toes that can extend up the foot and leg and often there is little that can be done except amputation.

Recently some very exciting research and treatment of diabetic foot infection has been reported from the Veterans Administration Medical Center in Buffalo, New York. Dr. Thomas Beam and associates treated forty-one patients suffering from severe chronic diabetic foot infection with a new quinolone antibiotic called ciprofloxacin (brand name Cipro) that can kill "a broad range of bacteria" and is reported to be well tolerated. The forty-one patients were started on the intravenous form of the ciprofloxacin and later put on the oral (by mouth) tablet. Three to ten days later they were discharged from hospital and then treated as outpatients on the tablet every twelve hours.

Result: Of the forty-one patients, thirty-eight "were either cured or significantly improved," reported Dr. Beam.

Ciprofloxacin is available by prescription both in the U.S.A. and Canada.

A Case of Diabetic Neuropathy

Dear Dr. MacInnis:

My father, age 70, with long-standing diabetes, has come down with pain and burning sensations in both feet and lower legs that the doctor calls "diabetic neuropathy." Although he is under good sugar control with insulin, the symptoms persist. Painkillers, including a strong one called Tegretol, were not very helpful and made him dopey. Another drug, used for mental depression, called imipramine was tried without success. The neuropathy is getting worse. Is there anything else to try?

Mrs. A. D., Ithaca, New York

Answer

Nerve and vascular complications of diabetes are an accelerated version of the aging process itself on these structures and, such being the case, usually defy specific treatment. There are reports that lidocaine, a local anesthetic and a drug used to treat cardiac rhythm disorders showed some promise. However, it can only be administered by vein, which limits its usefulness outside the hospital.

Based on lidocaine's success, a Danish medical group has experimented with mexiletine (brand name Mexitil) another antirhythm drug similar in action to lidocaine, but available in pill form. Their double blind study was recently reported by Dejard and others in the British medical publication *Lancet,* vol. 1 (1988): 9–11.

Nineteen diabetic patients with painful neuropathy (from no other causes) and of more than six-month duration, were treated with mexiletine oral tablets for ten weeks. *Results:* Oral mexiletine significantly reduced symptoms in all but one of the treated patients. The placebo was ineffective. They found that mexiletine could relieve the pain, tingling, itching, burning, and numbness without troublesome fall in blood pressure or any effect on tendon reflexes. It was safer, they felt, than either imipramine or Tegretol.

A word of warning: Patients must be rigidly selected for treatment with mexiletine, which may adversely affect those with associated heart disease. Side effects such as nausea and tremor are dose related, requiring careful monitoring. I would advise that only physicians thoroughly conversant with the drug undertake initial therapy.

Further investigation of mexiletine involving much larger patient populations is indeed warranted to conclusively prove its worth in the treatment of the heretofore considered intractable symptoms of diabetic neuropathy.

Please discuss the progress of this medication with your doctor.

Diabetes and Aging

What do diabetes and old age have in common? Both suffer the ravages of excess sugar. So say scientists at New York's

Rockefeller University, who believe that in diabetes, particularly advanced diabetes, excess sugar circulating in the system reacts with normal tissue proteins, generating all sorts of abnormal reactions in the body. Examples are "hardening" of the arteries, causing cardiovascular, kidney, and retinal diseases. And there's often impaired nerve function and gradual clouding of the lens leading to complete opacity (cataract). In the aging process, the same tissue changes occur, however, slowly and insidiously over a lifetime of tissue exposure to excess sugar. Diabetes, then, with its many complications, presents as a form of accelerated aging.

This reaction between certain sugar chemicals and body proteins is called "cross-linking," whose main effect on problems is to transform them from separate, flexible bodies to linked, stiff, and inflexible ones. This is especially true in the walls of arteries and contributes to the so-called hardening and narrowing, causing increased resistance to blood flow and higher pressure required to force the blood through. Cross-linked body cholesterol can change in structure from the "good" soluble kind that flushes itself out of the body systems, to the "bad" insoluble kind that hangs around artery walls, narrowing and often permanently plugging them.

It can be seen, then, that this cross-linking of sugar and protein contributes to the degradation of cells and eventual loss of function so apparent in the natural course of diabetes mellitus and indeed to the process of aging itself.

Any chemical, then, that could slow down or prevent the process of cross-linkage would provide a valuable agent in the amelioration or prevention of diabetes complications or even the ravages of mortality.

The Rockefeller scientists feel they have discovered such a chemical, called "aminoguanidine." Reporting on their newly found chemical in the June 1986 issue of *Science* magazine, the authors declare that aminoguanidine (already appearing to block cross-linking in laboratory animals) "may some day become an important drug in preventing illness common among the diabetic and the aged."

Exciting as these developments are, both in diabetes research and gerontology, there's a long, complex, and tortuous road ahead before successful human application is realized. Nevertheless, the Rockefeller scientists are optimistic that the results so far achieved in animal research will be paralleled in human testing to begin later. So don't run to the phone! Success, if achievable, is many years away.

But even now, there are interesting spin-offs, evolving from basic aminoguanidine research. For instance there's a test being developed to determine the amount of cross-linking in a person's blood which would indicate in earlier life, susceptibility to various diseases of aging that it is hoped might call on a cross-link blocking agent like aminoguanidine for remedy.

And ladies, if that oft-quoted platitude "your lines are your legend" contorts you in rage, here's a message of cheer from the Rockefeller group. They're working on an aminoguanidine ointment that they hope may block cross-linking in facial collagen (tissue building blocks) said to be the cause of wrinkles.

Perineal Itch

Dear Dr. MacInnis:

I've been reading and enjoying your column for some time and thought perhaps you might be able to assist me, as you have done for so many others.

What can be done for "perineal itch"? I have tried a few of the "over the counter" medications without much success. They seem to bring relief for a few days and then it's back to that itch. It doesn't usually cause a problem during the daytime but at night it really disrupts my sleep. I am awakened at least once during the night by the incessant itch and the severity often results in minor bleeding from my scratching. I suppose the end result of all this is the continuing disruptions to my normal sleeping pattern causing me to become irritable during daytime.

I presume there are other people also in this situation. If printing this along with your response would help them in any way, by all means feel free to do so. Thank you for any assistance.

J. M., Ottawa, Ontario

Answer

For the benefit of readers not conversant with the term "per-ineal," it refers to the perineum, that area between the legs extending from the anus to the genitals (in both sexes). Severe perineal itching—perianal (around the anus) itching and vagi-nal itching—are often a manifestation of diabetes. So my recom-mendation is for you to see your doctor for a diabetes test. If it turns out to be diabetes, treatment for it will cure the itching. If it's not caused by diabetes then your doctor will probably prescribe a steroid (cortisone) ointment. My favorite ointment for the severe itching you describe is fluocinide (brand name Lidex) ointment or cream in 0.05 percent strength. (I find the cream a bit messy.)

June 1993: Diabetes Breakthrough Announced

The ten-year Diabetes Control and Complications Trial is now completed with its momentous conclusion announced by the American Diabetes Association at their June 1993 meeting in Las Vegas. The objective of the study, the largest ever conducted, was to determine conclusively which is the better way to help prevent the near- and long-term complications of insulin depen-dent diabetes—by our usual, so-called conventional treatment or by a rigid insulin intensive regimen. Some of the well-known complications of diabetes are blindness, heart and kidney dis-ease, and neuropathy (nerve disease) that is particularly damag-ing to the legs and feet.

"Conventional" treatment meant the usual routine of tak-ing insulin twice daily, checking the blood sugar daily, and mak-ing regular visits to the doctor. "Intensive" treatment meant taking insulin three or more times a day, checking one's blood sugar four or more times a day, taking regular exercise, and making monthly visits to the doctor.

Over the years it was noted in small clinical studies that the above-noted intensive approach to treatment resulted in much fewer and less severe complications than with the usual conventional treatment, but it became clear that a much larger trial would be needed to prove it conclusively.

So in 1982 a consortium of twenty-six universities and teaching hospitals in the United States and three in Canada (Mount Sinai Hospital, Toronto; University of Western Ontario, London; and the University of British Columbia in Vancouver) inaugurated their ten-year study under the sponsorship of the U.S. National Institute of Health.

The study involved 1,440 insulin dependent diabetics, the largest trial ever and the ten-year result was nothing less than dramatic!

Patients treated intensively (as described above) had a 76 percent decrease in eye complications; diabetic kidney disease was prevented or delayed by 35 to 56 percent; and diabetic neuropathy (nerve disease), the main cause of ulceration, gangrene, and lower limb amputation, decreased by 60 percent.

However, the strict regimen is not without its complications. The four or more daily doses of insulin may lead to hypoglycemia (low blood sugar), a serious medical emergency that if not treated quickly can lead to coma and death. (Fortunately most "experienced" diabetics can "feel" hypoglycemia and take corrective measures before the condition progresses.) Nevertheless, it now emphasises the necessity and urgency for research to develop a better agent than insulin to control diabetes.

How will this new treatment routine work on our large non–insulin dependent diabetic population, the majority of whom are the elderly? This question is answered by Dr. Bernard Zinman of Toronto's Mount Sinai hospital and one of the principal researchers. According to Dr. Zinman, it should also benefit this class since they, too, develop the same complications, albeit at a slower rate. But Dr. Xavier Pi-Sunyer, head of the American Diabetes Association, points out that such an insulin intensive routine might not be appropriate for all aged non–insulin dependent (Type 2) diabetics, who often have a number of other medical conditions superimposed on the diabetes.

The implications of this discovery are far reaching, not the least being financial. Although it will require a great deal of extra provincial funding (in Canada) to implement this new approach to the treatment of diabetes, it will certainly in time drastically reduce the present cost of diabetic care, now estimated to be $2.5 billion a year. (In the U.S. it is approximately ten times this figure.)

Chapter 17
Nutrition, Vitamins, Megavitamins, and Quackery

This chapter will address a number of contentious issues where controversy has waged for many years and no doubt will continue. As a "balancer" I have included two columns dealing with two popular and less controversial topics, herbal medicine and dietary fiber.

Nutrition as a science has traditionally been poorly taught in medical schools, leaving us often at the mercy of charlatans and self-appointed "nutritional experts," to whom our patients fall easy prey. This is particularly the fate of the elderly, who consume on the average four times the quantity of prescription and nonprescription "remedies" than younger folk with much of the "over-the-counter" purchases being vitamin and nutritional products that virtually guarantee a return to the Fountain of Youth!

Readers often are confused about the benefits of vitamin and megavitamin supplements espoused by the health food industry and just as vociferously denounced by the scientific community.

It was all so easy to understand in my medical school days and indeed in my practice for many years after. We were taught that vitamins in our food were necessary for good health and even life itself, and if you were deprived of any one particular vitamin, you developed, in time, a *predictable* deficiency disease which, if not corrected by replenishing the vitamin in food or pill form, death was not a possibility but a certainty.

If your diet was deficient in vitamin C (ascorbic acid) you came down with scurvy. The same with vitamin B_1 and beriberi, vitamin B_3 (niacin) and pellagra, vitamin B_{12} and pernicious anemia, vitamin D and rickets—and so on. These were taught as irrefutable scientific facts, and still are, as well as milestones in medical discovery and progress. Prescribing was easy, too, because the average medical practitioner saw few of the abovementioned deficiency diseases (with the exception of pernicious anemia).

But it wasn't to last. The 1950s ushered in new ideas on vitamins. We were told that our patients did not need to have advanced deficiencies to enjoy the fruits of vitamin therapy. Indeed, they didn't have to be sick at all. Vitamins could make well people feel even better than well!

Then came multivitamins for so-called multiple vitamin deficiencies that along with the megavitamins (vitamins in superdosage) now hold center stage, and a very controversial one at that.

That, in brief, is the "vitamin story" experienced by all our country's medical practitioners over the past fifty years.

In the past twenty-five years, vitamin research has reached new heights of controversy and debate. No sooner had a highly respected two-time Nobel Prize winner, the late Dr. Linus Pauling, presented to the world his success in preventing his common cold and other virus infections with vitamin C in megadose, than it was completely refuted by the Food Sciences Department of the University of Toronto. As for vitamin C in cancer treatment (again espoused by Dr. Pauling), the Mayo Clinic, using 10,000 milligrams daily in advanced cancer cases, could not detect any improvement in their prolongment or quality of life.

Still the controversy rages on!

And this chapter only "skims the surface."

Herbal Medicine

Consider that more people in our world rely on herbal remedies to cure their ills than on all other medication, prescription and over-the-counter drugs combined!

The thought occurred to me on a recent visit to a Shanghai hospital, a huge institution of 3,000 beds but totally inadequate to serve the needs of that great city with a population half that of Canada!

In the well-stocked pharmacy (of proportionate size) there were ample stores of "Western" medicines. All of the latest psychotropic (mind changing) drugs were there, all with familiar names—Largactil for schizophrenia, Elavil and lithium for depression, and the omnipresent Valium, just to name a few. And for one of mankind's physical scourges of the elderly, osteoarthritis, there was not only ASA (aspirin) but also numerous brands of non-steroid anti-inflammatory drugs (NSAIDs) that I have mentioned so many times in these columns.

If I was surprised at their huge array of modern pharmaceuticals, I was totally unprepared for what I saw next. It was another similarly stocked pharmacy of herbal remedies, thousands of them, all minutely catalogued for every conceivable mental and physical ailment.

This immediately begged the question: "How," I asked my escort and interpreter (the pharmacist), "do your herbal medicines work in mental disease?" To which he replied without being too evasive, "Both work sometimes but not always." He then explained that in many cases herbal and Western drugs had common properties, and when one didn't work, the other was available. Truly, the best of both worlds!

But such therapeutic luxury is available only in the larger metropolitan hospitals. Rural China, comprising 90 percent of that vast land mass of a billion souls, is mainly dependent on herbal medications, a healing legacy, like acupuncture, backed by the experience of thousands of years. This fact was not lost to the university medical schools where "traditional medicine" comprises an important place in their university teaching curriculum.

These remarks can serve as a background to this announcement released by the American Rheumatism Association on June 12, 1987:

Chinese Herbal Remedy Found to Improve Arthritis

"A Chinese herbal medicine has been described as an effective treatment for people with rheumatoid arthritis," doctors reported. According to Tao Xue-Lian, Associate Professor in Internal Medicine at Beijing, China's Academy of Medical Sciences, an herb grown mainly in South China has been found to improve the condition in people with rheumatoid arthritis. The remedy that goes by the botanical name of *Tryptergium wilfordii hook,* and named T2 for short, was reported to have been effective for arthritis in ancient Chinese medical books.

Dr. Xue-Lian said that the herb has become more widely used in China in treating several kinds of rheumatoid arthritis and lupus, both due to malfunction of the body's immune system.

The seventy people studied were split into two groups. In the double blind study, one group was given T2 for twelve weeks and the other group a placebo [inert dummy look-alike]. Then the two groups were switched for four weeks.

Results: At the end of sixteen weeks, 90 percent of the group given T2 showed "significant improvement." How T2 works is still not clear.

Cautions a spokesman for the American Rheumatism Association, "Until many questions are resolved, T2 must be considered highly experimental. . . . People with rheumatoid arthritis should continue their regular prescribed treatment programs and contact their rheumatologists if they have questions."

Note: It's 1994 and still no word on T2. But in ancient China, that repository of medical knowledge for four thousand years, the world seems to turn a little bit slower than our frenetic pace.

Vitamin E, Antioxidant

Dear Dr. MacInnis:

I take supplementary E and C vitamins to prevent cataracts, which seem to run in my family. Although I am now 70, the optometrist tells me I have no sign of them. I can recall my mother having cataracts in both eyes at the age of 45, requiring operations. As I have not received any congratulations from my medical

*doctor (who thinks I'm just "lucky"), I am writing to you for
another opinion. In other words, could I be on the right track?*
                                        Mrs. M. M., New Brunswick

Answer

There was a time in the forties and fifties when vitamin E
was touted as the cure-all for every malady of mankind, or so
it seemed! The medical establishment almost universally
shunned it and woe to the medical doctor who was known to
secretly "self-dose" to prevent coronary heart disease, a dogma
wildly proclaimed to the medical world by the Drs. Shute and
their co-workers of London, Ontario.

And vitamin C had an equally inauspicious early history.
Remember vitamin C prevention of the common cold and cancer,
with its foremost proponent, the two-time Nobel Laureate, the
late Dr. Linus Pauling, who reportedly dosed himself with
12,000 milligrams a day regularly, and upped it to 40,000 milligrams when signs of a cold appeared. Although Vitamin C's role
in preventing or curing the common cold has been scientifically
repudiated, it is still used in huge quantities for its "drying"
effect on the early "sniffle stage."

But all is changed. I'm sure the medical world winced and
swallowed hard when it read the report of a symposium on the
biochemistry and health implications of vitamin E, sponsored
by the New York Academy of Sciences. Writing in Canada's
Medical Post, Kristen Jenkins stated, "Although many of the
findings need to be confirmed by larger double blind trials, early
results in clinical testing of the impact of vitamin E on various
disease processes indicate that this fat-soluble vitamin may (1)
improve immune response in the healthy elderly, (2) prevent
cataracts, (3) combat some of the effects of cigarette smoking,
(4) slow the progress of Parkinson's disease, and (5) prevent skin
ulceration in chronic venous insufficiency (as in varicose veins)."
Due to space limits I'll comment only on 2 and 3.

Scientists believe that free radicals (highly reactive chemicals, the result of high-energy radiation as well as oxidation
reactions in our bodies), if uncontrolled, can cause mutations,

cancer, loss of tissue elasticity, and many of the clinical manifestation of aging, such as cataract formation.

It has long been known that vitamin E is a powerful antioxidant capable of neutralizing these destructive free radicals, and, as I recently stated, researchers at the University of Western Ontario have found that of 175 cataract patients and an equal number of patients without cataracts, those without cataracts were heavy users of vitamins E and C (another antioxidant). It was also found that cataract patients had lower levels of E and C than non-cataract patients. Much more scientifically controlled investigation is warranted, the University of Western Ontario study suggests.

It is believed that free radicals may play a role in the genesis of degenerative brain disease and that antioxidants such as vitamins E and C may be useful in slowing the downhill progression of disorders like Parkinson's disease. The New York Symposium heard a study revealing that Parkinson's patients taking large doses of vitamins E and C (E 3,200 I.U. and C 3,000 milligrams daily) were able to go on an average of two and a half years longer than normal without having to take Sinemet.

Yes, indeed, vitamin E is finally coming into its own, due mainly to its scavenging property of policing, arresting, and finally wrestling down these uncontrolled free radicals, hell bent on destroying us.

Has Vitamin C Finally "Arrived"?

At long last, it looks like vitamin C has "arrived," having received an official nod of recognition and approval from the "medical establishment" (which includes yours truly).

In my medical student days we were taught that vitamin-C deficiency in the diet caused a dreadful condition called scurvy characterized by extreme debility, bleeding gums, general hemorrhages, and death. Early observers of the condition surmised (correctly) that the cause was from something lacking in the diet and one astute naval surgeon eradicated scurvy on his ship by feeding his sailors a daily ration of lime juice. The regulated administration of lime juice in the British navy began in 1795 and virtually eliminated scurvy from the naval service where to this day the British sailor is still called a "limey."

The mysterious curative agent in the lime juice (as well as fruits and vegetables) was, of course, ascorbic acid or vitamin C.

Over the years, scientists have attributed many other important life-giving functions to vitamin C, including its role in hormone production, maturation of cartilage, the synthesis of collagen, and the production of so-called memory receptors in the brain (said to be lacking in Alzheimer's disease).

More recently, research scientists believe that vitamin C plays an important role in human immune function and many studies attest to its ability as a "scavenger" to attack and neutralize free radicals, where it is thought to be more effective than either beta-carotene, vitamin E, and other antioxidants. (I have written several columns on the role of antioxidizing agents like vitamins E and C in the possible prevention of cancer, heart disease, and senile cataracts.)

But despite its ever-increasing importance in physiology, cancer research, immunology, and biology (particularly the biology of aging), the medical profession's recognition of vitamin C has been up to now somewhat less than enthusiastic.

It is refreshing, then, to see in the May 1991 issue of the *Annals of Internal Medicine* a well-researched editorial titled "Vitamin C: A New Look," where it reported on a symposium on vitamin C at the National Institute of Health (Bethesda, Maryland, September 1991).

To give readers some idea of the extent of the two-day program, I will quote from the editorial where it reports on the presentations dealing with vitamin C and cancer: "A review of seventy-five epidemiologic studies found that fifty-four studies provided statistically significant evidence of a reduced risk for cancer in persons with a high dietary intake of vitamin C."

Best Food Sources of Vitamin C

Dear Dr. MacInnis:

I am a bit confused about the proper amount of vitamin C to take daily. Would you please advise. And would you please tell me the best food sources of vitamin C.

Mrs. K. L. (87), Vancouver, British Columbia

Answer

The latest recommended dietary allowances (RDA) (released in October 1989) still advise 60 milligrams daily for healthy adults. For the first time the RDAs recommend that smokers, because they excrete vitamin C faster than non-smokers, should take 100 milligrams daily.

Here is a list of the best sources of vitamin C and the amount of milligrams found in *one cupful*. The vegetables are cooked.

Source	Milligrams of Vitamin C
Baked Potato	26
Tomato Juice	44
Cauliflower	68
Cantaloupe	68
Grapefruit juice	83
Strawberries	85
Brussels Sprouts	96
Orange Juice	97
Broccoli	98

What might happen if, over a prolonged period, you received much less than 60 milligrams of vitamin C (ascorbic acid) per day? You would be risking scurvy, long the scourge of sailors until a British navy surgeon found the cure by giving them lime juice. (Lime juice, like orange juice, is high in vitamin C and only 10 milligrams daily is necessary to prevent scurvy.) The rest of the daily RDA is necessary to carry out many key biochemical functions to maintain health, e.g., synthesis of hormones; repair of all connective tissues, teeth, bone, and cartilage, and maintaining an efficient immune system—just to mention a few.

Possible Vitamin B₂ Deficiency

Dear Dr. MacInnis:

I am a male, 78 years old. My problem is a red, sore tongue and chapped lips and cracks around the corners of the mouth. Otherwise I am in good health. The doctor took blood tests for anemia, particularly pernicious anemia, but they were all okay. I forgot to mention that I have dry, scaly, red skin around the nose and ears. I live in a very dry climate. Could this be due to the low humidity or am I lacking something in my diet?

Mr. F. M., Penticton, British Columbia

Answer

Although some of your symptoms may be due to a dry climate, I believe you should see your doctor again for possible vitamin B_2 (riboflavin) deficiency. And although you state you are "healthy," you should take a good look at your diet. Is it adequate for lots of dark green vegetables, milk, and meats, enriched cereals, and bread—all good sources of Vitamin B_2. If there's the slightest possibility that you are not eating well, you should consider taking riboflavin (vitamin B_2) 25 milligrams daily to supplement your diet.

For the information of other readers, vitamin B_2 deficiency may cause a sore, red tongue (glossitis) as well as deep fissures or ridges. Another prominent symptom of possible B_2 deficiency is burning eyes with a cloudy cornea and sometimes impairment of vision.

I should point out that B_2 deficiency is rare except in cases of severe malnutrition. Occasionally, however, so-called healthy elderly people may be malnourished and not know it, as witness the tea and toast ladies' syndrome—common amongst social recluses.

Bad News for Megavitamin Pill Poppers

It's a case of shooting the messenger, for megavitamin pill poppers, that is. For today I bear them bad tidings. Spare me, I beg of you!

411

According to a National Research Council report out of Washington, "Megavitamins and supplements of calcium and fiber are apparently useless in maintaining health." *Note:* Do not confuse supplemental with *dietary* calcium and fiber.

The 1,300-page report titled, "Diet and Health: Implications for Reducing Chronic Disease Risk," maintains that there is "no conclusive evidence of any healthful effect from the supplements now taken by 40 to 60 percent of people and that an excess of some vitamins, such as vitamin A, can be harmful."

The study recommends that when dietary supplements are taken they should not exceed the RDA (recommended dietary allowance) in any one day.

What is the RDA?

RDAs are the recommendations of a panel of scientific experts called the Food and Nutrition Board of the National Research Council. They are defined as the levels of intake of essential nutrients considered, in the judgment of the Committee of Dietary Allowances of Food and Nutrition on the basis of available scientific knowledge, to be adequate to meet the known nutritional needs of all healthy persons.

Please note that RDAs are average daily amounts of minimum daily requirements and are deliberately set to exceed the estimated requirements of most individuals.

It is well known, however, that much clinical research is being done in vitamins and supplements, and some scientists have recommended relatively high doses (many times greater than the RDA) per day on an experimental basis. In fact some researchers are on record as testifying to the safety of a certain dosage when used over a period of time (on an experimental study). I can recall reporting that a researcher stated that 200 milligrams of vitamin B_6 daily could be considered a safe dose. In the same column I mentioned that the RDA for this vitamin was 2 milligrams. This prompted a reader to write that the 2 milligrams must have been a typographical error! This indicates that the average person is not aware of "recommended dietary allowance" and is influenced solely by a variety of dosages either used in experimental medicine or by non- or quasi-medical people purveying food supplements in megaproportions.

Writing on the subject of vitamin B_6 or pyridoxine (for carpal tunnel syndrome where in one study 100 milligrams a day produced beneficial results), I made this general statement on B_6 dosage: "Although there are some studies indicating no side effects after pyridoxine dosage up to 500 milligrams per day, it is the general feeling of research scientists using pyridoxine (for whatever reason) a more conservative 200 milligrams should be the dosage of choice."

My correspondent was taking, I believe, 200 milligrams of B_6 a day but did not state the reason. He asked me to be specific. Is 200 milligrams of B_6 the accepted dosage or is it 2 milligrams as I stated? My answer went something like this: "If you are taking pyridoxine on an experimental basis for some condition, research scientists recommend a more conservative 200 milligrams per day. On the other hand, if you are a healthy person (with no disease) your RDA is 2 milligrams per day. The corollary to the last sentence is that if you are a healthy person you can obtain an adequate vitamin and mineral supply in your food." (Problems such as premature birth, inherited metabolic disorders, infections, chronic diseases, and the use of certain drugs may require special dietary allowances that are not covered by RDAs.)

Vitamins: Pros and Cons

Dear Dr. MacInnis:

I have been a devoted reader of your column for many years and have never written to you before. I am sorry that this has to be a "beef" and ending in a question I would like you to answer.

It has to do with your apparent attitude towards the use of vitamin supplements not only in the aged but for all ages. Although you were especially rough on those of us taking multivitamins to ward off various illnesses such as the common cold and even cancer, you didn't spare those of us who take vitamins even though we may be healthy. However, in a column written some months ago you wrote at length on the use of vitamins C and E in the prevention of cataracts in elderly people. Here you seemed to concur with current research and even offered to send more complete information in the way of "cataract papers," which I would like to receive if you please.

As you can see, I am getting mixed messages from you and would appreciate clarification on how you stand on the use of vitamin supplements in general for all ages.

Mrs. M. L. (RN), Ontario

Answer

Thank you for your kind sentiments which I appreciate as well as your critical concerns regarding my seemingly contradictory attitudes toward vitamin supplements.

In my many years of medical practice and more recently in the field of geriatric medicine, I have never dispensed nor have I recommended the prescribing of vitamins to healthy people eating a healthy diet. And in a decade or more of medical journalism I have not deviated from this attitude. Since you say you are a long-time reader of my columns, you may recall an especially spirited one on the subject of multivitamins and, particularly, mega-vitamins where I stated that the good citizens of this country are guzzling hundreds of millions of dollars in the form of vitamins annually that pass in virginal purity through their kidneys, rendering their total urine output analogous to a golden mother lode—the most expensive in the world!

The question of vitamin C for the prevention of the common cold and even cancer is still controversial with the majority scientific opinion that it is useless on both counts. As you correctly state, I wrote at length on all aspects of the subject but could not recommend it.

On the other hand, I have always recommended vitamin D as a supplement in winter for housebound children, and in a column on vegetarianism I recommended for its adherents vitamin B_{12} (which is also essential for patients with pernicious anemia and those who have had surgical removal of part of the stomach). In my many columns on elderly nutrition, I've stated that while the healthy senior citizen on a good nutritious diet doesn't usually need a daily vitamin supplement, the frail older

414

person frequently does, and this also goes for people of any age on a rigid reducing diet.

Again on the subject of vitamins as prevention therapy, I reported on vitamins C and D in the prevention of senile cataract. The reason I devoted a full column to this subject recently was because of the promising research being currently conducted in many parts of the world. I will continue to provide my senior readers with progress reports on this field of vitamin research.

Finally, in the July 21, 1990, issue of the *British Medical Journal* the principal researcher, Dr. S. Truswell, critically evaluated the current status of vitamin supplements. The consensus of this report was that "the ingestion of vitamins in nutritional doses results in no benefit or detriment for the general population." The article reported in passing that people who already eat well are the most likely to take vitamins while those needing them most are least likely to be on them. I recommend this *BMJ* article to all health professionals.

Thanks But No Thanks

Dear Dr. MacInnis:
Some of my friends take gobs of vitamin pills daily and urge me to do likewise. Should I go along with them? I am in good health, my appetite is good and I am healthy as far as I know.
Mrs. D. Y. (60)

Answer

If you are in good health with a good appetite, Mother Nature provides you with all the vitamins you need. However, if any of you reading this are on an extreme reducing diet, or are an alcoholic or avoid certain foods because of religious conviction or other reasons, you should consult your doctor about vitamin and mineral supplements in your diet. This also applies to frail elderly people, newborn infants, and pregnant women.

Getting back to yourself, if I were you, I would say to my friends, "Thanks, but no thanks."

Medical Quackery: Part 1

I often hear from readers, mainly up in years, who are worrying about their nutrition. Some are on the honored "sucker lists" of so-called nutrition counsellors who bombard them with the hard sell; others are confused by the bewildering array of vitamin and "food supplement" ads in popular magazines. Their corner bookstore abounds in questionable health literature plausibly presented by self-acclaimed nutritional "experts" who daily tout their theories, nostrums, and books on TV talk shows. And many of our health food stores may regularly display for all to see and buy the literary avails, sometimes of downright charlatans—all calculated to promote their wares, be they "food supplements," "natural" foods, or vitamins in extraordinarily high and dangerous dosage.

No wonder they are bewildered. And there's so little I can do except to warn them, as I've done so often before, that much of what they hear and read about nutrition in the media is nonsense—and maybe dangerous nonsense at that. A Congressional hearing in May 1984 heard testimony that what's spent on medical quackery each year amounts to $44 for every man, woman, and child in the land. Compare this to the measly $4.40 per person spent that year on legitimate cancer research.

Dr. Victor Herbert, chief of the Hematology and Nutrition Laboratory at the Bronx, New York, Veterans Administration Medical Center, is a world-recognized expert on quackery. He co-authored, with Stephen Barrett, M.D. (equally eminent in exposing medical frauds), the well-known book *Vitamins and Health Foods: The Great American Hustle* (Philadelphia: J. B. Lippincott Co., 1981).

In a feature article in the January 1986 issue of the *Observer* (an American College of Physicians publication), Dr. Herbert tragi-comically recounts how easy it is to become a nutrition "consultant." For a fifty-dollar fee he applied for a nutrition certificate in the name of his dog, Sassafras. He likes to display this elegantly calligraphed, framed document which reads, "The American Association of Nutrition and Dietary Consultants—Professional Member—Sassafras Herbert." Not to be upstaged, Dr. Herbert's cat, Charlie, applied for and received a similarly "prestigious" certificate, this time from "The International Academy of Nutritional Consultants," again at a cost of fifty dollars to Charlie Herbert's master!

Both of the above-noted organizations were closely associated with one Kurt W. Donsbach (he was board chairman of the former and founder of the latter). The two are now melded into the American Association of Nutritional Consultants that publishes a monthly magazine *Nutritional and Dietary Consultant*. And one of the editors was Donsbach, who according to the May 1985 *Consumer Report* on "Foods, Drugs or Frauds?" (May 1985) is "America's leading proponent of nutritional supplements for preventing and treating disease." In his booklet on alcohol (co-authors Durk Pearson and Sandy Shaw)—one I randomly picked from a dozen—Donsbach's curriculum vitae includes his position as "Chairman of the Board of Governors of the National Health Federation"—a politically powerful 17,000 member group that lobbies successfully for the health food industry. It's difficult indeed to wander through a health food store without encountering the well-recognized garish display of Donsbach's and similar books.

Kurt Donsbach's first brush with the law was in 1971 when he pleaded guilty to illegally practicing medicine. In 1973, a female undercover agent for the California State Bureau of Food and Drug Inspections was told by Donsbach that his strictly prescribed diet of vitamins, minerals, and an herb tea (chaparral) would control her "breast cancer." As this is written, he is being sued for $6 million by an Illinois boy who allegedly suffered liver damage after following Donsbach's booklet for treatment of his acne. For over two years he allegedly took 50,000 international units of vitamin A daily (recommended limit 10,000 IU). This booklet suggested 150,000 IU.

Nutritional fraud in all its many guises is estimated to cost in the U.S. $6 billion annually, not to speak of its danger to public health. So readers beware and always consult with a dietician registered by the American Dietetic Association. In Canada, contact your Provincial Nutritionist. (My thanks to the American College of Physicians, for permission to extensively quote from Dr. Herbert's article in the *Observer,* Jan. 1986 issue.)

Medical Quackery: Part 2—How to "Smell" a Quack

"Quackery is a multibillion dollar industry. To sell themselves, its promoters must undermine public confidence in doctors, government, and medical science itself," states Dr. Stephen Barrett, nationally acclaimed author, editor, consumer advocate, and America's best-known expert on health and nutrition fraud.

How can you "smell out" a quack? "It's not easy," says Barrett, "because quacks pretend that there's a scientific basis for what they do; they use scientific terms and suggest they are scientists ahead of their time. And an M.D. or Ph.D. title can be very misleading."

Here are a few warning signals for starters. Be suspicious of:

1. Anyone who says that everyone needs vitamin supplements "to be sure they get enough." (Most people can get all the vitamins they need by eating a varied and balanced diet.)
2. Anyone who suggests that unsuspected yeast infection is a widespread cause of many diseases.
3. Anyone who says diet is a major factor in behaviour. (There's simply no scientific evidence to back it up.)
4. Anyone who advises to "strengthen your immune system" with vitamins, minerals, amino acids, etc. (This is the latest "in" fad stimulated by the fear of AIDS. It is heinous to exploit our modern day's greatest medical and social tragedy to promote a book.)
5. Anyone who suggests that most diseases are caused by faulty nutrition and that large doses of "nutrients" are effective against a large number of diseases.
6. Anyone who suggests that emotional stress and stresses of everyday living are reasons to take vitamins. (There's no scientific proof whatsoever for this assumption, despite that

some of our nation's giant pharmaceutical companies are heavy vitamin supplement advertisers.)

7. Any practitioner who diagnoses most patients as suffering from hypoglycemia (low blood sugar). True hypoglycemia is uncommon.

In a previous column I incurred the wrath of health food people when I suggested that they might be aiding and abetting all sorts of charlatans by promoting their books. Lest I be accused of prejudice or of being a lackey running-dog of the "Medical Establishment," I will quote directly from a twelve-page booklet published by the Nutri-Books Corporation, the largest distributor of health related books and magazines in the nation. This is what they say about themselves and their books:

"Books are your silent sales force," they tell their retailers (health food stores). "Books are the 'cutting edge' of growth and direction for the nutritional food industry.

"Millions of dedicated users of health food and supplements were persuaded to make their first nutritional purchases by the books of Adelle Davis, Dr. Carlton Fredericks, Dr. Richard Passwater, Dr. Lendon Smith, Dr. Earl Mindel, Gayelord Hauser, and others.

"Books and magazines are designed like billboards. They reach out and 'grab' the customer.

"They tell your customers what your products will do for them. They explain the ways your products can be used. Very often this is information you may not be able to give or be permitted to discuss.

"Sell a pound of wheat germ and it satisfies your customers. Sell a book and it creates a whole new set of needs for your customers."

In the face of such tremendous high-pressure sell, it's little wonder that the majority of our citizens (including senior citizens) ingest millions of dollars of unneeded vitamins that are simply flushed out of the urinary system intact and down the toilet drain. (My thanks to Dr. Victor Herbert, co-author of *Vitamins and Health Foods: The Great American Hustle* [Philadelphia: J. B. Lippincott Co., 1981].)

It's Ginseng All the Way

Dear Dr. MacInnis:

I have been appointed by a group of senior club members (male) to write to you in the hope you can settle an argument among us regarding the effect of ginseng on sex. Three have reported what they term "excellent" results with the dried root, with little or nothing from the tablets; three others have been reporting success (bragging?) with ginseng tea, having got nowhere with the root. As for myself, I've given up, having tried every form of ginseng. The same thing (nothing) happened as well with elixir of antelope horns. I believe it's all in your head, but, still it's hard to argue with success. Is it or isn't it? What's your opinion, doctor, from your own experience or the experience of others?

"Born Loser"

Answer

Dear Loser:

My travels in the Orient convinced me long ago that there must be something to this ginseng thing. A billion people couldn't be all wrong. So when I asked a Chinese lady clerk what kind of cigarette I should buy for my "geriatric friends back home," she knowingly and without hesitation replied, "Ginseng," and I've never regretted her choice. (Those were the days when cigarette smoking was a semi-respected, self-pleasuring preoccupation, even in my country.)

So that's how I personally felt about it despite the bad mouthing it received from our prestigious, erudite, and somewhat staid "Medical Letter," which gravely proclaimed, "Ginseng has been described as an aphrodisiac and promoted as such, but no aphrodisiac effects have been demonstrated," and concluded that "there's no good evidence that it has any beneficial effects, and any harmful effects and possible interactions with other drugs are unknown" ("Medical Letter," August 22, 1980).

This is hardly a damning indictment but more of a verbose and neutral scientific conclusion. But no matter how you read it, I'm not concerned, for ginseng, with the oriental mystique of

420

centuries behind it, will be always a good stimulant, yea, an aphrodisiac, if only you wish it to be. And there'll always be winners and losers.

I Want to Be a Vegetarian

Dear Dr. MacInnis:
 I plan on becoming a vegetarian. Are there different types of vegetarians? Is it a safe practice?
 K. M. (60), Saint John, New Brunswick

Answer

Yes, there are at least four different kinds of vegetarians, classified according to the extent that animal sources of food are excluded. *Vegans:* These exclude from their diet *all* animal sources of food, including milk; they are *true* vegetarians. *Lacto-vegetarians:* These allow milk and other dairy products. *Lacto-ovo vegetarians:* These include eggs as well as milk and milk products in their vegetarian diet. *Semi-vegetarians:* These are casual vegetarians; they consume poultry and fish but reject saturated fats; the bulk of their diet is plant food, however.

Well-planned and prepared vegetarian diets generally pose no health hazards, particularly if milk is added to the diet. Vegans may have to take supplements of vitamins B complex and D and maybe iron and calcium.

Nutritional "Mythinformation"

Getting tired of the overwhelming barrage of nutritional "facts" and fallacies? Are you confused about cholesterol, "the good, the bad, and the ugly"? Then it's time to separate myth from reality.

To celebrate National Nutritional Month (March), Diet Center, Inc., has prepared:

421

The Five Most Common Nutritional Myths

Myth 1. "Light" or "lite" products are always low in calories. Not always. "Light" or "lite" have no legal definition. They may refer to color, texture or even taste. "Lite" products may be high in calories.

Myth 2. Avoiding eggs is the *best way* to lower cholesterol. The biggest culprit is saturated fat found in fatty cuts of meat.

Myth 3. Butter contains more calories than margarine. Both are fat, containing 100 calories per tablespoon. Margarine has no cholesterol.

Myth 4. Drinking water inhibits weight loss. Wrong. The body eliminates excess water immediately. Drink at least eight water glasses daily.

Myth 5. Taking calcium supplements will prevent osteoporosis. Wrong. Osteoporosis prevention starts with adequate calcium in the diet, but other important factors include regular weight-bearing exercises and cessation of cigarette smoking. Taking calcium pills may be beneficial if your diet should, for some reason, fall short of calcium.

Chapter 18
Hurtin' Feet and Burning Soles

Whoever dreamed up that old medical maxim "As your feet go so go you" most certainly had the old in mind and, more than likely, was a fellow sufferer!

As I mention in one of the columns in this chapter, whenever I write on old and hurtin' feet and casually mention some possible remedy, I can always expect a torrent of reader mail requesting more information or offering another remedy that worked wonders for the reader, but didn't often turn out to be the universal panacea it was thought to be. Nevertheless, I have always respected readers' "research" and many times gave them space in my columns because I feel that "nothing succeeds like success" and even if one more reader was helped, then the whole exercise was not in vain.

Take "burning feet." This is one of the commonest complaints I receive from old people, and medical science has no remedy for it let alone an explanation of what causes it. Yes, I've searched my modern medical references and geriatric textbooks, but nary a word have I seen about this scourge of the aging foot. Is it a variant of the well-known and minutely described peripheral neuritis (neuropathy), where vitamin B_6 (pyridoxine) is sometimes prescribed? Well, over the years, I've received the testimonials of many older readers and long-time burning feet sufferers who have finally found relief using that very same vitamin B_6!

Since there are a myriad of causes for hurtin' feet, many of them are dispersed throughout the book and only a few carefully selected columns have found their way into this short chapter. So heed them well!

****

Burning Feet

Burning feet is one of the commonest ailments of older people, surpassed only by constipation, gas, and waning sex. I've treated the first three with varying success but have failed miserably in the management of burnin' feet, that is, until recently.

Readers may recall the many "testimonials" I printed from grateful patients who found comfort in 50 to 100 milligrams daily of vitamin B_6 (pyridoxine). You may also recall I expressed some reservations on their enthusiasm but had to concede that one just doesn't argue with success.

That was a year ago, and letters still come in, like the one from Mrs. M. M. of Honeoye Falls, New York

Dear Dr. MacInnis:

Re your request for reaction to the use of vitamin B_6 for relief of burning feet.

After years of trying everything from soaks, powders, and cotton soles to relieve my discomfort (suffering), your recommendation seemed worth a try. Walking on my hands seemed the only alternative (at my age not practical)!

I tried 100 milligrams of B_6 (1 tablet) daily and within a week the burning was gone—like a miracle. At a cost of about one and a half cents a day I can walk through a twelve- to fifteen-hour day without discomfort.

I am an old nurse doing private duty on weekends and operating a kennel full time, so I am on the run constantly.

Thank you for the opportunity of being a "delighted guinea pig."

Answer

And thank you, Mrs. M., for your delightful letter.

The majority of patients with burning feet complain that the problem is worse at night, and many are the methods they use (usually futile) to cool off their burning soles, such as sticking their feet out from under the bed covers, playing an electric fan on them, cold water soaks, etc., etc.

I should point out that burning feet is a subjective, or "felt," sensation because the soles are not overly warm. In a previous column I have theorized as to the cause of this phenomenon. (It has not, as far as I know, ever been discussed in medical literature.) Since it occurs almost always in the soles of the aging foot where there's little padding left, I speculated that the sensory nerves in the soles become irritated and eventually damaged to the extent that they send bizarre stimuli to the brain that interprets it as a "burning" sensation.

Well, "scientific" explanation or not, the fact remains that practitioners of medicine, particularly geriatric medicine, have this formidable problem of burning feet on their hands, and it behooves them to do a bit of office clinical research with vitamin B_6, which, if successful, just might attract attention from the "research boys" out there for a scientifically conducted study.

The same mail brought another letter from Honeoye Falls, New York. Here Mr. J. M. (43) describes his experience with a condition where his feet became "red and raw, swollen and intensely itchy. . . . It would occur primarily in the wintertime," writes Mr. M., who sought medical advice and was told that since cold seemed a factor, he should try to keep his legs and feet warm. "But since my workplace was so poorly heated and insulated," says Mr. M., "this wasn't feasible."

It happened that Mr. M. later spent a winter in England. He mentioned his problem to a British friend who said, "Oh yes, chilblain—you want to take niacin (nicotinic acid) for that." Mr. M. reported a "90 percent relief of symptoms."

Chilblain is caused by the action of cold, damp weather on the circulation of the extremities (feet and hands), maybe, it is thought, in "susceptible" people. I really don't know. And why it's so prevalent in the U.K. and relatively unknown in similar climatic areas in North America, I also don't know. Is it the paucity of central heating over there?

Perhaps. But what I'm pretty sure of is that the reputed benefit from niacin (vitamin B₃) is probably due to its vasodilating (expanding) effect on the capillaries (tiny blood vessels) under the skin.

Burning Soles

Dear Dr. MacInnis:

For several months now, I have suffered from a burning sensation on the soles of my feet, irritation that is constant day and night. Tests for circulation and diabetes are normal. I am 70 and have angina but had the foot problems before my angina was diagnosed in January 1991. I would appreciate any advice.

Mr. B. W., Rochester, New York

Answer

The sensation of burning feet is one of the commonest complaints I receive from elderly people. Several years ago I wrote a full column on the subject and even proffered my "theory" as to its cause. Due to space restriction here, I can only synopsize the all-important part of that column, the treatment.

Many grateful readers with burning feet found comfort in taking 50 to 100 milligrams daily of vitamin B₆ (pyridoxine), the same dose recommended by some authorities for peripheral neuritis from "age-damaged" sensory nerves in the sole due to lack of protective padding. As I mentioned in a previous column, the brain then interprets these bizarre sensations as a burning feeling. I suggest that you give vitamin B₆ a trial for a month and see for yourself.

Hurtin' Feet: Bunions

Dear Dr. MacInnis:

I'm sure you get lots of letters from senior people complaining about their hurtin' feet and here's another for you, please. I am a firm believer in walking to keep fit but my feet can't hoof it any more with my bunions.

I hear the operation is a very painful one and a person is laid up for a long time afterwards. Can you recommend any measures short of an operation to help this condition? I am a woman 55 years old and in otherwise good health.

Mrs. A. B., Saskatoon, Saskatchewan

Answer

You're as old as your arteries and young as your feet!

I get so many foot complaints that I must soon devote a couple of columns to the subject of corns and calluses, hammertoes, metatarsalgia (pain and tenderness on ball of foot), painful heels, and, of course, your bunions—just to name a few of life's miseries. No matter how well you are otherwise, bad feet age you long before your time.

I have no way of knowing just how bad your bunions are or if there is any degree of hammertoe (usually of second toe) present or if there are calluses on the bunion or the ball or foot.

If your bunions are of the mild variety, you might get relief from bunion-last oxfords. But I have the feeling somehow that yours are quite bad and will most likely require custom-made shoes with removable innersoles so that any plantar (sole of foot) problems can be corrected if necessary.

My function as a medical communicator is to inform and advise, and here a clear-cut recommendation is necessary. See a good podiatrist (foot doctor). Don't try treating yourself. Remember the old saying that even a physician who "treats" him/herself always has a fool for a patient!

Restless Legs Syndrome

Dear Dr. MacInnis:

Can you please help me. I suffer from a peculiar condition affecting my legs for which I am told there is no cure. Just as I start to fall asleep, I get a sensation of aching and a feeling of worms crawling deep under the skin between the knees and ankles.

There is always a great urge to get up out of bed and walk and that usually gives relief. It doesn't happen every night, maybe on the average twice a week. If I am tired and can go to sleep quickly it doesn't usually occur. Have you any information on this condition? Is it a common ailment?

Mrs. K. L.

Answer

From your description it would appear that you have a condition known as restless legs syndrome (RLS). It is fairly common. In some cases it can be the result of anemia, and fortunate indeed are those who can cure it with iron medication. It can be caused by peripheral nerve complications of diabetes and chronic alcoholism, which usually defies treatment. But in many instances the cause is unknown and yours is a case in point. Classical restless legs syndrome, as you describe it, usually occurs at night, whereas the type caused by diabetes, alcoholism, anemia, and certain drugs can be present throughout the day and night. (Some mild parasthesias [nerve sensations] occur only in the still of the night when the patient is not distracted by daytime stresses.)

In a former column I stated that two antiepileptic drugs, carbamazepine (brand name Tegretol) and clonazepam (Klonopin) were often successful in suppressing some of the unpleasant, distressing symptoms of the restless legs syndrome regardless of cause. They are still prescribed, but another drug, L-dopa (used for treating Parkinson's disease, but in lower dosage), has been found successful in treating RLS on what seems to be a rational scientific background.

In *Neurology* 38 (1998): 1845–48, Dr. C. Brodeur and associates postulated that central dopamine (lacking in Parkinson's disease) might also be deficient in the restless legs syndrome and periodic sleep movements. Most patients with restless legs syndrome, they observed, exhibited periodic sleep movements, suggesting that the two conditions were manifestations of the same central nervous system disorder and akin to Parkinson's disease. Accordingly, in a scientifically controlled study of six patients over a period of seven weeks, they administered 100 milligrams of L-dopa twice a night (one hour before and three hours after bedtime).

Results: Parasthesias (restless legs sensation) recorded by the patient and confirmed by electrical muscle testing fell from 45.4 per hour after placebo (dummy pill), to 9.4 after L-dopa. Periodic sleep movements were also markedly reduced—from 236 in two nights on placebo, to 73 on L-dopa.

Although the researchers used a drug called benserazide to neutralize the side effects of L-dopa alone, others have combined L-dopa with carbidopa, which are the ingredients in Sinemet used in Parkinson's disease. I would suggest Sinemet 100-10 given at the aforementioned time schedules. Please discuss this with your doctor.

I would also strongly suggest that all patients receiving Sinemet for restless legs syndrome be under medical supervision during the trial period. It should be remembered that although Sinemet is a scientifically established treatment for Parkinson's disease, it is still only an experimental approach to the management of restless legs syndrome.

And only time will eventually prove its worth.

Leg Cramps

Dear Dr. MacInnis:
What can be done about leg cramps at night? The doctor gave me quinine for it, but it didn't help. I am 72 years old.
Mrs. L. T., California

Answer

Nocturnal leg cramps are a common affliction of the elderly and for years quinine sulphate has been the treatment of choice, indeed the only treatment for this disorder where, when you're just on the verge of slumber, your legs cry out in cramping pain.

Every time I write about nocturnal leg cramps, I can expect a flood of letters all extolling the virtues of quinine, massage, calcium, vitamins, and a host of other remedies that seem to work only on an individual basis but always fail the general test.

In the *Archives of Internal Medicine* 148 (1988): 1969–70, Dr. L. Baltodano and colleagues report on the beneficial effect of the heart drug verapamil on a group of eight elderly patients age 62 to 87 suffering from nocturnal leg cramps. All eight had been on quinine sulphate, 260 milligrams at bedtime without any benefit. Instead of quinine they all received 120 milligrams of verapamil at bedtime for eight weeks. Results: Leg cramps disappeared in seven of the eight patients under study during the eight-week trial period.

The patient sample is admittedly small, and further controlled studies are necessary. In the meantime, any patient wishing to give verapamil a trial for nocturnal leg cramps should do so only under the guidance of a physician.

The cause of nocturnal leg cramps is unknown, as is verapamil's mode of action.

Burning in Arms and Legs from Peripheral Neuritis

Dear Dr. MacInnis:

I am a male 67 years old and have been diagnosed as having peripheral neuritis with burning in arms and legs. I am presently taking two capsules of Dilantin, 100 milligrams per day.

Could you please comment on this condition and how effective this drug might be over the long run.

Mr. M. M., Ontario

Answer

"Peripheral neuritis," now more commonly termed "peripheral neuropathy," is really not a diagnosis in itself but rather a symptom or complex of symptoms involving a nerve or group of nerves affected by some existing disease. A good example is in far-advanced diabetes, where the disease over time can cause a degeneration of nerve cells in the upper or lower extremities or both (as well as the muscles they supply). It is termed "peripheral" because the nerves and muscles of only the extremities are involved. In a full-fledged case of peripheral neuropathy there may be signs of distal weakness and wasting of the muscles, loss of sensation, pain from nerve irritation, and loss of tendon reflexes when tapped with the reflex hammer.

Peripheral neuropathy (or polyneuropathy when all extremities may be involved) can be caused by literally a score of diseases. Apart from diabetes already mentioned, such conditions as hypothyroidism (low thyroid function), kidney failure, and malignant disease, for example, may all be associated with various degrees of peripheral neuropathy. Exposure to toxic agents like drugs, solvents, heavy metals, pesticides and other chemicals are examples of extraneous agents causing this type of neuropathy.

The treatment, then, of peripheral neuritis or neuropathy is the treatment (if any) of the condition causing it. Vitamin B_6 is sometimes helpful for "burning" sensations in the feet. I have no information on Dilantin as a treatment for peripheral neuropathy; in fact, I've not heard of it being prescribed as a remedy.

Plantar Heel Spur Syndrome

Dear Dr. MacInnis:

I have what my doctor calls a spur in my heel. It is very painful, and I like to walk a mile or two per day for exercise. I am a senior. I have been advised by my doctor to wear a good athletic shoe but it doesn't help much. Have you any suggestions?

Are there any (over-the-counter) medications to relieve the pain? I am not on any medication. Would Indocid help? And what are the side effects? I am very healthy otherwise.

Mrs. M. J., Saskatchewan

Answer

The commonest type of hind foot pain in men is the so-called plantar heel-spur syndrome. I stipulate "in men," because it occurs less frequently in women except in the much overweight. The heel-spur syndrome is characterized by often severe pain in the heel that is worse on initiating weight bearing, especially on getting out of bed. In over half the cases there is tenderness on pressure in the middle of the sole of the heel. In other cases tenderness may be elicited by exerting pressure on a bony prominence on the inside back edge of the heel. It is said that 15 percent of all cases of heel-spur syndrome develop into arthritis. X ray of the heel may reveal a bony spur but I should point out that normal painless heels may show large spurs; so it would seem that the bony spur, while picturesque on an X ray film may have little or nothing to do with the pain and tenderness.

According to some authorities, and this is of particular interest to female patients, wearing high-heel shoes can sometimes be helpful because they cause the foot to be thrust forward with weight bearing shifting to the ball of the foot and the heel relieved from pressure.

Treatment: First, what *not* to do. Do not have the spur removed. It will not help. Treatment is conservative. A well is cut out from the inside of the (shoe) heel under the painful site. The well is then filled with sponge rubber. Then the entire shoe heel area is covered with three-eighth-inch foam rubber. This provides a nice comfy cup for the patient's heel to rest in. The procedure is called "Steindler heel-spur correction" and if you cannot do it yourself, see a podiatrist. Some practitioners do a little more correction by a tapered heel elevation causing forward thrust (like the high-heel shoes idea).

The Steindler procedure is considered to be the best management for the painful heel. But if after two or three weeks there's little or no relief, arthritis must be considered and, if diagnosed, appropriate treatment will be prescribed by your doctor. Very occasionally, inflammation of the large toe tendon (tenosynovitis) at its insertion in the heel can imitate the symptoms of heel-spur syndrome.

You ask about Indocid. This is an exceedingly potent anti-inflammatory drug that is used only in severe cases of arthritis that doesn't respond to standard treatment with other non-steroid anti-inflammatory drugs (NSAIDs). Side effects such as headache and digestive disturbances can be quite severe. I would not recommend it.

There are a number of OTC (over-the-counter) NSAIDs for arthritis such as Advil, Medipren, Nuprin and Motrin (IB) (all brand names for the generic parent drug, ibuprofen) that may aggravate existing kidney disease. Please check with your doctor.

I'm Losing My Big Toenails

Dear Dr. MacInnis:

I am losing the nails on both my big toes. I didn't injure them in any way I'm aware of. They are just slowly loosening from the top of the nail down and are no longer growing.

I am 75 years old and in fairly good health. I'm wondering if my system is lacking something and is there anything I should be taking to treat this problem?

I will be watching for your answer in the paper.

Mrs. T. V., Edmonton, Alberta

Answer

Chronic fungus infection in aging toes can wreak havoc with nails causing all sorts of deformities, e.g., hypertrophy (nail overgrowth) with a ram's horn appearance and ingrown toenails with or without secondary infection.

In your case, Mrs. V., the chronic fungus infection has caused detritus (disintegrated nail material) to form under the nail causing it to lift off as far down as its matrix (nail bed).

The treatment is surgical involving excision of the entire matrix along with the removal of the nail itself.

I advise you to consult a podiatrist (foot doctor).

Chapter 19
Skin Problems in the Elderly

While many of the subjective manifestations of aging, besetting us all in senior years, are insidious, concealed, and often suppressed *inner* feelings, skin changes are visible for all to see. Indeed, the ravages of time are more clearly portrayed on the skin than anywhere else.

Aging causes thinning and reduced function of all three layers of the skin, namely the epidermis, the dermis, and subcutaneous (under-skin) fat. For example, the epidermis (outer layer) contains the so-called Langerhan's cells that provide the skin's immune defenses. These cells are said to be reduced by 50 percent in the aged, which may account for their well-known loss of sensitivity to allergic skin trauma and may also, by this loss of protection, render the aging skin more susceptible to cancer than that of younger folk.

The most conspicuous aging change in the dermis, or true skin (beneath the epidermis), is about a 20 percent loss of thickness, manifested by its thin, transparent texture, particularly conspicuous on the face and hands of old people. Aging, too, reduces the under-skin fat, affecting its role as an insulator against injury and cold, which explains why the elderly are easily traumatized and are singularly susceptible to the cold, leading sometimes to a state of hypothermia.

Superimposed on these skin changes of old age is a lifetime of exposure to the elements like sunlight, with its damaging ultraviolet rays, and the cold of dry winter winds. Both can play havoc with the exposed skin and are at least partly responsible for wrinkling and sagging of facial skin as well as spotty pigmented areas on the face and exposed areas of the arms.

The collection of columns making up this chapter is *not* truly representative of the aging skin conditions you will find in a textbook of dermatology. The reason for this, I believe, is that old people tend to take their skin changes for granted as inevitable, and only when they become exceedingly bothersome do they see a doctor or write in asking for help. You may wonder why I have devoted so much space to two topics, namely poison ivy and cold sores, neither particularly rampant maladies in the field of geriatric medicine! But in actual fact, both items were introduced by letters from senior readers and provoked a flood of responses from people of all ages. My second and most imperative reason for featuring them is that I believe "plausible" therapy is offered for two heretofore medically "untreatable" conditions. So thanks to our aboriginal shamans for pioneering immunization for poison ivy and to my widely dispersed readership who presents a compelling case for the amino-acid–L-lysine treatment of cold sores to the scientific community for evaluation.

******

"Dishpan" Hands

Dear Dr. MacInnis:

I have a chronic dermatitis of the hands that my doctor tells me is "occupational," that is, caused by certain household agents—soaps, detergents, bleaches, etc. He put a name on it—"housewife's eczema," which I think is rather sexist, don't you?

I have tried to prevent this condition by avoiding as much as possible the apparent causes of it all, but this is easier said than done although it would be a pleasant diversion to give up practically all my household chores and let my husband do them!

Have you any information on this condition, which, by the way was given another title by another doctor—"contact dermatitis of the hands."

Mrs. K.M., Sun City, California

Answer

A more down-to-earth, non-sexist diagnosis is "dishpan hands," which is not only picturesque but immediately incriminates the *commonest* cause for this very common household skin problem—hand washing with soaps and detergents. To this add bleaches (which you've mentioned), oven cleaners, ammonia, furniture polishes, and just about every chemical irritant known to mankind. Remember, the offending agent may not announce its irritating properties immediately and you may continue to use it. On the other hand, some people are exquisitely sensitive (allergic) to very brief exposure to such common agents as rubber or nickel.

Ironically enough, rubber gloves, so often prescribed to "protect" the hands during dishwashing can themselves cause an allergic contact dermatitis. Allergists tell us that if you do use rubber gloves do not use them in hot water so as to avoid perspiration which aggravates the condition.

A common (and effective) prevention suggestion is to buy rubber gloves a size too large and wear *underneath* next to the skin, thin cotton gloves which absorb the perspiration as well as protecting the hands from rubber.

As you can see, Mrs. M., there's no magical preventive remedy for your dishpan hands short of abrogating completely your household duties (which you alluded to in your letter). I would suggest, however, that this important transition be thoroughly discussed with your husband before you embark on your contemplated life of luxury and ease.

Acne Rosacea

Dear Dr. MacInnis:

I have a red rash on my nose, which has been there for some time. Perhaps I should not call it a rash, it's just a red spot that covers the top of my nose. I have been to the doctor and also to a skin specialist who told me it was not cancer. He gave me some cortisone ointment to rub on my nose which helps, but does not take the redness away. Sometimes red pimples come on my nose.

Have you had any experience with red noses? Have you any advice that would help me?

Miss K.M., Edmonton, Alberta

Answer

As I specialize in geriatric medicine, diagnosing red noses is not exactly "my cuppa tea." I have a hunch though. You're *relatively* young, no more than a middle-aged adult at most.

And from your statement, "Sometimes red pimples come on my nose," you provide me with another hunch and it's this—you may have the acne-like condition associated with areas of skin flushing and the presence of tiny dilated blood vessels giving the area a rose-colored appearance. Sometimes there are super-imposed eruptions of pimples or pustules. The fancy name I bestow on your red nose is "acne rosacea."

But I may be completely off the mark—I mean the mark on your nose, which makes me wonder why the skin specialist didn't tell you what you had instead of what you didn't have.

My advice: Go back to him again and this time pop the question.

Poison Ivy

Dear Dr. MacInnis:

Re your column on poison ivy—Democrat & Chronicle, Rochester, New York.

Shame on you! I sent you a letter on this problem a couple of years ago and you wrote me a nice letter promising to use mine later. At the time I pointed out that there was a wonderful treatment for the itch of poison ivy, far superior to calamine lotion. (My husband is a doctor.)

We are currently using Diprosone (Schering), which is wonderful for small burns and things like the itch from poison ivy. This is slightly different from whatever I mentioned to you before, but my husband tells me that there are a variety of drugs, some over the counter (OTC), that also work. Diprosone is a spray, but

I believe there is an ointment. The important point is that they should contain cortisone or a cortisone type. I guess I've got that straight; I'm not the doctor!

As you say, there is no cure for the poison ivy, but who cares if you can just stop that awful itch.

As for the poison ivy itself, we too live in the country and my husband follows a program of spraying the stuff with Roundup.

Mrs. D. R., Upstate New York

Answer

I was remiss in not mentioning certain topical steroids either in spray or ointment form and I thank you for bringing Diprosone to my attention. On further investigation, I found that I did publish your letter of several years ago. You must have missed it. In that letter you mentioned Meti-Derm spray, at the time your favorite steroid. You also mentioned in your previous letter about a friend of yours taking "shots" to prevent getting poison ivy. I checked up on this and, indeed "immunization" has been achieved, not from shots but from the oral ingestion (by mouth) of urushiol (the toxic ingredient in poison ivy) in gradually increasing dosage over a three-month period. This form of immunization must be repeated annually *(Scientific American Medicine)*. You should consult a dermatologist or an allergist about this procedure.

I would like to thank several other readers who recommended steroids in ointment form and Chlor-Tripolon tablets. Stokgard Outdoor Cream is also recommended by the *Scientific American Textbook of Medicine* to be rubbed on the skin prior to possible exposure to poison ivy. A reader from Arnprior, Ontario, sent me a Stokgard wrapper and wrote on it "it works," price $3.69. It should be available in the U.S. without prescription.

Next week watch for another *Democrat & Chronicle* reader's results from using the stem juice of the wild touch-me-not or jewel weed that he grows in his vegetable garden amongst the raspberries.

Dear Dr. MacInnis:

I have a perfect cure for poison ivy. A native Indian told my father to crush the leaves of the mullein weed and rub it on the itchy parts of the skin. If anyone does not know about mullein write to me and I will tell you what to look for. It is gone with one rub of the juices, in a second!

You will be surprised with the result. If the weather is hot and dry and mullein leaves are dried up, make a tea by boiling water and let leaves soak. Wash with this.

Sincerely,
Earl Beatty, RR #2 Lanark, Ontario, Canada K0G 1K0

Answer

I haven't been able to find a description of the mullein weed in my reference books. Interested readers should accept Mr. Beatty's invitation to write to him at the above address or phone (613)-259-5499.

Dear Dr. MacInnis:

Your column that appeared in our daily Democrat & Chronicle *on poison ivy suggested that I write to you concerning the jewel weed or wild touch-me-not to treat poison ivy for relief or cure.*

My father, who came from Cape Vincent, New York, on the Saint Lawrence River (about a mile from Canada) showed me this jewel weed when I was a child and I have much respect for it! I have some growing in my vegetable garden (among my raspberry bushes).

I dug out my All about Weeds *book by Edwin R. Spencer and am enclosing a copy of the section re jewel weed in the treatment of poison ivy for your files.*

A few years ago, one of our daughters who lives in San Diego, California, got poison oak and had a difficult problem with it. So I mailed some stems of this plant (jewel weed) to her. She was cured!

We enjoy your column in our morning paper very much.

Art Mance, Rochester, New York

Answer

Thank you for a your kindness in sending me a copy of the intriguing section of your *All about Weeds* book dealing with the curative property of wild touch-me-not or jewel weed in treating poison ivy.

For the benefit of many interested readers, here's a synopsis of this section: "There is but one reason for including the wild touch-me-not in this *All about Weeds* book. It is the weed everyone susceptible to poison ivy should know. Rubbed on the affected skin, the juice of this plant (found in the stems) frequently brings almost immediate relief and a complete cure is likely to result in twenty-four hours.

"The stems of the plant are almost glassy in appearance. When crushed, they're found to be gorged with a watery juice and the peculiar swelling of the nodes of the stems seem to be reservoirs for the storage of this juice. It's useless to look for this weed except where it grows—a shaded little glen, perhaps shaded by only a few shrubs and a tree or two, a glen made rich by the washed-in dirt from the fields above. It seldom grows by a running stream unless it be a mere rill from a spring.

"If you are susceptible to the poison of the ivy you should spot a natural habitat of the wild touch-me-not before the growing season starts. Watch the place and if there appear to be weeds that are 'glaucous, succulent annuals' and if the leaves are ovate with petioles and stems seem filled with a watery juice, shout '*Eureka*' and go back there whenever you find yourself 'breaking' with the poison pimples.

"Of course you may find the plant ineffective in your case, but it may be the very remedy you require, and if it is, you will be forever grateful for the quirk that placed this harmless plant among the hundred or more weeds treated and illustrated in this book."

All about Weeds, by Edwin Rollin Spencer, Ph.D., is the updated version of *Just Weeds* and is published by Dover, New York City. It may be available in your public library or can be ordered from your book store. Price U.S. $7.95.

Natural Immunization against Poison Ivy?

Dear Dr. MacInnis:
Re your columns on poison ivy.
My dad's family were farmers in the Churchville area, west of Rochester. In the 1930s he worked in a lumber yard and also was a hunter and fisherman. Every spring he would eat poison ivy leaves! He always said, "You have to know which ones." He could literally roll in the stuff (poison ivy) and never have a problem! Unfortunately, wherever he got the idea is now lost. He claimed his grandmother was an American Indian.
Was it Indian lore or farmer's lore? Who knows? I suppose he was lucky he didn't get an allergic reaction.

M. L., Rochester, New York

Answer
I have received several letters like yours relating the protective value (protection from poison ivy) of eating certain parts of the plant. (Another reader referred to "certain buds or nodes that should be eaten to confer 'immunity'." I regret I no longer possess this letter).

At any rate I am becoming more and more convinced that what those people were eating for protection against poison ivy was the part of the plant containing *urushiol*, its toxic ingredient. Readers will recall that I recently wrote on how the oral (by mouth) ingestion of urushiol taken over a period of time could immunize against poison ivy for about a year, when it had to be repeated. It is interesting that our native Indians practiced this form of immunity to poison ivy centuries before our so-called Age of Enlightenment!

Nail Polish Allergy

Dear Dr. MacInnis:
I do hope you can help me. I am a 64-year-old woman and like to wear nail polish, but when I do, my eyelids get red and very itchy.

When this happens, I take the nail polish off right away, the redness and itchiness goes away in a couple of days but as soon as I put on the nail polish again it starts all over. I have had this for years.

My eyelids almost look as if they are transparent. I have tried different brands but they all do the same thing to me. This can make me feel pretty miserable, especially when I am all dressed up to go out. Thank you for any help you can give me. There must be others with the same problem.

Mrs. R.V., Ontario

Answer

No question about it, you are allergic to an ingredient in the nail polish you have been using. Since your eyelids have perhaps the most delicate and allergy sensitive tissue in the body, they are often the first and sometimes the only area of skin to manifest allergic signs and symptoms, namely, redness, swelling, and itchiness. Constant allergic assaults over the years can play havoc on delicate skin causing the transparent look you mention.

My advice to you is to quit using nail polish unless you can find a brand you're not allergic to, but that may be difficult if not impossible, for all brands are pretty much the same.

Your best option, in my opinion, and one I heartily recommend, is to wear artificial nails. I suggest that you see a manicurist and get her advice on the type of artificial nails appropriate for you.

"Geographic" Tongue

Dear Dr. MacInnis:

I have a problem and would like to get your opinion on it.

After seeing three doctors I was told I have a "geographic" tongue. It started one and a half years ago with red spots surrounded by a white edge—in all, the size of a dime. It would stay for a few days, then would go away and reappear in a different

443

*place on my tongue. I was told not to fear as it wasn't cancer. I
was given medication that did nothing but make it worse. My
family doctor told me not to use mouthwash (Cepacol). My tongue
now looks better. I would appreciate your good advice if possible.
Thank you.*

Mrs. J.S. (73), Ottawa, Ontario

Answer

Geographic tongue (wandering rash) is well described in
your letter. I am pleased to assure you that it requires no treatment. It's quite common in the elderly and is in the class of
anatomic variants like ridged scrotums and lobed tongues—both
benign.

Acute Shingles

Dear Dr. MacInnis:

*Is there any good cure for acute shingles? Two of my aunts
came down with it and both suffered intense discomfort and pain
for about three weeks at which time the blisters dried up. But one
of them, the older (76), after a year and a half, is still plagued
with a painful neuritis where the blisters were.*

Mrs. B. R., Edmonton, Alberta

Answer

Shingles (herpes zoster) is frequently followed by intractable pain in the area where the shingles previously appeared. In
some cases it can go on for years. The medical name for this
nerve pain is post-herpetic neuralgia.

I have written on herpes zoster many times, so my remarks
this time will be brief.

It has been established beyond doubt that acyclovir taken
by mouth is effective therapy for acute herpes zoster (shingles).
This was the conclusion of a recent double blind placebo controlled trial. It was found that acyclovir accelerated the virus

shedding, crusting, and healing of the blisters. It was also demonstrated that 800 milligrams of acyclovir five times daily for ten days was superior to a regimen of 400 milligrams five times a day for ten days. Furthermore, patients on the higher dosage experienced less incidence of post-herpetic neuralgia than the controls (who received placebo). In fact those who received the lower dosage didn't do much better than the placebo group.

Just about everything has been tried for the pain of post-herpetic neuralgia without much success. It is thought that this intractable debilitating pain is due to the accumulation of a chemical irritant called "substance P" in the (zoster) damaged sensory nerves. Recently, I mentioned a product called capsaicin cream 0.025 (brand name Zostrix) that prevents the reaccumulation of substance P, thus relieving the pain of post-herpetic neuralgia.

Vitamin D from the Sun

Dear Dr. MacInnis:

In your columns on the long-term effects of prolonged sunbathing on the skin (premature wrinkling and skin cancer), you didn't mention some of the benefits—the most important being the production of vitamin D. At 75 I'm probably as wrinkled as I'm ever going to be, so what's the harm in getting my supply of that important vitamin—and cheap, too, as no pills are necessary. I always keep an eye out for suspicious skin spots and years ago I detected a skin cancer that the doctor said was an early melanoma. And he got it all, so he said. He must have been right. I'm still alive and well.

Mrs. B. R., Edmonton, Alberta

Answer

Your point is well taken. Everyone your age should take heed of what you, Mrs. R., are doing. There's scientific proof it's the right thing.

Increased exposure to sun may be essential for many elderly persons to insure that they receive adequate vitamin D, according to research conducted by Dr. Michael F. Holick of the USDA Human Nutrition Research Center on Aging at Tufts University, Boston, Massachusetts.

Because elderly people lose a significant degree of their capacity to produce vitamin D, they can often offset this loss by increased sunbathing, Dr. Holick said at a Bristol-Myers Pharmaceuticals news briefing in New York City on June 20, 1985.

"To measure vitamin D production," explained Dr. Holick, "we measure the amount of a substance called previtamin D_3 which is formed in the skin after exposure to the sun's ultraviolet radiation. Once pre-vitamin D_3 is formed, the body converts it into vitamin D over a period of two to three days."

In Dr. Holick's study, skin tissue from subjects who were 8, 18, 77, and 82 years old was exposed to ultraviolet radiation and then measured for pre-vitamin D_3 content. This was found to be twice less frequent in the skin of the 77 and 82 year olds than in the younger subjects. Dr. Holick and his colleagues estimate that the average Caucasian young person living in Boston in the summer will obtain adequate vitamin D nutrition from sunlight by exposing the face, hands, and legs to the sun for fifteen minutes twice a week.

Because of their decreased capacity to produce pre-vitamin D_3, Dr. Holick believes that elderly or dark-skinned people living in Boston during the same season may require longer exposure of more skin area or both. For those, he recommends an exposure of fifteen to thirty minutes twice weekly, stopping short of becoming sunburned. Note: Sunscreen lotions should not be used when one is sunning for Vitamin D. They should, however, be used at all other sunbathing times.

"By increasing the amount of skin they expose to the sun, like sunbathing in a swim suit," said Dr. Holick, "elderly people can fulfill their vitamin D requirement without taking vitamin D pills. But those who expose only a limited part of the body, like the face, hands, and legs, would probably require a vitamin D supplement," he stated.

446

Vitamin D is the regulator of calcium in the body. And inadequate calcium can cause the loss of bone mass—in other words, osteoporosis.

A twofold decrease in vitamin D production capacity (from sunlight) can be serious for elderly people who are not receiving adequate vitamin D in their diet.

Angular Cheilitis

Dear Dr. MacInnis:

My father, age 82, has troublesome cracking, wetness, and inflammation at the corner of the mouth (both sides). Sometimes the cracks bleed and are quite tender and sore. What causes this and what is the best treatment for it?

Mrs. M.M.

Answer

Your father has a very common skin condition in the elderly called "angular cheilitis" caused generally by irritation in those areas. And the cause of this irritation is nearly always misalignment of the aging jawbones (resulting in misaligned mouth angles) of poorly fitting dentures, or both. The soggy, macerated skin gives rise to infection from bacteria or yeast (candida albicans), or both.

In people who are eating poorly, there's always the possibility of vitamin deficiency, particularly of riboflavin (vitamin B_2), that in itself can cause angular cheilitis.

Treatment consists in (1) reducing the inflammation and promoting healing with a combination antibacterial, antifungal and steroid (cortisone) ointment applied three times a day; (2) vitamin B_2 (dosage to be determined by your physician); and (3) consultation with a dentist.

Dry Itchy Skin

Dear Dr. MacInnis:

What can I do about my dry itchy skin, especially on my legs, although it can at times be anywhere? It's worse in the winter when I'm mostly in the house. The only relief I can get is by rubbing alcohol, but that doesn't last long.

Mr. O. A. (81)

Answer

As you live in a cold climate, your dry itchy skin goes under the label "winter's itch" and is caused by reduced humidity from the cold weather outside and from dry central (hot air) heating inside.

In younger people, such a dry environment may be only mildly bothersome, if indeed at all. But in the aging skin, such a lack of humidity can certainly increase the misery, and you have a full-fledged case of winter's itch to cope with.

And how do you cope with it? When you're outside in winter, wear suitable protective clothing. When inside keep the heat below 70 F. (20 C.) and humidify the air with pans of water on or near heat registers, or better still by humidifiers.

Go easy on tub baths and showers because they remove the little bit of protective natural skin oil you have left. Once a week is plenty. At other times hand-sponge the face, hands, legs, and private parts. And watch out for that soap! Use only superfatted soaps and sparingly at that.

What about oil applications? Always after the wash. This helps to contain the skin moisture. A good oil preparation contains a substance called urea (a moisture retainer).

Winter's itch, like most cases of pruritus, is often worse in the still of the night (when you've nothing to concentrate on but yourself). Here an antihistamine, with its combined anti-itch and sedative properties, is often helpful.

448

Capsaicin Ointment

Dear Dr. MacInnis:
In a recent column you mentioned a topical ointment for pain relief after shingles.
My mother had a very severe case of shingles about four years ago. It lasted the better part of one year. Ever since, certain parts of her chest and shoulder are terribly sensitive. Even soft clothing gives her pain.
I would very much appreciate finding out the name of the medication that you recommended and where I could obtain it.
Thanks for this and your column, which is very helpful.
Mrs. G. N., Ontario

Answer

The medication you are referring to is capsaicin whose brand name is Zostrix. It is by no means a "cure-all" for postherpetic neuralgia, your mother's affliction, but as you describe her symptoms it might be worth a trial for the pain. Zostrix is quite expensive, so don't continue using it as a skin rub unless you are satisfied that is helping and then use it sparingly, as it can be irritating to sensitive skin. This is because capsaicin is derived from red peppers.

Zostrix is procurable by prescription in most pharmacies in Canada and the United States in a 1.5 ounce tube (0.075 percent strength). It comes with full directions for application. Be careful to wipe your hands clean after rubbing it on the afflicted areas. If it should irritate your eyes, apply milk—a good antidote. So try it for fourteen days as directed. If there's no improvement by that time, quit. It's not for you.

Other "remedies" recommended over the past few years have been (1) an antidepressant (in small dosage) combined with Tegretol, and (2) an antidepressant (in small dosage) along with Zostrix ointment application, as described above.

I have written many columns over the years on shingles and whenever I have the opportunity and the space I like to

449

quote what Sir William Osler, in his 1906 textbook, *Practice of Medicine,* said about post-herpetic (after shingles) neuralgia.

"Severe cases of shingles in elderly people are often followed by *the most intractable neuralgia.*" Now that was written nearly ninety years ago and nothing really has changed very much.

Cold Sores

Dear Dr. MacInnis:

I have a problem with cold sores. I get a cold sore on my lower lip about every four months on the same spot and it usually lasts a week or ten days. I treat it with camphor spirits and Polysporin ointment. A number of my family members get cold sores occasionally. Does this means they are hereditary?

What causes cold sores? And what if anything is there to prevent them? What would you advise for treatment?

Mr. B. S. (age 60), Saskatchewan

Answer

The cause of cold sores (herpes simplex) is a virus that tends to erupt in the form of a blister or group of blisters usually around the corner of the mouth but can be anywhere on the lips. It is said that this cold sore virus "just waits around" for something to trigger it off, like exposure to strong sunlight, infection with fever, and sometimes a period of emotional stress. After a few days the blisters dry up and a yellowish crust appears. There may be a family tendency.

Treatment: The initial symptom is frequently a tingling and sometimes an itchy sensation at the site. If drying lotions such as calamine or just plain alcohol (70 percent) are applied to the site sometimes the blister can be aborted. Bathing the site with very hot water can be just as beneficial. As you have observed, cold sores have a tendency to recur, usually in the same place. There is, as far as I know, no way to prevent them.

Canker *versus* Cold Sores

A canker sore is an ulcer occurring on the mucous membrane of the mouth. It starts out as a burning sensation for a day or so followed by a round yellowish spot surrounded by a red ring. The pain may last for several days and then subsides. When you accidentally bite the inside of your mouth it may develop into a canker sore. The actual cause is not definitely known but an immune reaction may be the culprit. They tend to recur. Cold compresses or ice help lessen the acute pain. I have found that lidocaine local anesthetic in the form of a viscous solution applied frequently to the sore may be helpful.

A "cold sore" has nothing to do with a cold. It is caused by a virus, and unlike a canker sore, may be catching from towels, eating utensils, etc., used by another person with the infection. The usual sites are the mouth, lips, and nose. Occasionally they can occur on the cheeks and even the hands. They start out as blisters, occurring as late as twenty days after exposure. Cold sores tend to recur and can be associated with such varied events as menstruation, sunburn, and fever. Your doctor may occasionally prescribe antiviral medication in stubborn cases but most infections last only two or three days.

L-Lysine Control of Cold Sores

Everytime I write a column on cold sores, I can expect a rash of "cures" ranging all the way from ice cubes to biofeedback. Although they all lack scientific substance, the users have found them successful and often take the trouble to share their good fortune with others. Although I usually can't even imagine how they work, I take the attitude that "nothing succeeds like success" and sometimes print the "recipe" in the hope that even one reader may derive some benefit.

Well, I got a surprise from my last column on cold sores. On one day I received two letters—one from the east coast, the other from the west—both extolling the value of the amino acid

L-lysine in the rapid successful treatment and prevention of chronic, recurrent cold sores, which most readers know is caused by a virus.

As the content of both letters is practically the same, I'll print the one with the earlier deadline and use a bit of dietary material from the other.

Dear Dr. MacInnis:

I do enjoy your column in our area newspaper. Let me say that right off the top.

You spoke about cold sores (herpes simplex) this past week, and in that regard I am a 64-year-old woman who has had recurring cold sores ever since I can remember. In my teen years I discovered that too much sun caused an ugly breakout, so I never got in the habit of sunbathing. (Today I'm glad about that; I have very few wrinkles.)

Later, when I was extra tired or stressed I might get one, but then I decided it was because I was getting a cold that made me distressed. I never knew which came first! Of course, when every a big dance came 'round or on any occasion when I wanted to look my best—bingo. The fact that they hurt was insignificant; the bother was that they were ugly. They were mostly on my upper or lower lip, but often they would "pop" just inside my nostril. There would always be a few hours' warning—a tingling sensation.

In my forties I received a smallpox vaccination after which my attacks were much less violent. About ten years ago, I discovered L-lysine and at first took 325 milligrams daily, cold sore or not. Remarkable! I would get the tingling feeling about once every six months and would take an extra couple of tablets immediately. Often the sore didn't appear or, if it did, it would be small and gone in a day or two. (Until L-lysine, a cold sore would last seven to ten days.) I'm aware that some medical folks laugh at this, but I know it has made a difference for me. Not having cold sores has changed my life. I'd be happy to have your comments.

Mrs. H. M. M., Spencerport, New York

Answer

I agree with you, but not many of the medical establishment would be very impressed. I consulted my medical references in vain—nothing, repeat nothing, about L-lysine, although it is readily available at your pharmacy.

As I mentioned, my other correspondent's experience was similar to yours. She was kind enough to send along a list of high lysine foods—the foods to eat: fresh fish, shark, canned fish, chicken, beef, goat's milk, cow's milk, and lamb (in descending order). Foods high in arginine *should be avoided*. Here are a few of them: hazel nuts, brazil nuts, peanuts, walnuts, almonds, cocoa powder, peanut butter, and sesame seeds (in descending order of strength).

Testimonials like Mrs. M.'s and others are of course anecdotal and as such are unacceptable to the medical profession. But over the years, I've heard so many compelling reports of the virtues of L-lysine in the treatment and prevention of herpes simplex (a universal malady still without a cure) that I believe it should be put to the scientific test by our research colleagues to determine its value one way or other.

After all, what's there to lose?

Cold Sores: L-Lysine Treatment Explained

Dear Dr. MacInnis:

I read your column on the L-lysine treatment of cold sores with interest. Just last week I was discussing this very topic with a friend who is a Ph.D. chemist and takes a great deal of interest in health and nutrition.

The explanation for the success of L-lysine is actually quite simple. Both L-lysine and arginine are amino acids, the building blocks of protein. All living organisms need protein. The herpes virus (which causes cold sores) utilizes mostly arginine; hence, your advice to avoid arginine-rich foods. Now, L-lysine, and arginine have similar chemical structures, so if you load up on L-lysine, the herpes virus tries to use it, but fails and is inactivated in the effort.

This probably isn't the precise explanation, but at least it answers the question. I hope it clears things up!

V. S., Kincardine, Ontario

Answer

Sounds good to me. The herpes virus actually dies from starvation! Right? Thanks for writing.

Vitiligo

Dear Dr. MacInnis:
I am quite an active, healthy 68-year-old woman and do everything possible to stay that way. But I have a problem.
I have developed large white areas on the skin of my arms and hands. I now look like a spotted leopard and am constantly being asked about it. There is no history of this condition in my family. Could you tell me what it is and is there any treatment for it?

Answer

You most likely have a disorder of pigmentation called vitiligo. It usually occurs in healthy people and is present in one percent of the population where it can start in childhood and young adulthood and usually intensifies as age progresses up to and sometimes past middle age. It is thought to be an inherited skin disorder.

Vitiligo is characterized by skin depigmentation (loss of natural pigment) and often begins on the back of the hands and arms, on the neck, skin folds, and the nail-skin junction of the finger. Lesions may be single or multiple, and can be bilateral (on both sides of the body). Frequently, several areas of depigmentation join together to form a single large white patch. Very rarely the whole body becomes depigmented—a condition known as "vitiligo universalis."

Vitiligo may be psychologically and socially disabling especially when the face is affected. It is therefore expedient to reduce the contrast between the white and normal skin areas by the use of sunscreens and the avoidance of sun exposure. This is especially important for fair-skinned individuals. For dark-skinned people certain prepared aniline dyes are helpful as a make-up to mask the white areas.

The treatment of vitiligo is prolonged, tedious, and not for the undedicated! The therapy currently gaining favor is the so-called PUVA treatment. Here 0.1 percent psoralen (a photo-sensitizing drug) lotion is applied to the affected area or areas which are then exposed to artificial long-wave ultraviolet light. A typical course of three times a week may take a year or more depending on the severity. Another treatment uses a high potency cortisone, again for a long period. Note: Both require specialized supervision.

Psoriasis—and Bad!

Dear Dr. MacInnis:

I have psoriasis and bad! I have it all over except my face. There are also big patches on my chest, abdomen, legs, arms, and the back of my hands. It goes without saying, I can't wear a swim suit and it's always a problem wearing suitable clothing to at least cover the worst parts. People often ask me how I have lived with it so long without going crazy! (I am 50). No question about it, you just can't put it out of your mind. It's always a part of you and, would you believe it, I suffer more not so much from the frustrations of having it but from what I feel people think of it and the way they look at me. I've been refused service in a restaurant, for example.

People with bad psoriasis will try literally anything in the hope of a cure. I've tried just about everything, and strange as it sounds, just about everything seemed to help at first, the best being H-cortisone ointment, which turned out to be the worst in the long run, for it had a rebound effect. Tar ointment would be somewhat tolerable if it didn't smell so bad and stain my underclothing and bed linen.

I'm not being melodramatic when I tell you that it has ruined my life. But, again, I always hope that there's "something big" coming up that will change things for my time left.

Miss A. L. (50), Ontario

Answer

Readers can now appreciate how it feels to be a victim of intractable psoriasis. And what Miss L. says is right—it can definitely affect every aspect of living.

It's with some temerity that I suggest a new topical drug, calcipotriol (brand name Dovonex), a vitamin D derivative, that is now available on prescription in Canada and the U.S. Although recommended only for "mild to moderate" psoriasis, it might be still worthwhile to consult a dermatologist.

Is It Pityriasis Rosea or Not?

Dear Dr. MacInnis:

I find your weekly column very interesting and informative. The column I have in mind in the paper was titled "Hot Pepper Derivative (Zostrix) Helps Shingles Sufferers."

One of the questions asked was "Is it [Zostrix] used only for post-shingles neuralgia? Your answer was, ". . . . and it appears that what it does for post shingles neuralgia, it can do even better for the pain of arthritis." This answer is very interesting to me as I have both rheumatoid and osteoarthritis.

My main concern is, "Would it be helpful for pityriasis rosea?" Or have you some other suggestions for this dreaded skin rash problem? My husband, who has good skin but is of fair complexion, has avoided long periods in the sun. In fact, when this first appeared in (February 1990) he hadn't been in the sun for many months.

It is now May 26, 1992, and there still isn't much improvement. My husband has been seeing a skin specialist, then another,

456

and neither knew what it was. Neither did our family doctor know until a skin biopsy was done. And then they decided it was pityriasis rosea. My husband is 75 years old and is otherwise in good health. I will ask him to add a footnote to this letter telling you what medication he has been using. I found that after his last visit to the skin specialist last week, he seemed to be depressed as there were no further suggestions offered. As well, he was asked to attend (briefly) a conference of dermatologists. The group had never seen a case as bad as this. This alone was not encouraging.

Have you any suggestions? We would appreciate any help you can give us regarding pityriasis rosea.

Husband's footnote: "I am presently taking methotrexate, 2.5 milligram tablets, and have just finished my fourth week. I was told that there would not be much change before three to four weeks. I really have noticed an improvement within the last few days. I realize that this condition is most unusual and that it does take some time to improve.

"As my wife has stated, it would be very interesting to hear your comments. . . ."

Mr. A. L.

Answer

You ask if Zostrix might be useful for treating a condition like pityriasis rosea? My answer is "no."

Pityriasis rosea is one of commonest skin diseases encountered in the general practice of medicine. It begins as the so-called herald patch, a raised, red, scaly patch looking much like ringworm. The herald patch in five days or so gives birth to a multitude of itching smaller patches that usually appear on the trunk and upper extremities but rarely above the neck and below the knees and elbows (a distinguishing feature by which any doctor can usually diagnose this skin condition at a glance). It lasts six to eight weeks, disappearing completely. Ultraviolet (sun lamp) treatment may hasten recovery. It usually affects the relatively young (15 to 35 years).

There is a very rare skin disease called pityriasis rubra pilaris that can affect any age. I've read of a case in a 25-year-old man who responded to intravenous methotrexate but not to the tablet.

Resistant cases of psoriasis (not responding to the usual measures) have been successfully treated with oral methotrexate (your husband's current drug). In fact it may be the only reasonably successful treatment of such cases. Psoriasis can affect people of all ages.

I do trust that you will derive some information from my comments on pityriasis rosea and two allied conditions. I will not comment any further from "long distance" except to hope that your husband continues to improve on the methotrexate treatment for his psoriasis.

Nail Ridging

Dear Dr. MacInnis:

What causes longitudinal ridges in the nails and is there any treatment for this? Has it anything to do with diet? And what causes puffiness below the eyes?

Thank you kindly for any information you may be able to give me regarding the above conditions.

Mrs. L. S., Saskachewan

Answer

Longitudinal ridging of the nails is quite common. It is caused by damage to the matrix or nail bed. In younger people this damage may be the result of chronic infection or actual injury from an accident. In elderly people it is usually the result of "aging" of the matrix and of course occurs on all the nails. Some people seem to have a hereditary disposition to the condition.

If the tissues below the eyes were as tough and rigid as skin elsewhere, a slight excess of tissue fluid would not show up. But the infraorbital (under eye) skin is exceedingly thin and fragile reflecting minute retention of body fluid. Cutting down on salt might help in decreasing fluid retention and in turn decrease the puffiness. Of course, heart and kidney disease can cause excess body fluid (edema) and these conditions can be easily diagnosed by your doctor.

Dry Itchy Skin Again

Dear Dr. MacInnis:
What would you suggest for a 72-year-old woman with very dry skin? I was advised to bathe frequently and follow this up with a skin lotion. I try to do this daily but it doesn't seem to help much.

Mrs. T. L., Sun City, California

Answer

If that was *medical* advice you received, think seriously of getting another doctor or at least another opinion. As we get up in years our sebaceous (oil producing) skin glands slip into second gear and the skin shows it. And the condition is compounded by frequent showering or bathing in *hot* water. So my advice to you is to bathe every other day or so and make it brief in tepid (not hot) water. Follow up with a skin moisturizer and shun the midday sun. And unless your house humidity is high, you should have a humidifier in your bedroom at night.

Burning Mouth and Tongue

Dear Dr. MacInnis:
I am a woman, age 58, with a complaint of persistent burning pain in my mouth and tongue. This has been present about five years and I have seen many doctors about it but to no avail. The five other doctors were quite interested in my case, did a lot of tests, including X rays of the jaw, but came up with nothing.
As a last resort I'm writing to you to see if you have any suggestions, which I will be glad to try out.

Mrs. G. H., Ontario

Answer

I don't know how to handle this "doctor of last resort" business. I would like to think it identifies me as final arbiter of medical mysteries but, alas, it looks as though I'm just number six on the diagnostic totem pole.

"Burning mouth" is a common complaint, particularly of post-menopausal women. It may present itself as a pure burning sensation in the mouth and/or mouth-tongue pain.

The causes are many: denture problems, dry mouth, anemia, vitamin and hormone deficiencies, and psychological disturbances.

In one study of burning mouth published in *Oral Surgery, Oral Medicine, Oral Pathology* 64 (1987): 171–74, psychiatric assessment revealed that while 16 percent of burning mouth cases had identifiable physical causes, 44 percent were associated with mixed anxiety and depressive symptoms. You should note this and see your doctor again.

Shingles and After-Shingles Neuralgia

Over the years I have written numerous columns on herpes zoster, commonly known as "shingles," and an equal number on the often intractable pain that persists after the wet blistering shingle vesicles have dried up, scabbed, and disappeared. The medical term for this after-shingles pain is *post-herpetic neuralgia* and, until recently, defied treatment. Shingles is a very common affliction of past midlife with the incidence of cases increasing with advancing age.

In acute shingles there is usually a prodromal or initial period when the patient feels out of sorts and develops pain along the course of a nerve, usually somewhere on the trunk but it can be practically anywhere on the body. (One of the most debilitating forms of acute shingles involves the ophthalmic (eye) nerve with the pain and vesicular rash attacking the eye.) But no matter what nerve chain is affected, the pain and rash is almost invariably limited to one side of the body, neither crossing the midline. The herpes zoster (shingles virus) is the "adult" version of the chickenpox virus that after "hibernating" for years in the spinal cord cells emerges as a cluster of chickenpox-like vesicles on the skin over the affected nerve. What incites the onset of shingles is uncertain but since it is far more common in the aged, it may be due to a weakening immune system allowing the chickenpox virus to express itself as a shingles infection. It is estimated that 50 percent of people over 80 develop shingles and 50 percent of them will develop post-herpetic neuralgia.

Sir Williams Osler in his 1906 *Textbook of Medicine* wrote as follows: "Severe cases (of shingles) in elderly people are often followed by the most intractable form of neuralgia." That was over eighty-eight years ago and only recently have some treatments become available and I have previously reported on several of them. Before commenting on them again, I should tell you what is considered the cause of post-herpetic neuralgia. Substance "P" (a chain of amino acids) is normally contained in small nerve endings. When nerves are damaged (by the shingles virus) they release this substance "P" which, in turn, triggers the pain. Treatments are as follows:

1. Tegretol-Elavil combination. Tegretol is an anti-epileptic drug and Elavil an anti-depressant. It is said that their mode of action is to suppress either the release of substance "P" or the pain it produces. It doesn't always work, however.
2. Transcutaneous electrical nerve stimulation (TENS). This is a popular device for alleviating the pain of sprains, strains, and other sport injuries. It is sometimes helpful in post-herpetic neuralgia.
3. Capsaicin cream (brand name Zostrix). Capsaicin is the pungent element in red peppers and other plants of the solanaceous family of vegetables. Although its precise mechanism of action is not fully understood, it is thought that capsaicin rubbed on the skin renders it insensitive to pain by depleting and preventing the reaccumulation

of substance "P" in the sensory nerves damaged by the herpes zoster virus.

Zostrix is manufactured by GenDerm Corporation of Northbrook, Illinois, and Montreal, Quebec, and is procurable in 1.5 ounce tubes. Directions: Adults and children 2 years and over: Apply Zostrix not more than three or four times daily. It may cause transient burning on application. Avoid contact with eyes or broken or irritable skin. Apply for fourteen days. If no improvement, quit. Zostrix treatment should be supervised by your doctor. It is quite expensive.

For the lesions and pain of *acute shingles,* the anti-viral drug acylovir (brand name Zovirax) in a 5 percent cream is recommended for topical (skin) application over a period of fifteen days. This treatment, too, should be given under the supervision of your doctor.

Chapter 20
Insomnia and Other Sleep Problems in the Elderly

O sleep! it is a gentle thing,
Beloved from pole to pole!
To Mary Queen the praise be given!
She sent the gentle sleep from Heaven,
That slid into my soul.

—Samuel Taylor Coleridge
"The Rime of the Ancient Mariner"

One of the most prevalent and persistent myths concerning sleep is that the aged need more of it than younger folk. Why this legend still prevails, I'm not sure but may be from the general observation that they *seem* to be sleeping or dozing a great deal of the time when in reality they often choose a state of semi-oblivion from sheer boredom. This is particularly seen in some chronic-care institutions where there's little motivation for social interaction and where often distorted sleep patterns cause patients to sleep in fits and starts at night and doze the next day. And then there is often the need to get up to urinate one or more times a night. It is said that in men around age 60, one in four need to get up to the toilet, but when they reach 85 it's nine out of ten. The pains and aches of arthritis are another bugbear, preventing a normal "getting to sleep" and when "blessed sleep" at last arrives, it's light and fraught with vivid dreams, often awakening the sleeper. This is why older people, more than any other age group, frequent the doctor's office seeking sleeping pills and stand a good chance of getting their request fulfilled. And if the sleeping pill happens to be a long-acting hypnotic, the patient is virtually guaranteed a long period of dozing the next day.

This chapter will stress the non-drug approach to elderly insomnia, and when it is explained that difficulty getting to sleep and frequent awakenings are a part of normal aging, elderly patients will comply much better with the program. But we must always remember that there are a great many of the "old old" (over 80) age group who are so firmly "hooked" on their nightly "fix" that it would be difficult as it would be hazardous to attempt a so-called weaning program.

Finally, there are, in my view, legitimate occasions to use hypnotics on a short-term basis and these are outlined in several columns in this chapter.

Insomnia in the Elderly: Part 1

In preparing this column I had to research the relevant literature on sleep disorders and found that every authority on the subject agreed that insomnia is prevalent in persons over 65. In fact, the elderly are about six times more likely to have trouble falling asleep and to experience more night awakenings than people under 45.

These are the *normal* changes in sleep patterns due to aging and no kind or amount of medication can alter very much this natural reality. Most medical practitioners are aware of this and should therefore not make the mistake of prescribing "medication" for a normal situation.

In investigating a patient with insomnia, the doctor should not attempt treatment without a thorough evaluation of possible causes. This involves a careful history and physical examination to determine whether or not a medical condition like painful arthritis is responsible for the sleep disturbance. Other disorders might be heart trouble with shortness of breath or palpitation or a prostate gland causing frequent getting up at night. Psychiatric disorders like depression and the behavioral problems of senile dementia can frequently cause insomnia.

Drugs are frequent offenders. Some elderly patients are so stimulated by caffeine that as little as one cup of coffee in the morning is enough to disturb sleep that night. Alcoholics are always troubled with insomnia. Heavy smokers sleep better after quitting.

There are many drugs that cause insomnia, such as medications for heart rhythm disorders, hypertension, and thyroid conditions, to name a few.

In most cases, determining the type, cause, and relative severity of the insomnia is not difficult. Occasionally, however, in problem cases, your doctor may require the specialized assistance of a sleep laboratory (available at most university hospitals).

Once diagnosed, how is insomnia treated?

Some readers will be immediately disappointed to hear I'm not tabling a list of drugs for chronic insomnia. In fact I'm not going to mention drugs at all in this column. What I'm going to stress is the *non-drug* approach—the *first line* of treatment. It may surprise you to learn that most sleep researchers feel that sleeping pills should play little or no part in the treatment of *chronic* insomnia (see next column).

Most older people are unaware that their changing sleep habits (difficulty falling asleep and frequent awakenings) are a part of growing older. Once they accept this fact, they seem to relax and feel less stressed about these features of insomnia. So education is my rule number 1.

2. The elderly person should establish and maintain the habit of going to bed and arising at regular times. Even if you have a "bad night" don't try to sleep in. Get up at your usual time. Don't toss and turn for what seems like hours in bed. Get up and read or watch TV until you're sleepy again.

3. Getting up several times a night to the toilet is exhausting. Restrict fluids after 4:00 P.M.

4. Older people tend to catnap frequently during the day. Try *not* to indulge; you'll retire sleepier—and that's good.

5. As before mentioned and worthy of repetition, avoid stimulating beverages such as tea, coffee, and colas after 4:00 P.M. No big night meals.

6. Certain medications are stimulating. Consult with your doctor re taking them before noon if practical.
7. If you have arthritic pain at night that keeps you awake, take something for it. There are good long-acting pain-killers. Symptoms of heart/lung conditions should be kept under control.
8. A daily program of walking exercises is fine, but don't exercise late in the evening.
9. Finally, make your bedroom conducive to sleep—a comfortable temperature, a good mattress (not too soft), spot-lighting from a table lamp instead of a glaring ceiling light. You might benefit from controlled background noises, like a fan or air conditioner to "mask" disruptive sounds.

Insomnia in the Elderly: Part 2

Those of you who read the previous column on sleep disorders in the elderly now know that the *non-drug* approach is the *first line* treatment of chronic insomnia. You will also recall that most sleep researchers decry the use of drugs in all but transient types of insomnia.

The current literature on sleep disorders tells us that approximately one-third of the general population complain of some degree of insomnia. About half of these (15 percent of the population) suffer sufficiently that they seek medical aid and about half of these (7.5 percent of the population) are prescribed sleeping pills.

And here's something to note well. Of this 7.5 percent of the population prescribed sleeping pills, only 60 percent (5 percent of the population) take them for longer than a month, and only 20 percent of these (1 percent of the general population) take a sleeping pill *every night*. This is considerably lower than most people think.

I have no statistics for the elderly, but I know from long experience that their usage of sleeping pills is higher than that of the general population, with an extraordinarily high consumption in geriatric nursing homes and chronic care hospitals.

The main reason for this increased consumption in the elderly is their higher incidence of insomnia—about six times that of the general population. As mentioned in my previous column, their main sleeping disorders are (1) increased falling asleep time, (2) light sleep (elderly people almost never attain the deepest, stage four sleep), and (3) frequent night awakenings. Although these are normal changes due to aging, they are *perceived* by the elderly person as sleep disorders for which they consult a physician. Unfortunately, more often than not (and particularly in many nursing homes) sleeping pills are freely prescribed and dispensed.

I believe the older (over 60) patient who consults a physician for *chronic* insomnia should be treated the same as a younger person. After determining the type and probable cause of the sleep disorder, the doctor should initiate the no-drug sleep hygiene program listed in my previous (part 1) column. If time is taken to educate the elderly patient on what are the normal changes due to aging (see 1, 2, and 3 above) half the battle is won. Many times the other half is won because an educated, enlightened patient will fully cooperate with the total program.

I believe also that sedative/hypnotic drugs, if prescribed at all, should be given only for transient (short-term) insomnia brought on by acute illness, bereavement, sudden environmental change from travelling, and the like. An effective, safe, and inexpensive hypnotic for transient insomnia (lasting a week or so) is chloral hydrate. However, it can sometimes cause excessive flatus (gas) and should not be given to someone on an anticoagulant (blood thinning) drug. The bedtime dose is one-half to one gram. (Chloral hydrate may lose its effectiveness over time.)

When a hypnotic drug is necessary for a longer time (up to a month), I would recommend a benzodiazepine. There are short-acting benzodiazepines like trialzolam (Halcion) that is advocated by some for the elderly because it does not produce daytime sleepiness. However, it can cause early morning insomnia after a week or two. In addition, it possesses the bothersome property of occasionally causing amnesia both retrograde and antegrade (loss of memory for events before or after taking the drug). For these reasons, I would not recommend triazolam for the elderly. On the other hand, flurazepan (Dalmane) with its very long "half-life" is classified as a long-acting hypnotic and can build up in the system over a few weeks causing excessive daytime sleepiness.

The ideal hypnotic for the elderly would be an intermediate acting drug that would not cause excessive daytime sedation or early morning insomnia while sustaining sleep for four to five hours. The benzodiazepine nearing that ideal, I believe, is temazepam (Restoril). The dose of temazepam for the elderly insomniac is 15 milligrams one-half hour before bed time.

They Need Their Nightly Fix

Dear Dr. MacInnis:

In your column on insomnia in the elderly you gave me the impression that hypnotics (sleeping pills) should only be used when the insomnia is of a transient nature caused by strange sleeping quarters when travelling, for example, and that they should be discontinued when the episode is over. The same would apply to transient grief reactions and other equally disturbing events. This sounds reasonable, but what about the elderly person who has been taking sleeping pills over a long period—perhaps years and is in effect, totally "hooked"? It would be difficult, indeed dangerous, to deprive this person of his nightly "fix." What's your opinion?

And would you call a person an "insomniac" if she does just fine on three to four hours' sleep a night? By this I mean she remains quite active all day and never complains of feeling sleepy, nor do I ever hear her complain of "not getting enough" sleep.

R. N., Seneca Falls, New York

Answer

Question No. 1. Many elderly patients, especially in nursing homes, receive routine night sedation and before long, they become dependent. As long as they get their "fix," as you say, they are not fearful of the long night ahead even at the expense of next day sleepiness. In my experience it has been next to impossible to wean elderly patients off the habit without causing serious physical and emotional withdrawal symptoms that they simply cannot cope with. I agree with you. Sometimes we must accept the lesser of two evils where quality of life is the all-important thing.

Question No. 2. There is a well-recognized, though small, part of the population who seem to "program" themselves to be short sleepers. Sleep experts don't classify them as "insomniacs." An outstanding characteristic of these people is that they do not consider themselves as poor sleepers and consequently never complain about it.

Should I Stay in Bed or Get Up?

Dear Dr. MacInnis:

Re your article on insomnia. My problem at night is having to get up to go to the bathroom two, three, and sometimes four times a night. I go back to bed and after tossing and turning to get back to sleep, I finally doze off. Then I get the urge to urinate and up I am again. Sometimes I just lie in bed all night without sleeping. Is this insomnia? Should I stay in bed or get up?

Mr. H. J. (77), Ottawa, Ontario

Answer

From your complaints, I would make an educated guess that you have prostate enlargement. If you haven't already seen a urologist you should do so at once. In the meantime you should cut out fluids after 4:00 P.M. and have no coffee or tea except for breakfast. Sleep specialists advise that you should use your bed for rest and sleep, never for tossing, turning, and ruminating over events of the day. When this happens, leave your bedroom and retire to a quiet and comfortable place, and don't return to your bedroom until you are relaxed and sleepy again. Yes, you have insomnia and the cause seems obvious.

Insomnia in a 90 Year Old

Dear Dr. MacInnis:

I am a woman almost 90 years old and now get around in a wheelchair, so of course can't go for a walk; but you would be surprised at what I can do around the house. So I am not idle.

For years I have hardly slept at all. I just lie awake hour after hour all night long and although I also lie down in the afternoon I do not sleep.

I have been to three different doctors and two of them are against me taking sleeping pills. They say sleeping pills are addictive. The third doctor says I can take temazepam but only one at bedtime and that's all. This temazepam sometimes puts me to sleep but not always and then I only sleep for one or two hours and for the rest of the night I lie awake. I need sleep and it's beginning to tell on me. My appetite is poor and I am under-weight.

I have had a slight stroke lately and for that I take warfarin and aspirin. I also have mild heart trouble. My home life is happy and I am well cared for. I need your advice.

Mrs. W. E. C.

Answer

Yes indeed, sleeping pills are addictive and some more than others. But there always comes a time in life—and 90 is getting close—when one must decide what poses the greater harm, endless nights or insomnia with no hope of reprieve (that you so vividly describe) or getting some sleep and running the risk of "getting the habit." If I were in your shoes at your age, I would run that risk, for quality of life remaining is what matters most. I believe your doctor would agree.

My attitude toward sleeping pills for insomnia is well known to anyone who has read my many columns on the subject. Put briefly, I would never prescribe sleeping pills for more than ten days or so to tide the patient over a sudden change of environment, such as traveling, sleeping in strange surroundings, temporary stress situations, e.g., a death in the family, and so on. My recommendations were mainly directed to the elderly who are exquisitely sensitive to sleeping pills and who "get hooked" quite readily. But in actual geriatric medical practice, I soon learned that I must relax the rules in my 90- to 100-plus patient age group.

My favorite hypnotic (sleeping pill) for the elderly elite like you, Mrs. C., would be the tried and true, time-tested chloral hydrate. Chloral hydrate, unlike some other sleeping medications, is usually not associated with worsening of insomnia after it is discontinued for whatever reason—a very important point in its favour. And here is the clincher. It's the least expensive of all hypnotics! One note of caution though: Do *not* take chloral hydrate if you have gastritis or duodenal ulcer. It will make these conditions worse. Chloral hydrate is available in either capsule or liquid form. Each gelatin capsule or 5 cubic centimeters of the orange-flavored liquid contains 500 milligrams (1.2 gram) of chloral hydrate. Like another old timer, Buckley's Cough Syrup, the liquid "tastes awful, but it works"! Chloral hydrate may lose its effectiveness over time, but not in transient insomnia. The dose is 1–2 capsules at bedtime.

And finally, Mrs. G., I recommend that you try not to nap in the afternoon and to stay up as late as you can before retiring. This helps to make the long dark night a little shorter with perhaps a brighter day tomorrow.

Halcion

Dear Dr. MacInnis:

Would you please give me some up-to-date information on the sleeping pill called Halcion. There's a lot about it in the papers and TV lately, and some doctors claim that it can cause mental problems. I have taken Halcion on doctor's orders on and off for short periods of time (a week or less) and as I am 67 years old the doctor prescribes it in half-dosage (one-half pill) at bedtime. I must say that over the past five years on this sleeping pill I've never really had any problems. I believe this is because I take it only when I really need it and then only for a very short time.

Mr. H. G., New York

Answer

Evidently you missed my latest column on Halcion printed some months ago. As I pointed out, Halcion is the most widely prescribed sleeping pill in the world, and for the last decade it has been the subject of continued controversy in medical circles. In fact, quite recently it was ordered off the market in Britain for its alleged capability of causing excessive anxiety, depression, paranoid tendencies, and, in some cases, suicidal ideation. In Canada the regulatory authorities have recommended that it be prescribed only for short periods (ten days to two weeks). In my previous column, I reported on a study done at Tufts New England Medical Center where it was found that in the elderly, bothersome side effects of Halcion and other benzodiazepines were dose related. The researchers recommended the geriatric dose be halved, and specifically that Halcion be prescribed in a dose of 0.125 milligrams at bedtime (*Johns Hopkins Medical Letter,* "Health after 50").

The very latest news on Halcion is that the U.S. FDA (Federal Drug Administration) has ruled that the drug may be prescribed but suggests short periods at a time, again I believe, about two weeks.

As for your personal regimen, I believe it is excellent and I commend your doctor for being far ahead of the researchers and regulatory bodies on this one!

Long-Term Use of Halcion

Dear Dr. MacInnis:
    I have just read your columns on "Insomnia in the Elderly" in the Rochester, New York, Democrat & Chronicle.

I have a sister, age 88, who is the victim of dementia brought on by a stroke seven years ago.

For about two years she had been taking Halcion (triazolam) 0.125 mg, regularly at bed time (as prescribed by her physician). With this, she had been sleeping very well at night.

My question is: What are the possible side effects of the continuous long-term use of Halcion?

Any information and possible advice will be greatly appreciated.

Mrs. L. J., Penn Yan, New York

Answer

The serious side effect of prolonged usage of *all* hypnotics (sleeping pills) is addiction. In addition, short-acting benzodiazepines like triazolam (Halcion) and lorazepam (Activan) sometimes can cause bothersome amnesia. In the elderly they can also cause early awakening due to their short-acting property.

Having said this, I must now state that there are notable exceptions to the rule and your sister's precarious condition is one of them. It is ludicrous to be concerned with addiction in such circumstances. My advice is to carry on with the Halcion and be thankful it is so effective in such low dosage.

Low-Dose Anti-Depressants for Sleep and Good Sex

Dear Dr. MacInnis:

I am 69 and would like to comment on my experience with two problems often mentioned in respect to age and aging. One is insomnia and the other is diminished libido (sex drive). In my particular case both these problems have responded to very small doses of antidepressants.

At times I tended to awaken early and had difficulty getting back to sleep. I was given amitriptyline (25 milligrams) to be taken as needed. I started out using it twice a week, or spaced three or four days apart, with good results. However, I got quite sleepy the next afternoon or early evening, so began cutting the tablets into three milligram pieces (before getting dust!) and still had beneficial results with much fewer side effects.

The larger (25 milligram) dose diminished my libido for a day or so, but it came back strong a couple of days later. The smaller dose (three milligrams) improved my sex drive the next morning.

Also, I've found that if I awaken early and cannot sleep, I eat just one graham cracker (or a slice of bread), do a few stretching exercises and then will have no trouble sleeping again.

I am not taking amitriptyline now after hearing better things about another anti-depressant called trazodone. My doctor put me on 12 to 25 milligrams of this drug just twice a week and I obtained the beneficial results on sleep and libido with fewer side effects than before on the other drug.

Please excuse this long letter, but I wanted to make the point that seniors often need much smaller doses and longer intervals of medication to get the same results as do younger folk with minimum side effects.

Sincerely,
Mr. J. C., Upstate New York

Answer

I've printed your letter Mr. C., not because of its claim to scientific validity but because of its strict observance of a principle that I wish more practitioners of medicine would practice when treating the elderly. It is well known that old patients—particularly the "old old" (85 plus) always react adversely to medications prescribed in adult dosage. As a rule of thumb, one should initiate dosage of most drugs in the order of one-third to one-half the recommended adult doses. This will in most cases prevent bothersome side effects and get the elderly patient off to a good start. Dosage may then be cautiously increased, but in my experience the drug is usually effective in its fractional dosage. On this score, Mr. C., I salute thee.

But "Simon Purists" are going to take issue with you for ingesting an anti-depressant drug for its well-known sedative side effect. I would call it "therapeutic opportunism" as long as the "side effect" of drowsiness takes place at the proper time, i.e., at bedtime. You, Mr. C., must possess extraordinarily sensitive receptors for amitriptyline in such minuscule dosage. And just as I was about to wish you well on this mini-regimen, you switched to trazodone! One of the well-known side effects of trazodone is drowsiness, which you are again taking advantage of at about one-quarter to one-half the usual dose taken at bedtime.

I'm afraid that I cannot generally endorse an antidepressant drug for enhancing the sex urge. But it's your libido, Mr. C., and who am I to argue with such success achieved with a minimum of pharmacological effort?

Do Old People Need Less Sleep?

Dear Dr. MacInnis:

Do old people need less sleep? My grandmother, age 81, spends most of the night up, and come late afternoon, she starts "catnapping" and sometimes falls asleep at the supper table. My theory is what they lose in sleep at night they make up during the day. She never takes sleeping pills.

Have you any suggestions about changing her sleeping habits?

Miss N. T., Ontario

Answer

According to specialists for sleep disorders, the prevalent idea that older people need less sleep is "just another myth." It's been said that the ability to sleep decreases with age much more than the need to sleep.

Many elderly people and especially men with prostate trouble have to get up two, three, or more times a night to go to the bathroom and women, too, with urge incontinence may lose several hours of sleep. Various physical and mental illnesses like arthritis, dementia, and depression may all cause sleep disturbance. In contrast, healthy old people sleep rather well through the night.

In a recent column on insomnia in the elderly (part 2) I may have surprised a lot of readers by not recommending sleeping pills when it's well known that they consume 30 percent of all sleeping pills produced in the nation. Your grandmother should do well on my "non-drug" program as she is not a pill-popper.

Sleep Apnea

Dear Dr. MacInnis:

My husband, age 55, is quite obese, 240 pounds, and has high blood pressure under treatment. But this is not his problem. It is a condition the doctors call sleep apnea (SA). Sometimes I feel I suffer from it more than he does, especially when he stops breathing during sleep and I just have to wait and wait until he emits a loud grunt and gets his breathing back. Some nights his sleep is so interrupted with his breathing problems and night restlessness that he can't function the next day due to sleepiness, excessive tiredness, and mental depression.

My question: Is there any medication you know of to help him? None so far has been of help. What about an operation on the throat area (where the trouble is). It seems that most doctors don't know much about this condition.

Mrs. J. K., Vancouver, British Columbia

Answer

There are many causes for sleep apnea (which literally means "without breath during sleep") but by far the most common is upper airway obstruction that occurs most frequently in obese men who have a short neck and a narrow pharynx. Add to this an excessive growth of throat tissue including that of tonsils and adenoids and you have all the ingredients for sleep apnea that you so ably describe. It is said that hypertension (high blood pressure) can be an added aggravation and this your husband has, too. Alcohol and hypnotics worsen sleep apnea.

There is no specific medication that I can recommend for sleep apnea. Weight reduction and in your husband's case, drastic reduction, is an absolute must. The throat surgery you refer to is often beneficial in appropriate cases. Dr. Dickson's Division of Otolaryngology at the University of British Columbia has an excellent operative record and should be consulted.

Many sleep apnea patients are now using a device called the continuous positive airway pressure (CPAP) system for night sleep. This will be described in the next column.

Sleep Apnea, Again

Dear Dr. MacInnis:

I am writing in regard to the lady whose husband suffered from sleep apnea. My husband (60) also has this problem, and three years ago he was flown to the University of British Columbia Hospital (Vancouver) to see a specialist who recommended that he use a continuous positive airway pressure (CPAP) system at night, which we find works very well. For two years we rented it for $70 a month and then we bought it for $500. Many have not heard of this device but it has helped.

Mrs. R. I., British Columbia

Answer

Several readers have written to me about CPAP and how it helped.

My medical reference, the *Scientific American Textbook of Medicine,* has this to say about CPAP: "This technique called 'continuous positive airway pressure' has been tried most often and appears to be sufficiently successful and well tolerated to be the currently recommended choice among mechanical aids. Unlike drug therapy, where beneficial effects may be delayed for weeks, nasal CPAP has the advantages of immediate onset of action. It also differs from surgical corrective procedures [mentioned in my column] in that it is neither invasive nor necessarily permanent. . . . The technique involved a tight-fitting mask designed to fit comfortably over the nose. Tubing is attached from the mask to an electric blower device that applies an adjustable positive pressure to the airway sufficient to prevent inspiratory collapse of the airway during all phases of sleep. The positive pressure also forces the soft palate to come in contact with the back of the tongue preventing leakage of air out of the mouth. . . ." (Mrs. I's husband used the "Sleepeasy" CPAP system.)

Another reader relates the dramatic beneficial effect of CPAP on her husband's sleep-apnea syndrome, how he quickly falls into long periods of deep (rapid eye movement—REM) sleep and awakens "wonderfully refreshed."

"He has a new lease on life," she writes. "He is rested, is no longer depressed, and is rid of allergies. He must sleep with the aid of the CPAP but it's worth it. He can now handle his farm work, drives vehicles and farm equipment, and is able to think and enjoy life again."

Mrs. P. G., Saskatchewan

Chapter 21
Lookin' Good

Over the years, I have received ever-increasing mail from female readers requesting information on various aspects of cosmetic and reconstructive surgery. Most letters gave plausible and realistic reasons for their decision to improve on their present physical features rather than aspiring to create some "new image," an idealistic goal always doomed to failure. It was a most heartening experience, for it seemed to dispel the last vestige of the "geriatric stereotype." Perhaps it could be better described as a formidable expression of "geriatric liberation"!

Most men over 60 have philosphically accepted their balding tops with grace and humor, as evidenced in many of their letters making up this chapter. In fact, there's the tendency to idolize and pamper their deficit and make it a thing of beauty—and male vanity!

Cosmetic Surgery

Three years ago I wrote a column on cosmetic surgery for the older person. It was sparked by a letter from a lady "close to 60, happily married, financially comfortable, and still very attractive." But she had a problem. It was her ever-increasing facial wrinkles that reached the point "where no amount of cover-up artistry will conceal them." She was "seriously thinking of a face-lift" and wanted an outside and unbiased opinion.

My answer to this lady was swift and sure. "Do it," I advised (almost commanded!), "and it will provide immeasurable satisfaction to you. What better gift can you give yourself? And if in a few years you need another, so what? You can afford it and you're certainly psychologically mature about it."

I received an unexpected barrage of brickbats and bouquets for that column—kudos from the ladies and a not-so-enthusiastic response from the men.

Nearly all of the ladies were eminently satisfied. They spoke of "a new lease on life" and "feeling good" about themselves. It is interesting to note that those who felt the best about it were the ones who had it done "for themselves alone" and not to achieve some pie in the sky aspiration, so often destined to failure, disillusionment, and dejection. "Impossible dreams" included the salvaging of a hopeless marriage or regaining the wanton and wonderful days of youth! Emotional maturity, then, is the key to successful cosmetic surgery.

One lady, believe it or not, came up with the old saw that "you can't beat nature" and "your lines are your legend." I cannot help wondering if, after three years, she's still contemplating the "wonders of nature" and still feeling good about it.

The "male" letters were mainly of the "Gloomy Gus" (she didn't have to do it for me) type. This self-accusatory male stance often refers to his wife's breast reconstruction after a mastectomy. It may come as a surprise (and relief) to these men that their wives didn't do it for them (their husbands) at all. They did it for themselves and they feel good about it. Now that hubby knows, the feeling becomes contagious.

One solitary male was certain that his wife's nose reconstruction job was to impress and eventually capture and marry an imaginary suitor. Several complained about the cost but reluctantly conceded that it might have helped their marriage. All agreed that their wives were happier, and (again from contagion) so were they.

So what's the score on my "mini-Gallup"? A landslide success rate for those women correctly motivated for cosmetic surgery. In short, the psychologically mature—something that experienced, discerning cosmetic surgeons continually tell us.

480

This year an estimated one million Americans and Canadians (women and men), many of them past middle life, will undergo face-lifts, eyelid and tummy tucks, chemo-surgery (face-peeling), breast reduction, breast rebuilding, body sculpting—indeed anything it should always make us "feel good" about ourselves. And it always helps to be rich.

What Causes Wrinkles?

Dear Dr. MacInnis:
Why do we develop wrinkles as we age?

Mrs. K. G. (59)

Answer

Aging affects both the deep and superficial (surface) layers of your skin. The deep layers of the skin have a protein substance called collagen that gives your skin that elastic quality enabling it to bounce back into shape when it's pinched or stretched. As you age, chemical changes take place in the collagen, causing the skin to lose its elasticity so that it sags and creases. As the surface area of your skin thins out, fine wrinkles are formed around the eyes (crow's feet) and mouth and other places that are temporally creased by smiling, grimacing, pouting, and other facial expressions.

Prolonged sun exposure over time virtually guarantees premature wrinkling. Keep this in mind all ye now ravishing sun goddesses!

I'm Thinking of Getting a Face-Lift

Dear Dr. MacInnis:
I'm thinking of getting a face-lift and maybe a nose job. Could you please give me some idea of the cost of these operations? Thank you. (I also have a weak chin.)

Mrs. V. F. (70), Ontario

Answer

Many readers have written in about fees. Here they are. Costs vary from city to city. The following is the fee range for some procedures in Toronto. These are 1988 figures and should now (1994), *serve only as a guide.* It's pretty pricey, I assure you!

Face-lift, $3,000 to $4,000; breast augmentation, $1,800 to $2,500; nose reconstruction, $1,500 to $4,000; eyelid surgery, $1,000 to $3,000; body fat reduction (liposuction) $1,500 to $2,000 per area; chin augmentation, $1,000 to $1,500 or more.

Some (average) U.S. fees (from American Society of Plastic and Reconstructive Surgeons, Inc., 233 North Michigan Avenue, Suite 1900, Chicago, Illinois 60601).

Abdominoplasty ("tummy-tuck"): Where excess wrinkled skin and fatty tissue from the middle and lower portions of the abdomen is surgically removed, $2,000 to $6,000.

Breast lift: Where sagging breasts are raised and re-contoured (in some cases it is performed along with breast augmentation), $1,000 to $4,000.

Chemical peel: Involves application of a chemical solution to peel away top layers of the facial skin, which will be replaced during the healing process with a fresh new skin surface, $250 to $3,000 or more depending on the time and complexity of the procedure.

Post-mastectomy reconstruction: Reconstructive plastic surgery to restore the form and appearance of a breast following total or partial removal. Fee not given. But since the breast has been lost due to illness, surgeon's fees and other costs may be partly or fully covered by your insurance carrier.

Fees for plastic surgery vary greatly. The actual cost will depend on a number of factors including the extent and complexity of the surgery, the skill and experience of the surgeon, where the surgery is done, the type of anesthesia used, and whether or not a hospital is involved.

These are 1988 figures and are now (1993) only relative, but will serve to give you a rough idea of what to expect.

For the free twenty-page booklet *A Guide to Facial Plastic Surgery*, write to American Academy of Facial Plastic and Reconstructive Surgery, 1101 Vermont Avenue NW, Suite 404, Washington, D.C. 20005.

Note: Cosmetic plastic surgical procedures are not generally covered by insurance carriers in the United States or by the Provincial Health Insurance Plan in Canada. However, in both countries, surgical fees and other costs may be partly or fully covered, as in the reconstruction of organs lost or impaired due to disease or physical dysfunction.

Oh, for That Brigitte Bardot Pout!

Dear Mr. MacInnis:

I read your column on cosmetic surgery with great interest and even sent away for the booklet you recommend. You wrote about face-lifts, tummy-tucks, nose jobs, eyelid surgery, chemical peeling, etc., and so did the book but not a word about my affliction—thin lips. I just can't get up the nerve to ask my own doctor about referring me to plastic surgeons, especially at my age. He would think I'd gone bonkers if I asked him for the sensuous Brigitte Bardot pout. But since I don't know you and nothing seems to bother you, I don't mind asking and expect to get a sensible answer. Is there a good operation to fill out my lips and what does it cost? Thank you, sir.

Mrs. F. W. (74), Kelowna, British Columbia

Answer

Most thin-lipped ladies would kill for that sensuous, sultry pout, and it makes me feel real good that you ask. For it's people like you who can make geriatric medicine such a stimulating specialty. Let's hope that query is a harbinger of even more exciting and challenging questions to come my way.

Yes, there's a very satisfactory "lip lift" operation available. The procedure involves increasing the vermillion or darker colored segment of both upper and lower lips. The surgeon first uses computer imaging to show you what you'd look like with various degrees of lip pout, and with that decided, he makes a small linear incision along both lips. The incision is then stitched so that the lip is pulled up to exposed some of its under surface. The stitches are removed in four to five days. The scar is minimal and can be completely concealed with lipstick.

Some surgeons enhance the surgical pout with injection of fat cells (from the patient's own body) or collagen (derived from cowhide).

The cost? About a thousand dollars (minimum). Dr. David Ellis, a plastic surgeon at Toronto Western Hospital, has pioneered this operation and consulting him could be your first step. Good luck!

I Did It for *Me*

A column I wrote about a year ago on cosmetic surgery for seniors brought an unexpected response from readers 50 or better. No longer do they anguish over what people think. I recall one very liberated lady of 55 frankly confess that she had her face-lift done not for her husband (although he thought so) but for herself. "It made me look younger and prettier, and that made me feel young and good about myself. If my husband thinks I did it for him," she wrote, "that's what he thinks and so let it be!"

Once a person decides cosmetic surgery is the way to go, the second most important decision is the choice of surgeon. In a previous column I advised readers to make sure the surgeon is well qualified to do the job.

The American Academy of Facial Plastic and Reconstructive Surgery (AAFPRS) is the world's largest association of cosmetic and reconstructive surgery of the face, head, and neck. The academy's bylaws provide that AAFPRS fellows be board-certified surgeons with training and experience in facial plastic surgery and be fellows of the American College of Surgeons. Many Canadian cosmetic and reconstructive surgeons are members of AAFPRS.

In a June 15, 1989, press release, the AAFPRS provides interesting statistics attesting to a tremendous increase in facial plastic surgery in the United States since 1986.

Here's a synopsis of a study conducted by the University of North Carolina for the AAFPRS:

More than one million persons in the United States had facial plastic surgery in 1988. Based on this figure, cosmetic surgery has, on the whole, increased 17 percent since 1986.

While rhinoplasty (cosmetic and functional surgery of the nose) remained the number one procedure performed by facial plastic surgeons, blepharoplasty (surgery of the eyelids) ranked number two and face-lifts were number three. Mentoplasty (chin augmentation), frequently done along with a rhinoplasty, was the fastest single growing procedure (26 percent). Otoplasty (surgery of the ears) showed an overall increase of 19 percent.

U.S. readers wishing to learn more about any of these specific operations can obtain a free booklet dealing with the above-mentioned topics by dialling this toll free number: 800-332-FACE.

Canadian readers may dial this toll free number: 800-523-FACE. If you prefer not to phone, please write to: FPSIS, 1101 Vermont Avenue N.W. Suite 404, Dept. CSG-NR, Washington, D.C. 20005, and ask to be mailed this free booklet.

I Dreamed I Looked like Harlow

Dear Dr. MacInnis:

Ever since I was a teenager, I dreamed of looking like a movie star (at that time, Jean Harlow). When I was crowned beauty queen at the local Cornhusker's Ball (1941), a judge told me that all I needed was a bit of touching up here and there (meaning cosmetic surgery) and I would "really go places." Of course nothing ever happened, but I can't help daydreaming of what might have been if I had gone ahead with it. I was wondering if a face-lift now at my age (60) would fulfill my girlhood dreams? I'm still basically good looking but could stand some improvement.

Mrs. E. T., California

Answer

You're a cosmetic surgical catastrophe just waiting to happen!

I say this because you are planning a face-lift for entirely the wrong reason and it's doomed for disaster. Discerning cosmetic surgeons warn us never to have cosmetic or reconstructive surgery with the hope of looking like someone else (usually a movie idol). However, if you would just settle for being a younger-looking version of your "basically good-looking" self, then go for it with my paternal blessing—for what it's worth.

It's Easy for Angie

Dear Dr. MacInnis:

In a recent column you advised a lady (presumably well-to-do) to go ahead and have a face-lift and a second one if necessary, like certain time-ravaged movie actresses.

Well, I'm not in that lady's money class and Medicare won't pay, so what's left? I read about a twelve-day treatment in the States where they apply a special cream made in Egypt and wrap your face in bandages, which are removed and re-bandaged every two hours.

The "before" and "after" pictures are out of this world! I'd certainly go for it or if wasn't too expensive. Have you heard of this remedy? Or do you have something better and perhaps cheaper?

I'm not all that old.

Mrs. M. R.

Answer

No, I haven't heard of this clinical management of facial wrinkles but I've seen the results of similar treatment—in a mummy room of Cairo's Archaeological Museum.

You don't state your age (exactly) but if you happen to be hovering around the half-century mark then I'll let you in on

Angie Dickinson's secret. She is now "over 60" (in calendar years).

Ms. Dickinson attributes her spectacular complexion to lots of almond oil and nothing but! "And make the best of what you got," she advises.

All of which is still pretty easy for Angie Dickinson!

It's All in the Way You Hold Your Mouth

Dear Dr. MacInnis:

I am a woman aged 57 and trying of cope with what's called "the midlife crisis" and I'm thinking seriously of having a face-lift. Do you think it is a question of vanity for me to want to look younger? My husband is dead set against it. He tries to persuade me that I'm just fine the way I am, meaning good enough for him! What he doesn't realize is that I'm doing this for Missus Me—not him. If it makes me look younger, then I should feel and act younger, and that should make me feel good about myself. Isn't that what it's all about? Again, I ask you, Is this vanity?

Mrs. H. H., Upstate New York

Answer

I don't think any cosmetic surgeon would consider it vain of you to want a face-lift, as long as you didn't aspire to look like some beauty queen. I would not consider it vain of you to want to look like a younger version of yourself. (If you were a knockout then you'll reap the bonus now.) Wanting to look younger is not the same as wanting to be younger. However, one may follow the other as you argue in your letter.

I believe your motives are right and expectations realistic. So go for it!

Some readers have asked if there are any medical situations that would prohibit cosmetic surgery. The more important are (1) malignant disease, and (2) severe heart disease and uncontrolled hypertension that might result in excessive postoperative bleeding.

I Do Facial Exercises

Dear Dr. MacInnis:

The lady who would like to indulge in the luxury of a face-lift and who couldn't afford it, didn't get much help from your answer, although I agree that "treating" your face with various tanning agents will only result in a tanned hide.

As for myself, I started years ago doing a set of facial exercises every day for just ten minutes or so.

I am now 60 and have fewer wrinkles then most women have at 40. Another tip: Stay out of the midday sun.

Mrs. M.

Answer

You're years ahead of your time, Mrs. M. By coincidence, your letter arrived the day I came across a review of a book titled *Youth Lift* by Beverly Hills skin therapist, Joseph Saffin (Warner Books).

"No drugs or injections or applications," says the review. "Just straightforward easy-to-do facial exercises and lots of good skin care advice thrown in."

If you go along with the fifteen-minute-a-day routine, you'll achieve over the years the same effect as a first class surgical face-lift and escape the $5,000 tab (in California anyway).

"But hold on," you ask, "what about us who already have wrinkles? Are we left out?" "Not so," says Saffin. "True," he admits, "it's better to start in your 30s. But even if you're 50 with lots of wrinkles, it's worthwhile. And it works for men too," says the author.

Am I buying *Youth Lift*? No thanks, I'll continue grimacing!

I Shine My Dome in Vain

Dear Dr. MacInnis:

In regard to your recent column on what to do about a bald head, I would like to make the following recommendations and hope it doesn't offend you. Stop lowering yourself to the level of your frantic balding brothers by devising high-fallutin' nostrums that are either useless or so expensive (like hair transplants) that only your rich "Adonis" friends can afford them.

As for myself, I have a dome even Yul Brynner in his day would behold with envy. I'm very proud of my achievement and would be glad to describe in detail how I keep it nicely shined for the ladies. It really turns them on, so I'm told. But I shine in vain. Can you help?

Mr. A. T., Brandon, Manitoba

Answer

Talk about ambivalence. You start out scolding me for offering solace to my "frantic" fellow baldies and in the next breath you play the "frantic" supplicant imploring me for help.

Yes, I'm aware ladies go for a shining pate but it must adorn more than an empty sphere, which to the vulgar means "a hole in the head." Remember that oldie?

But there I go again, lowering myself to that "level" of yours when I should be offering you a completely new philosophy, which, if followed, will guarantee you a harem!

It's my personal motto right here on my desk: "Bald Is Beautiful. God Made Only So Many Perfect Heads. The Rest He Covered with Hair."

"Hair" Today, Gone Tomorrow

Dear Dr. MacInnis:

I've decided to join the "Baldie Organization" and I would like you to tell me where to write and any other particulars. You also mentioned that you were thinking of becoming a member also, as you would undoubtedly qualify.

Since I made my decision on accepting the inevitable and improving my self-esteem, my friends tell me that a macho image is emerging and although I'm not yet a Telly Savalas with the ladies, I certainly don't lack female admiration. And this trend is growing, something my hair has stubbornly refused to do. But I'm happy with my lot and hope we'll soon be fellow members.

Best regards,
Chrome Dome and proud of it, Toronto, Ontario

Answer

Like the president of the Bald Headed Men of America (BHMA), I have known only too well what's it's like to be lonely at the top.

John Capps presided as head of the BHMA at its seventeenth "Bald Is Beautiful" convention last fall in Morehead City, North Carolina, headquarters of the organization. According to news reports about 200 "bright and shining" members from as far away as England traded baldy jokes and held competitions, such as the Solar Dome Contest for the best tanned head. Winners were inducted into the Bald of Fame.

Paradoxically, the bleak economic recession has had a positive effect on the fortunes of this unique organization. "In fact we're growing because of lack of growth and are proud of every hair we don't have," said the intrepid president to his 20,000 members.

Like you, fellow Chrome Dome, I'm no longer interested in pills, potions, nostrums, and lotions to raise the dead. It's "hair" today and gone tomorrow!

Should I Buy a Head Rug?

Dear Dr. MacInnis:

I am a male, age 74, and balding fast. For a while I was able to cover it by overcombing. Now there's little hair to work with. I'm seriously thinking of buying a good hairpiece or getting a hair transplant. Could you give me some good advice on either of these two options?

Dr. J. M. (74), Bath, New Brunswick

Answer

If I were to pose as an expert on hair restoration, I'd first hide my mug shot! But since you asked, here's my opinion for what it's worth.

Most authorities would not recommend hair transplantation for men even in their fifties. Scalp infection is a problem and you have a large bald area at risk.

A poor hairpiece is instantly obvious, an excellent hairpiece hardly ever, for it's a custom-made, master-crafted work of art that matches the skin color and texture and blends into the natural hair.

Now, I've almost talked myself into buying one, but I can't afford to mortgage the house. Can you?

Chapter 22
Social Studies

This chapter is a collection of miscellaneous columns that don't fit into the anatomical or physiological format that I endeavoured to loosely maintain throughout this book. I'm titling the chapter "Social Studies" because for the most part it is a forum from which my correspondents, mainly elderly people, voice their opinions or vent their spleens on a diversity of behavioral aberrations of their fellow creatures, including their own.

From the thousands of letters I've received from seniors over the years, few have been dull and "run-of-the-mill." Most are exceedingly well written, so much so that I have often wondered (out loud, at times) if our senior generation could be the sole remaining repository of fine literary expression frequently laced with humor—skills often lacking in our so-called modern elementary and high school systems of teaching.

I hope you will find this chapter as enjoyable to read as I did to compile.

Ecclesiastical Disease

Dear Dr. MacInnis:

In church there is a custom of everybody shaking hands before receiving communion.

As you know, anybody who has a cough always coughs in his or her hand, and after the handshaking they go up for communion. The priest places the host in the person's hand and it's then put in the mouth and swallowed.

My question: Is there any health hazard in this custom? What if some one had a serious illness and started an epidemic of disease?

The priest says he doesn't worry too much about germs. I guess I just don't pray hard enough to ward off the little critters! So I will remain worried.

Most people I talk to get about the same charge out of this ritual as they would shaking hands with a sausage!

Mr. A. R., Edmonton, Alberta

Answer

Yes, many unhygienic things happen to us everyday in every facet of our lives. You have singled out a possible unhealthful aspect of a religious ceremony fervently practiced by hundreds of millions of one particular faith, and you could have added the custom of other religious persuasions who share the time-honored communal wine cup.

Can the practice spread disease? As far as I know, no scientific research has been done on this matter, although I can recall that during a particularly severe spread of influenza in England, the custom of sharing the communal cup was banned. So your query may have scientific validity.

What can we do about it any more than to complain? Probably not much. So rather than complain, which in turn begets fear, we should find solace in the comforting view of millions of communicants who believe (rightly or wrongly) that they are protected from contagion by Divine Providence.

Memo to a Granddaughter

Dear Dr. MacInnis:

My granddaughter (17) keeps telling me I'm too religious and that religion is only for old women and the birds!

Is it true that one becomes more religious in old age? I'm 77 and I don't think I've changed much over the years.

Mrs. M. K., Halifax, Nova Scotia

Answer

It's thought that the elderly are more religious, not because of their age but because of a more thorough religious upbringing than their grandchildren.

And speaking of birds, ask your granddaughter to consider their amazing homing instinct. What directs the yellowlegs who fly consistently and unerringly 10,000 miles from the southern tip of South America to their nesting place in the Canadian Arctic? Call it radar if you will, but then who made the radar?

It's puzzles like this that would serve to sharpen your granddaughter's rather dull one-track mind.

A World of Old People

Dear Dr. MacInnis:

Sorry, I have no complaints for you today; just a question. Are the number of old people increasing in our midst? As an oldster myself, I don't think I'm imagining this just because I socialize almost exclusively with people my age. When I was a youngster (I'm now 74) I can recall that there didn't seem to be a great many old people in our community (I suppose they had already passed on at an earlier age than now), leaving a preponderance of children and young and middle-aged adults. Nowadays, there seems to be no scarcity of old and very old people all around. Do you think it will ever get to the point where there will be nobody left in the world but old folks? A dull prospect indeed!

Do you have any figures to prove my point?

Mr. H. de L., Kelowna, British Columbia

Answer

You're right and I have the figures to prove it! According to longevity experts, the numbers and proportions of older people are increasing almost everywhere in the world. In industrialized countries where a census is regularly taken, the fastest growing segment of our population is the 85 year olds, and census analysts in the United States predict that the centenarian (100-year-old) population, which was only 25,000 in 1983, will increase to 110,000 in the year 2000, a tremendous increase in only fifteen years. Another telling statistic that slipped by virtually unannounced was that in June 1984 the number of elderly (65 plus) in the United States for the first time exceeded the teen-age population.

Ours has been dubbed "the century of old age" where we have witnessed an average twenty-seven years' increase in life expectancy. This is roughly equivalent to the previous 3,000 years (Bronze Age to 1900) where it's estimated that life expectancy increased about twenty-nine years.

Since you don't seem to be overly enchanted with the prospect of living in an overpowering "geriocracy," it should comfort you to know that by the year 2000, Father Time will have looked after most of us.

Our Senators, Bless Them

Dear Dr. MacInnis:

I'm confused about the term senile *and wonder if you could clarify some things for me. In school many years ago (I am 75) we were taught that it meant "being old" and that the word* senility *meant "the state of old age." Nowadays, it carries the added burden of mental decline it would seem. My question: Should I call myself a "senile" man at my age when I still have all my marbles—or would it convey the wrong impression?*

Dr. R. S., Belleville, Ontario

Answer

It would indeed give the wrong impression even though you are historically accurate. Over the years the word *senile* has assumed the connotation of mental infirmity and that perception, alas, is here to stay.

It all began with *sen,* the Latin root for very respectable words like "senex," meaning "old age," and *senium* and *senility,* "the state of old age." Over time all three have been bastardized, but curiously, the term *senescence,* meaning "the process of aging," has remained undefiled. Let's look at the word *senate* (from the Latin *senatus*) meaning "an assembly of ancient men." In the last years of the Roman Republic, Julius Caesar increased the senate to 900, a stupendous accumulation of old folks in an age when the average life expectancy (at birth) was about thirty years!

And how has the term *senate* fared over time? Never did it attain virginal purity, because even in Roman times the 10 percent dementia factor in such an aged population applied (like today), leaving about 800 or so with all their "marbles," an achievement that you, Dr. S., so proudly proclaim.

A note to my U.S. readers: The American Senate, I regret to observe, has totally disowned its noble geriatric roots. Yours is an assembly of the relatively young always girded for battle, for it takes the vim and vitality of relative youth to fight for their honor in the hustings.

But not the Canadian Senate and its hoary counterpart, the British House of Lords. With the exceptional presence of a few pediatric interlopers and female intruders, both upper houses have jealously guarded their treasured Roman traditions. Bless them!

What Have You Got against Bachelors?

Dear Dr. MacInnis:

What have you got against bachelors? I resent your remarks in that column about our "sad plight" in our declining years with "no progeny to leave behind." I think it was a very insensitive remark and hope you'll see fit to apologize.

Yours truly, still happily single at 60, and proud of it!

Mr. M. T., Vancouver, British Columbia

Answer

Sorry, no offence intended. But if you thought I was rough on you, lend an ear to what the American humorist Artemus Ward said on the subject: "The happy married man," quoth Ward, "dies in good style surrounded by his weeping wife and children. The old bachelor doesn't die at all—he sort of drops off leaving nothing behind, like the pollywog's tail!"

Bedpan Usage Bottoms Out

Dear Dr. MacInnis:

I know you get lots of complains from people and they all think theirs is the number one scourge of mankind. So here goes mine. It's the bedpan.

I just got home from the hospital, the second time in fifty-one years, and do you know, the bedpan ritual hasn't changed a bit.

I don't blame the doctors. They mean well but how many of them started out their day with a balancing act on a contraption that's not only demeaning and dehumanizing but nearly always fraught with the fear of failure. And how many of your readers, yourself included, could have sworn they overshot and "did it" on the clean bed sheet? And how right they were. "Failure" can also mean a half-hour of futile struggle. There I was in my cosy four-bed ward trying to perform, knowing full well that six other eyes were watching and secretly pulling for me. And I disappointed them, which added to my stress and maybe theirs, too!

A nurse told me in confidence that there's a movement to phase out the bedpan to virtual extinction. In my humble opinion, that would be an achievement in Medicine worthy of a Nobel Prize.

And I believe it would come to pass, if the illustrious committee of Nobel judges were required (for a week before awards) to exercise their "duties" in bed thrice daily on this precarious perch.

Dr. J. A. T., Ottawa, Ontario

Answer

I share your frustration but not your despair. Since the bedpan was patented in 1877, there have been only minor modifications in design, and plastic has replaced metal. But the breakthrough of the century was in the area of creature comfort, like the heated bedpan on cold winter mornings to warmly caress the buttocks. In an age not so long ago, when most maladies required almost total immobility, this innovation was indeed a godsend.

But times, Dr. T., are slowly changing for the better with bedpans utilized in the more enlightened hospitals for only the most serious debilitating disorders. The bedside commode is taking over, with potty patients wild in rapture!

We can thank World War II for the concept of early mobility after surgical operations and heart attacks. Recently, researchers at the University Science Center in Dallas, Texas, have added scientific support for early ambulation that will contribute greatly to the demise of the bedpan in favor of the bedside commode. They measured the heart rate, oxygen consumption, and blood pressure of ninety-five men and women, (sixteen cardiac outpatients) after using a bedpan and a bedside commode. The results indicated that using a bedside commode wasn't physically harder, produced no more cardiovascular stress then using a bedpan, and best of all the patients just loved it.

And there were other benefits, too. Said one nurse researcher, "There's the psychological thing about urinating (or even worse) on your bed that's so terrible with the bedpan; people just hate it." And she added, "A lot of men simply cannot urinate lying down. I've been in the recovery room with these big bruisers with full, full bladders, so full it raised their blood pressure before we could get them to a commode."

Indeed, all the right stuff for a Nobel Prize!

Saltpeter Is Getting to Me (I Think)

Dear Dr. MacInnis:
Would you kindly give me the scientific facts on the antierotic properties of that well-known sexual downer called saltpeter. My

wife tells me that she regularly laces my tea with it to "cool me off," as she puts it. I don't know whether to believe her or not. All I know is that I'm not the man I used to be. Is it getting to me? Please advise.

Dr. A. B., Fort Saskatchewan, Alberta

Answer

The "cooling" effect of saltpeter has historical validity but your wife simply misunderstood what it "cooled," because the medical books as far back as two centuries ago have reported this action as "physiological only."

Furthermore, the *American Dispensatory* of 1806 wrote that it "diminishes the heat of the body and the frequency of the pulse." (Sex never!)

How the saltpeter myth originated we do not know. Could it be due to its touted ability to cool the heat of sexual ardour? Scientifically, potassium nitrate (saltpeter) has no effect on sexual function. But no one will believe this, for old myths die hard.

Do you really and truly believe your wife is secretly feeding you saltpeter? If yes, here's a bit of information that will really shake you: Potassium nitrate is the principal explosive ingredient in gunpowder!

Forget Aerobics—Just Keep Laughing!

Dear Dr. MacInnis:

I'm going to ask you a silly question and I don't mind a silly answer. It's this: Is laughing conducive to good health? The reason I ask you is that ever since I started watching late night reruns of old slapstick comedy films (Laurel & Hardy and the like), I sleep better afterwards and awaken more refreshed. If it's just my imagination, well, so be it. I'm going to keep on laughing for my health's sake—and for once my wife agrees. She's doing it, too!

A Merry Christmas to you.

Mr. K. L., 76, Utica, New York

Answer

A silly question yours is *not*! So hike over to Saratoga Springs (New York) and see Dr. Joel Goodman. He has a very successful *humor* project going there whose slogan is, "He who laughs, lasts."

Dr. Goodman is one of an ever-increasing breed of specialists who believe that a daily structured program of laughter, like the daily apple, will keep the doctor away. The late Dr. Norman Cousins popularized the idea years ago in his book, *Anatomy of an Illness*.

Laughing one hundred times a day, experts tell us, is as good for you aerobically as ten minutes on a rowing machine.

The concept too has scientific substance. Laughing stimulates the production of hormone-like substances called endorphins in the brain that promote well being and relaxation, which may explain why you're now sleeping so well.

And belated Season's Greetings to you, Mr. L.

Which reminds me. Could Santa's tremendous vitality, endurance, and longevity be tied in to this "ho ho" laughing thing?

A Touch of Immortality?

Dear Dr. MacInnis:

This may sound like a preposterous question but I'll bounce it off you anyway. I've heard it's possible to freeze the human body at the time of death so that it can be thawed and revived at some appropriate time in the future for a day when the cure is found for, say, Alzheimer's disease. By now you know what I'm getting at. Long before my mother came down with Alzheimer's she often expressed such a wish and now with her condition far advanced (ten years), I keep wondering if when the time comes, I should fulfill her wish, providing it's feasible and not in science fiction!

Mr. H. W., Vancouver, British Columbia

Answer

"Cryonics" (the science of body freezing at the time of legal death) is what you're talking about and there are at least twenty-six frozen bodies in the United States awaiting a better (earthly) life in the future. The Cryonics Institute of Oak Park, Michigan, founded in 1962, is the oldest and best-known cryonic storage facility that along with its two California counterparts have over a thousand members (with six hundred twelve in Canada) presently on the waiting list to be frozen and who are prepared to shell out about $125,000 for the experience. (For the less affluent, a "head only" cryonics job is available.) Members usually take out an ordinary life insurance policy naming the facility as beneficiary to cover the costs.

If any reader is sufficiently interested in these shenanigans to want more details, I would suggest Dr. Robert Ettinger's book, *The Prospect of Immortality*, written over thirty years ago. Ettinger, now a retired Wayne State University physics and math teacher, founded the Cryonics Institute, and several deceased members of his family are frozen there in liquid nitrogen awaiting better days to come.

Decaf or Not Decaf?

Dear Dr. MacInnis:

My husband and I have been drinking decaffeinated coffee for several years, mainly because of the caffeine keeping us awake at night. Now we hear that it raises cholesterol. Is this true? If so, why decaf and not regular (caffeinated) coffee? Your opinion, please.

Mrs. R. T., Syracuse, New York

Answer

What you heard is correct. Spoilsport scientists at Stanford University have recently reported that in a study of 187 non-smoking middle-aged men, those who switched from regular to

502

decaffeinated coffee increased their low-density lipoprotein (LDL) cholesterol (the bad kind) by an average of 7 percent. The researchers estimated that this rise in LDL could increase the risk of a heart attack by 12 percent. Their report was presented by the principal investigator, Dr. Robert Superko, director of Stanford's Lipid Research Clinic, at the November 1989 annual meeting of the American Heart Association in New Orleans, Louisiana.

Why decaf and not regular coffee? According to the study, the LDL rise was not due to the decaffeinating process but to the coffee beans. Regular coffee is made from the mild *arabica* bean, while decaffeinated coffee uses the stronger *robusta* variety. One or more of the reported 500 ingredients in the *robusta* bean may be responsible.

But the story doesn't end here, Mrs. T. There was swift retaliation from the Tea and Coffee Association of Canada. The Stanford study, it claimed, made "serious misrepresentations" to consumers and "there was no confirmed medical evidence that consuming decaffeinated coffee increases the risk of heart disease." Their spokesman went on to say that the Stanford finding "focused on isolated instances of changes in levels of LDL cholesterol which are of little or no value in determining the risk of heart disease." (I'm sure this LDL putdown will be hotly contradicted by cholesterol specialists!) They also pointed out that "total cholesterol levels and high-density lipoprotein (HDL), which are more important markers of potential heart disease, did not change in the subjects studied. (This is not too convincing a rebuttal, for again, the statement is highly debatable.)

Finally, the Tea and Coffee Association cited an ongoing study at the University of Rotterdam indicating no effect on blood cholesterol from consuming either regular or decaffeinated coffee.

So there you have it, Mrs. T., the pros and cons so far.

My own feeling is that the Tea and Coffee people "doth protest too much" with weak argument.

The last word goes to Dr. Kevin Graham, a cardiologist with the Minneapolis Heart Institute, who said giving up decaf entirely would be "overreacting to the study . . . This isn't major league stuff," he said of the (Stanford) report. "These aren't conclusive findings," he added. "Often you'll find that, later, people do further research and come up with a completely different reading." Time will eventually tell.

Is Owning a Pet Good for You?

"Pets Can Cure What's Troubling You." "Pets May Be the Best Prescription." "The Two-Fold Joy of Keeping Pets: Just Look What It Can Do for You."

What's this? Pet shop ballyhoo? Not at all. They're newspaper headlines all proclaiming the therapeutic value of owning a pet.

Why do more than half the nation's households have pets whose owners consider them in a human light and as-part of the family? The most quoted answer is from Dr. Gerald Jay Westbrook of the Andrus Gerontology Center at the University of California.

"Pets," says Dr. Westbrook, "are nonthreatening, nonjudgemental, open, welcoming, acceptive, and attentive." And who of us, pray, possesses such qualities?

Many years ago I made my Sunday geriatric hospital rounds very special by taking along my two "assistants"—a pair of Scotties named Hamish and Haig. Sunday morning was always a happy time for the aged patients and the nursing staff, too, who often remarked, "If only they'd let us have a little dog or a big cat."

The "they," of course, was the administration—a bureaucracy historically opposed to animals in institutions. And there was the usual doubt expressed as to the validity of pet therapy itself, especially in the absence of scientific proof.

Admittedly, we then had no scientific evidence that pets were therapeutic. But we could see for ourselves what it did for our patients. First their loving recognition, then with their outstretched arms—beseeching, just for a touch, a stroke, or caress and with fulfillment, always the wistful smile. No manmade elixir could work such wonders. We were sure of that.

Happily, time has revealed our observations had indeed scientific substance. One example: In a landmark study at the University of Pennsylvania's Center for the Interaction of Animals and Society, it was shown that heart-disease patients who owned a pet had a significantly lower death rate (after a year) than those without.

Another example: At the sixth annual conference on "Animals and Us" held in July 1992 at Montreal, it was shown repeatedly that just about everyone who owned a pet—the chronically ill, the elderly, the handicapped, as well as the healthy—can benefit from animal interaction, with less hypertension, lower cholesterol, and other cardiac-risk factors.

Medical and lay literature now abound with evidence that animals, in their own way, provide the solace, the comfort, and love that's so often elusive or missing in our lives—and this they freely give with constant devotions. No wonder so many pet owners prefer them to some relatives!

Eighty-five percent of our elderly live at home, and many of them are alone and lonely and often depressed. They are depressed from having suffered many losses—a spouse, maybe, relatives, friends, and not the least, loss of responsibility and aim in life.

Pet ownership can provide the old and alone with a meaningful daily routine—a good reason to get up in the morning to feed the animal and take it for a walk. And walking with a dog is a wonderful door opener for conversation with other dog strollers. (Several studies have reported this social breakthrough.)

Many health care institutions and retirement residences are slowly overcoming their traditional pet prejudices and are now witnessing that so-called human-companion-animal bond in action, with all of its emotional and physical benefits.

I would be remiss in not mentioning two long-time objections to pets in institutions. In my view, the "allergic connection" is a legitimate one with the so-called infection concern open to question. I would say that if a patient was *truly* allergic to animals I would prohibit pet therapy on the ward as long as the patient was there.

But with humans as their most formidable competitors, pet animals play a relatively minor role in the spread of infection, be it in hospital or home.

Budgies Beware

Dear Dr. MacInnis:

As a "concerned grandmother-in-waiting" could you please tell me if there are any health risks in allowing pair of budgies to fly about the house?

My daughter-in-law has just got pregnant and my eldest son has asthma.

Mrs. A. M., Victoria, British Columbia

Answer

Birds such as budgies, parrots, parakeets, chickens, and pigeons are known to be a source of lung infection in humans, called psittacosis. This condition is quite rare, so if I were you or your daughter-in-law or your son, I would not be worried about the budgies flying around the house.

Frankly, of more concern to me is the health risk to the budgies should a hungry cat be on the prowl!

My Granddaughter Is a "Chocoholic"

Dear Dr. MacInnis:

My granddaughter, age 15, is a "chocoholic." I keep telling her that it's making her acne worse and it causes cavities as well. Of course, she doesn't listen to either me or her mother. We wonder if you can help us by providing some scientific evidence of what gorging on chocolate will do to her. Thank you.

Mrs. T. O., Ontario

Answer

For once, Grandma's wrong! There's simply no scientific proof that chocolate or, for that matter, any other food is a cause of acne. Cavities, yes. But don't blame that chocolate (cocoa bean) itself. The culprits are sugar and other carbohydrates found in chocolate products.

Cirrhosis of the Liver

Dear Dr. MacInnis:

We have a question for you—the result of an argument. The topic is cirrhosis of the liver. My wife claims that there's only one cause for liver cirrhosis, namely chronic alcoholism. I say she's wrong. Who is right?

Dr. G. C., Wolfe Island, Ontario

Answer

You are. Liver cirrhosis and alcoholism go hand in hand and sometimes either or both can be acquired quite innocently. I recall the story of a high official in a national temperance organization, well known for her vociferous tirades against demon rum, who was diagnosed as having cirrhosis of the liver. It turned out that the good lady was a chronic guzzler of a once extremely popular "tonic" called Lydia E. Pinkham's Vegetable Compound that (unknown to her?) was laced with 12 percent alcohol!

The basic or root cause of liver cirrhosis is unknown. The most likely hypothesis is that an autoimmune attack occurs by which (1) the bile duct system becomes damaged and plugged, causing bile (normally transported to the gall bladder) to back up in the liver and seep into the blood (resulting in jaundiced skin), and (2) damage to the liver cells results in *scarring* (the tell-tale sign of cirrhosis).

What triggers the immune system to act this way? We know two causes—alcohol and certain drugs. But undoubtedly there are other mechanisms. I'm surprised that someone so apparently sure of himself as you doesn't offer a reason. Anyway, you're right, at least technically.

The Doctors Just Look at Me and Stare

Dear Dr. MacInnis:

I read your ads a lot and can see that you are good with help to older people. I am having problems and half a dozen doctors won't or don't want to help me. I am 78 years old and am in pretty good health. I am overweight by forty pounds and have a slight touch of sugar diabetes. I am not taking any drugs of any kind, only trying to cut back on food to lose weight but so far with very little progress. I have hip joint problems and am waiting for surgery. I have very bad pain in the right joint and painkiller pills don't do any good. Have you any good painkillers to help me and at least make me sleep? I am just about helpless in walking.

The other problem I have is that I had two prostate operations—one eight years ago that didn't do any good and the other operation last year. What happened is that right after the last operation I started peeing every one and a half hours from eight o'clock when I go to bed till eight o'clock in the morning when I have half-filled a three-litre ice cream pail, and this regularly day after day.

So what has gone wrong? Where is all the water coming from? What can I do and where can I go? I can't go on this way. It doesn't matter if I drink water or not, I still pee a cupful every two hours, and if I don't go pee it starts coming out by itself. As I said, I have tried half a dozen younger doctors, and they just look at me and stare and say nothing.

I hope you can help me, and please write because the other doctors won't help. We have Medicare and the doctors get paid, and whether they help you or don't, they are always sure of their money. Please answer.

Mr. Nick, Alberta

Answer

I have carefully read your letter and have come to the following conclusions: It would seem that you have chronic osteoarthritic in your right hip joint and you are awaiting a hip replacement. You undoubtedly suffer pain in that hip and it's unfortunate that you are not improving from your current medication. I would recommend that you see one of your doctors again and explain that you are not getting relief and most likely he/she will change your medication.

I am concerned about your weight because it may interfere with your recovery from the hip replacement. The good thing is that you are aware of this problem and you are trying hard to lose that extra poundage. So good luck for your earnest effort.

Again, you have been very unfortunate in the results of your two prostate operations—the last one being done presumably to rectify the first. Urinary incontinence in varying degree can be a complication of a prostate operation and even after a successful outcome the symptoms may recur in some cases after several years and the operation has to be repeated. Although I cannot tell for sure (from long distance), this may have been your history. I can only advise you to get a consultation with a urologist who may be able to help you after hearing your story. There may be other help at hand in the way of collagen injections around the urethra (urine tube), but this is something only your urologist can decide. (I recently devoted a column to collagen injections in selected cases of stress incontinence in females and post-operative prostatectomy incontinence in males.)

I probably haven't assisted you very much but my advice and recommendations are the best I can muster and hope that you will follow them, for help may be at hand for you.

Jogging Jars Joints—Especially 64-Year-Old Joints

Dear Dr. MacInnis:

I am a 64-year-old man 5 feet 9 inches weighing 180 pounds. I am in good health and hope to stay that way. That is why I have been seriously thinking of taking up jogging. I read Runner's World *and have Jim Fixx's* Complete Book of Running *and his second book as well. But since Mr. Fixx's sudden death on the track, I've had second thoughts about it all. Is it possible to go overboard on this jogging thing, particularly for an older person? Also, what is your opinion on walking to keep fit? Thank you kindly.*

Mr. T. E., Montreal, Quebec

Answer

Is it possible to "go overboard" on this jogging thing? Yes.

Jim Fixx was the recognized guru of that compulsive company of joggers known as "obligatory runners," whose daily ritual of intense and often painful physical activity attains an overwhelming mystical significance that transcends their every other life activity.

The obligatory runner is defined by a University of Arizona Health Sciences Center study (that coined the term) as "those for whom running is a compulsive drive that preempts fulfillment in other life areas, or who run to the point of inflicting physical damage on their bodies." The study found that obligatory joggers start running seriously (forty plus miles per week) later in life than most and become "unequivocally committed to running in their third to fifth decade" (*New England Journal of Medicine,* February 3, 1983). Another study showed that this type of runner usually found life—social and professional—devoid of real meaning and used this form of activity to achieve fulfilment. It was estimated that 25 percent of all serious joggers may be obligatory runners, "neurotically attached to their sport" (Callen, Oregon Health Science study published in *Psychosomatics,* February 1983).

The neurotically compulsive jogger performs his daily rite to conquer the ravages of his own mortality. Thus, he mentally denies illness, aging, and even death itself. It is therefore easy to understand why an obligatory runner will not follow medical advice and will carry on in the face of acute physical illness or debilitation from chronic heart disease and may succumb, as you say, "on the track."

In the same University of Oregon study, Dr. Callen profiles the typical obligatory jogger who may literally run himself to death: "A middle-aged man, tortured by the prospect of growing old, troubled by the prospect of diminished attractiveness, and bored by the absence of job or marital fulfilment."

You ask about walking as a substitute for jogging. I have answered the question on numerous occasions in these columns. In my opinion jogging is not for the elderly, except in the rare instance where a senior has been running regularly, sensibly, and successfully for some years and "knows the ropes."

To begin jogging at your age or even younger can be a dangerous adventure, for you are inviting damage to your ankles, knees, and hip joints that does not repair kindly.

Only young, healthy, resilient joints can absorb the constant stress. And even here there may be a long, painful break-in.

A well-structured and consistent walking program will eventually result in the same aerobic (heart and respiration) benefits as jogging (non-obligatory style).

Remember: Jogging jars joints, especially 64-year-old joints!

Should I Jog or Just Walk?

Dear Dr. MacInnis:

I am 78 with a loving wife who is always after me to get out and start jogging. But I don't buy that and would rather do brisk walking instead. We've decided to put the question to you: What's better at my age, a jogging or walking exercise program? Who's right? Please be kind to me!

Dr. H. D., Rochester, New York

Answer

Who is right? You are, of course. And I'm not being kind to you. Most aerobic experts, I think, would agree because in your case the determining factor is your age. Remember the JJJ syndrome: Jogging jars joints, in your case 78-year-old joints.

511

When you walk one mile at the brisk rate of three and a half to five miles per hour, you burn just about as many calories as jogging it moderately. Furthermore, the experts tell us that this modest program can confer on the elderly walker aerobic benefits similar to jogging. You do not state your weight but if you happen to be overweight, add a low-fat diet to your daily walking program and you'll lose weight.

Once you get settled in with your walking program on a flat surface, you may want to start walking up and down hills, keeping up the same pace; hard at first, but you'll meet the challenge. And swing those arms. This will burn an extra 5 to 10 percent more calories, as well as giving your upper extremities a good workout.

So keep this up, who knows, you might want to graduate into the sport of racewalking where even if you don't achieve Olympic status, you'll have won the everlasting admiration of a loving wife!

Exercises for a Couch Potato

Dear Dr. MacInnis:

Do you have a simple exercise program that might interest my husband? Anything more than just walking to and from the car would be a plus for my beloved couch potato. I recently signed up for an aerobic program at the gym suitable for my age in the hope that he might take a hint, but all he did was offer to pay for my course on condition I would lay off and leave him alone.

Do you think there's any hope for him at all, or is he destined to spend all his evenings (and mine) glued to the boob tube and guzzling beer in his usual reclining posture?

Mrs. S. B., Edmonton, Alberta

Answer

Have you heard of "The Official Workout for Couch Potatoes, Illustrated in Six Easy Steps"? (1) Warm-up—a few minutes of easy regular breathing to induce a refreshing snooze; (2)

stretch—by which the left arm is gently lifted from the lap; (3) reach—by which the outstretched left hand r-e-a-c-h-e-s for a bottle of beer; (4) twist—where the right hand is exercised by deftly twisting off the bottle cap; (5) sweep—left arm transports bottle to mouth in sweeping arc-like motion; beer guzzled; and (6) repeat—over and over. Note: The right hand gets its exercise by constant fiddling with the channel changer.

Enough levity! I have a startling study to relate, Mrs. B., that will stimulate the most incorrigible lounge lizard to *sit* up, take notice, and maybe mend his errant ways. Read this to him. He'll like it!

Scientists at the Institute for Aerobics Research in Dallas, Texas, have discovered that even minimum levels of fitness improve one's chances for survival. Here's how they found out: Using a treadmill that was programmed to become faster and steeper, they tested 13,344 apparently healthy men and women. Each subject then received a fitness rating. At the end of eight years the mortality (death) rate was correlated with the initial level of fitness score.

Result: By the end of the eight-year test period, 238 subjects were dead. In men the least fit died two and a half times the rate of the most fit. In women the same difference in fitness yielded a much greater death rate of four and a half times.

The most tell-tale finding: Being *above* the bottom 20 percent of fitness proved to be a tremendous advantage. *But further improvement in fitness scores had little effect on survival.*

The researchers concluded that very little exercise is needed to greatly increase the odds for survival, which would translate into "a good brisk walk for half an hour a day," they said.

This study was published in the November 1989 issue of the *Journal of the American Medical Association:* 2395–401.

Garlic's Got Everything—but the Love of Your Wife

Dear Dr. MacInnis:
My wife and I are having an argument about garlic. I maintain that garlic is good for the health and can ward off many

conditions like the common cold and the flu, and there's nothing better to keep your sex up. But my wife will have nothing to do with it—or with me after I eat it.

This means that I must eat anything with garlic outside the house, which is not very good for family life even though we've been married for fifty-two years.

So would you please tell her something good about garlic. She just might listen to you.

Mr. H. D., age 75, Kelowna, British Columbia

Answer

After fifty-two years, I would think your wife's aversion to garlic is pretty well fixed in stone and nothing I can say in praise of its many virtues will have the slightest effect on her. Yes, it's true that millions swear by it, but it's equally true that many swear at it—like your wife.

The medicinal properties of garlic were well known to the ancient world. The Egyptians, the Greeks, and the Romans (and the Chinese thousands of years before them) all extolled its merits to the heavens for treating everything—from healing the wounds of battle, preventing bubonic plague, and exorcising vampires, to the cure of hemorrhoids.

Remind your wife (gently) that the great surge of well-being and physical power you experience after a garlic-flavoured food was well known to the royal Egyptian contractors building the Great Pyramid of Cheops. History records that they fed their workmen garlic at every meal to keep up their strength and morale.

I still feel I haven't impressed your lady, and it looks as though you'll continue to dine in the doghouse. But it should be consoling to know you'll always have history on your side.

Getting Pregnant Past 70?

Dear Dr. MacInnis:

I heard some ladies (elderly) talking about the possibility of getting pregnant past 70. Some thought it was possible; others disagreed. Would you please state your opinion? I'm curious and would like to know the facts.

Jennifer S., New York

Answer

I'm assuming you're not putting me on, so I'll answer in the spirit of your question.

There always comes a time in a woman's life when her ovaries cease to produce eggs for possible fertilization and pregnancy. In the United States and Canada, the average age for this ovarian "failure" (menopause) is 48 years. Note that 48 years is the average—meaning that the ovaries can function successfully for some years beyond this figure. This is attested to by numerous well-documented reports of pregnancy in the early 50's.

According to the 1983 *Guinness Book of Records,* the oldest authentically documented successful pregnancy occurred in a woman aged 57 years and 129 days (Glendale, California, 1956).

When God told Abraham (then nearing 100) that his wife Sarah (90) would bear a son, the old gentleman laughed so hard at the joke that he fell flat on his face (Genesis 17:17). But God had the last laugh, for Sarah conceived and brought forth Isaac.

Another old-age "biblical" pregnancy was that of Elizabeth, wife of Zachary. When the angel Gabriel announced to Mary that she would conceive and bring forth a son, he mentioned, in passing, that her cousin, Elizabeth, had already conceived "in her old age" and in fact was six months' pregnant (Luke 1:35).

So there you have it, dear reader. The medical (non-celestial) record is for 57 years and 129 days.

And the biblical record? Well, let's give the last word to an angel. "Nothing," says Gabriel, "shall be impossible with God."

Try Parsley after Garlic

Dear Dr. MacInnis:
Sometime ago a man wrote you about his wife not having anything to do with him after he ate garlic.

515

I have a lady friend who eats garlic a lot and I personally can never detect it on her. What is her secret? She tells me she always takes parsley after a garlic meal.

Maybe some garlic lovers would like to know this, including that poor gentleman who has to eat in the doghouse.

Yours truly,

Dr. B. B., Edmonton, Alberta

Answer

Thank you for your thoughtful note. I have received a number of letters from readers, both wives and husbands, none of whom had anything nice to say about garlic despite its many reputed virtues.

Afficionados of the celebrated clove will bless you for this timely information despite its lack of scientific validation.

Scientific or not, it's certainly worth a try.

Think of it (you poor man in the doghouse), a bit of parsley garnish may restore your rightful place at the dinner table or even in the marriage bed.

Oysters Are Full of Zinc (and Sex)!

Dear Dr. MacInnis:

We are having a bit of an argument about the value of zinc to make a person sexy. One of the "racy" lads in the lodge here says raw oysters are full of zinc and that's why he's sold on them. Another says it's all an old wives' tale and I'm inclined to agree with him. We've appointed you the judge. Who's right?

Dr. J. S., Midland, Ontario

Answer

Your dissolute friend has science on his side. An oyster is a good dietary source of zinc. So is the unerotic herring. But here's the clincher. It takes zinc to produce testosterone and the testes contain the largest accumulation of zinc in the body. So there!

I've Got B.O. and Love It!

Dear Dr. MacInnis:

As you seem to know a little bit about everything, I have a question that may stump you. It's about body odor. My wife tells me I smell bad and is always after me to apply deodorants (she buys them by the bushel!). I keep reminding her that my body odor is a natural aphrodisiac and neutralizing it with a pungent artificial perfume is robbing her of the best years of our lives!

My question is: Do you agree with me scientifically and do you think I'm attacking this problem in a responsible manner? I shower faithfully twice a week.

J. M., Olds, Alberta

Answer

This is a loaded question for sure! There is no doubt about the erotic effect of body odor on the opposite sex, so you score full marks here. It's ironical indeed that we spend countless millions on worthless aromatics in the hope of achieving a sexual come-on by destroying the "real bonanza" that has been known for ages. It is reported that Napoléon, on retreating from Russia, sent the following message to Josephine, "I'm on way home. Do not bathe."

As for your shower routine, why not step it up to every second day, whether you really need it or not?

B.O. Rebuttal

Dear Dr. MacInnis:

Regarding the man whose wife complained of his body odor. Oh, how many, many women must sympathize with her.

When will men ever get over the macho idea that women should like it? No woman thinks a man becomes more desirable because he smells bad. How disgusting that he should think so!

Any man who will not make his presence more pleasurable for his wife by using a deodorant just because it will affect his

517

manhood proves only one thing: He doesn't love his wife, he loves only himself.

Mrs. J. M., Kelowna, British Columbia

Answer

You were one of many wives to write similar letters. And just as I was enjoying the distinct impression that B.O. rates a miserable zero in the love department (according to the ladies), the following letter made my day.

Dear Dr. MacInnis:
I am the wife of a traveling man and can tell the world without embarrassment that when I know the night my husband comes to me, I prepare myself like Josephine awaiting Napoléon, which means I don't prepare myself at all! No fuss, no bother, no silly bathing and waiting. And my husband just loves it. We both think that rapturous aroma is absolutely odorific! Please write on B.O. more often.

Mrs. L. M., age 56, Vancouver, British Columbia

The Corpus Callosum

Why are people talking so much about the "corpus callosum"? Wire services across the continent are awash these days with the news.

It seems that a professor from McMaster University, Dr. Sandra Wittelson, did an autopsy on forty brains and found that the corpus callosum grows smaller in men as they age but remains unchanged in women. In other words, elderly women have a lot more corpus callosum than their male counterparts. Before gloating over their good fortune, I would enjoin the elderly ladies to contemplate what they really have that men haven't.

My medical dictionary says, in effect, that the corpus callosum is a band of neural tissue that serves as a bridge uniting the right and left hemispheres of the brain. Now that's what it is. But what is it for? I've read that in 1982, Yale and Columbia

518

researchers found that the back part of the corpus callosum, called the splenium, was bigger in women than in men. This inferred that if the corpus was larger in women that in men, then there might be more connecting fibers in the female corpus and, ergo, better communication between the right and left female hemispheres, with mind boggling implications of female mental superiority just around the corner! But nothing seems to have happened. Research is confusing and contradictory, but what's really important from all this is that we men haven't lost face, not yet.

So we men must plod on in the knowledge that we have a little less of something than our womenfolk, but we don't know what we're missing and the ladies only know that whatever it is, they may have more of it!

In Praise of "Power Naps"

Dear Dr. MacInnis:

I am a healthy man of 72 years, so why am I writing to you? It's because at 3:00 P.M. everyday I get drowsy and have to take a short nap. About a half-hour is plenty, and I wake up refreshed and raring' to go and can then carry on till bedtime which is around 11:30. At first I thought it was caused by overeating at lunch, but I found out that had nothing to do with it. My wife, who is very active and always on the go, is not too sympathetic with my napping and has even accused me of being a bit lazy, and that is hard to take. I know several other people quite a bit younger than I am who routinely nap and I certainly can't accuse them of laziness, because in the run of the day they accomplish much more work than most people.

Please tell me, if you can, if napping is a good thing and how prevalent it is. I hope you agree with me as my wife reads your column.

Dr. S. H. St. Albert, Alberta

Answer

Winston Churchill, an inveterate napper, used to say that it was his way "to press a day and half's work into one." So you are indeed in noble company!

Most people who are overcome with weariness and fatigue usually in the afternoon are unable to indulge in that refreshing nap because of work. But that doesn't stop some of them from stealing a wink in their office chairs.

When I was in active medical practice, I developed the habit of taking my "power nap" at noon, a twenty-minute office ritual that set me up for the rest of my long day. It was not a long sleep but a most refreshing one. But the ideal time for a good restorative nap is said to be eight hours after waking and eight hours before bedtime (at night). Why do I say this? Sleep researchers tell us that between 2:00 and 3:00 P.M. (your nap time), the body experiences a small drop in temperature and this initiates sleepiness. The experts also tell us never nap more than an hour. Some people can energize themselves just by lying down and resting (and sometimes dozing off just for a few minutes).

At any rate, you will be pleased to know you're doing the right thing. You can hold your head high, for you now have science (and I hope your wife) on your side again.

Bachelors Are Hard to Snag—Matrimonially, That Is

Dear Dr. MacInnis:

I am writing to you about our son, a bachelor, aged 40. His problem is that he shies clear of any romantic involvement with women. He is good-looking, and successful in business, but seems to be very suspicious, even paranoid, feeling that women are scheming to "hook" him.

Don't you think it's time he left the parental roof?

Mrs. L. H.

Answer

Once a bachelor reaches 40 he tends to remain single. This is the opinion of psychologist Charles A. Waehler of the University of Akron (Ohio). Waehler studied thirty never-married men who were white, heterosexual, and between the ages of 40 and 50. As a group, the subjects showed three primary modes of defense in relationships: avoidance, isolation, and distortion. Overall, the bachelors appeared reluctant to get involved, make demands, or assert their needs in relationships, particularly in the major areas of sexual expression, career undertaking, and significant relationships.

Isolation was evident in their lives. About 20 percent of those studied were described as "flexible and satisfied." They had a greater number of significant relationships through their adulthood but extended interdependence was threatening to them. Thirty percent were described by Dr. Waehler as "rigid and satisfied." They were content with their lives mostly because they were attached to their defenses. Half of the bachelors were disappointed with their limitations in relating to others and in forming meaningful relationships; 80 percent were involved in psychotherapy. This group wanted to get involved romantically but then vacillated between wanting to get close and wanting to be isolated.

"Only 5 percent of bachelors after aged 40 will ever marry," Dr. Waehler said, "and women with a marriage goal in mind should be aware of that when they enter romantic relationships with never-married men age 40 and over." He added: "These bachelors often make very good companions but if women push them too far or ask for more they are capable of giving, these bachelors will frequently push them away or end the relationship." (Mothers should note this too!)

Dr. Waehler presented his findings to a meeting of the American Psychological Association in Washington on August 16, 1991 (from *American Psychological Association News*).

When You Read This, I'll Be Gone!

Dear Dr. MacInnis:
My wife and I argue a lot about the benefit of a steam vapor-izer for a head cold. She claims the steam, especially if medicated, is just the right thing to un-plug plugged noses. She swears by it. I swear at it and say it's no good. Who's right?
Mr. G. J., Gloucester, Ontario

Answer

You are. It makes no difference whether it's plain steam vapor or medicated, it's still no good. But don't listen to me. In a recent issue of the *Journal of the American Medical Association* there's a scientifically controlled (double blind) study that bears me out. So break the news to your wife (gently as possible) that any perceived benefit is all in her head, like her cold.
P.S.: I'm leaving town when this comes out in print!

Alcoholism in the Elderly: Part 1

Dear Dr. MacInnis:
My father, age 63, has changed a great deal since my mother died two years ago. Whether he seems to be drinking much more than usual or is not able to handle it as he used to, I'm not sure. He becomes quite depressed after a heavy night out with his drinking friends. When he is confronted with the possibility that he has an alcohol problem, he denies it and always gets angry. He would much rather socialize with drinking companions than with his and my mother's old friends. He's developed a brand-new lifestyle that is out of character for him.
His changed personality and unkempt appearance are becoming quite apparent to his family and old friends, and we are going to do something about it but need some professional advice on how to tackle the problem.
Mrs. J. L., Rochester, New York

Answer

You give a good description of what we known as the "older alcoholic" of recent onset. As in your father's case, the older person very often takes to alcohol after experiencing one of life's most stressful events, and the death of a spouse heads the list. Other stresses are retirement, especially if unplanned, and chronic, disabling illness with depression.

There are in the United States an estimated ten million alcoholics of which three million are over the age of 60. With the senior population expected to double in the next fifty years, it is easy to see what an ever-increasing problem it is going to be.

Now, getting back to your father's situation, I must tell you at once that you and the family are making a mistake by "confronting" him (to use your own words) with this alcoholic problem. Nothing will put an alcoholic person off more than "confronting" him or her. It will surely evoke a denial or an angry response. You must not be judgemental; he doesn't appreciate being preached to. My advice is to have someone his own age, especially one whom he respects, speak to him—at first casually and, later, more to the point. Ideally, this person would be from Alcoholics Anonymous, but if not, he or she should strive to get an AA member to see him. This happily could be the beginning of his recovery. Older alcoholic persons, particularly those like your father, of recent onset, generally respond favorably to intervention such as AA coupled with the necessary medical and psychological care.

Alcoholism in the Elderly: Part 2

Dear Dr. MacInnis:

My husband, age 66, has started drinking quite heavily since his retirement from the railroad service last year. During his working life he could be termed an "occasional social drinker." What bothers me is that there are several alcoholics in his family history—his father, a brother, and a sister.

My question: Do you think we are dealing with another alcoholic problem here and, if so, is this the time to seek the help of Alcoholics Anonymous?

Mrs. L. Y., New York

Answer

I do, indeed, and would advise you to first contact AA yourself and discuss how to best approach your husband, knowing well that he will at first deny he is an alcoholic and may resent the intrusion. But leave this important decision with AA to handle.

The incidence of alcoholism in the elderly is increasing. It is estimated that 10 to 15 percent of older people have a drinking problem. And there need not be a history of alcoholism as in your situation, Mrs. Y. Fortunately, the older the age of onset, the better the chances of recovery, because older people follow the treatment programs better.

If any reader feels that he/she, a relative, or friend may be developing a drinking problem, the following test, called the Short Michigan Alcoholism Screening Test, will be useful. To score, you give yourself one point for each answer that applies to you. If you come up with two matching answers you may be a *possible* alcoholic. If you score three or more matching answers you are a *definite* alcoholic.

1.	Do you feel you are a normal drinker?	NO
2.	Does your spouse or other relative worry about your drinking?	YES
3.	Do you ever feel guilty about your drinking?	YES
4.	Do your friends or relatives think you are a normal drinker?	NO
5.	Are you able to stop drinking?	NO
6.	Have you attended AA meetings?	YES
7.	Has drinking ever created problems between you and your family?	YES
8.	Have you ever gotten into trouble at work because of drinking?	YES

9. Have you ever neglected your duty, family, or job   YES
for two or more consecutive days because of your
drinking?
10. Have you ever gone to anyone for help   YES
about your drinking?
11. Have you ever been hospitalized for drinking?   YES
12. Have you ever been arrested for drunken driving?   YES
13. Have you ever been arrested for alcohol-   YES
related problems?

(Adapted from *Journal of Studies of Alcohol* by *Johns Hopkins Medical Letter,* December 1992.)

Gravitationally Challenged and "Devastated"

Dear Dr. MacInnis:

My wife just heard on the radio that short people are more susceptible to heart attacks than tall ones. I am taking this very personally because I'm a short, pudgy five-foot three and my wife, alas, is a very attractive and statuesque five-foot ten.

Is there anything to this? Please say it isn't so. By the way, she's 60.

"Devastated at 52 in Toronto"

Answer

Dear Devastated:

Your glamour girl heard right. Some recent (Harvard University) research has found that people five feet seven inches or less were at higher risk for a heart attack than those six feet one inch or over. The researchers point out that "short, pudgy people" (you said it) are more likely to be overweight, more likely to be hypertensive and tend to have high cholesterol and diabetes—all risk factors—and there is an inherent risk in being "short" itself. Men under five feet seven inches had about 70 percent more heart attacks than those over six feet one inch according to the Harvard Study.

So what do you do? If you have any of the added risk factors mentioned, seek medical help to help the odds, and don't forget your wife is eight years your senior, which helps to even things up.

"Better Halitosis Than No Breath at All"—Shakespeare, or Was It?

Halitosis: An unlovely word with a thoroughly good Latin origin, from *halitus* meaning "breath" and *osis,* "a condition of." So there you have it—a "condition of the breath" that we all know is plain bad breath, and to make things worse, "even your best friend won't tell you."

About 75 percent of halitosis is caused by problems arising solely in the mouth and throat.

Morning "jungle mouth" is common enough to be considered normal. It occurs in normal mouths due to overnight putrefaction of retained food particles in the absence of saliva during sleep. It's worse in mouth breathers, smokers, alcoholics, and world-class snorers. This universal condition is easily remedied by your morning brushing, aided by the resumption of normal saliva production.

Here are the more common mouth conditions causing "true" halitosis: (1) Dental cavities (rotten teeth), (2) gingivitis (inflammation of gums), (3) pyorrhoea (inflammation of tissue around teeth), (4) dental plaque (a slimy film composed of bacteria and debris around the gumline) and (5) chronic inflammation sometimes with ulcer formation anywhere in the mouth and throat cavity.

Any of the above mouth and throat conditions produces a wide range of germs that act on food particles, the shredded mucous membrane debris, and even on the saliva itself. This decaying process produces the distinctive rotten egg odor of hydrogen sulphide that even your "best friend" suffers through and dares not break the dreadful news to an unsuspecting *you.*

And then there's the so-called "between periods" bad breath around ovulation time when the level of sulphur-containing chemicals in the saliva is reported to be ten times that of other times.

Certain foods and liquids can cause bad breath. Common culprits are alcohol, garlic, and onions. Breath odors they create don't originate to any extent in the mouth; they are eliminated through the lungs. (Garlic rubbed on the soles of the feet can be detected on the breath.) Many drugs emit distinctive odors.

So what's there to do? First of all you should have a mouth examination—not the quickie, "say ah" sort of thing but a thorough search for the aforementioned mouth conditions. If there's a even a suspicion of a dental cause, you should be referred to a dentist.

In the majority of cases the answer will be found right there in the mouth. The treatment is medical or dental or both, followed by an ongoing program of oral hygiene. This will include frequent brushing of the teeth (don't forget the back of the tongue) along with dental flossing to remove as much as possible the retained food particles between the teeth.

Mouthwash? Swish for taste only. Manufacturers of leading mouth washes have been ordered to desist from proclaiming that their products "effectively destroy bacteria causing tooth decay." "There's simply no proof," says the U.S. Federal Drug Administration.

Now suppose that after careful medical and dental examination nothing is found in your mouth and throat cavity to account for your halitosis. Then what?

This calls for a detailed history taking of your problems and a complete medical workup with particular reference to the respiratory and digestive systems. There are many ailments, some serious, whose only outward signal is persistent and severe halitosis.

To sum up: (1) Seventy-five percent of halitosis is due to treatable mouth problems; (2) the other 25 percent is found elsewhere in the body and may be treatable in whole or in part depending on the cause; and (3) in all cases, proper halitosis management calls for the combined efforts of your physician, your dentist, and above all—yourself.

Hot Chicken Soup

Dear Dr. MacInnis:

I'm sure many readers will recall, as children, being fed hot chicken broth on the first sign of sniffles. Mother said it was "good for you" and that was that! We took it and always got better—because of it or in spite of it, it's hard to say. Then came a generation of skeptics and it seemed to lose favor and I believe it went into disrepute.

But maybe Mother was right after all. I recently caught an item on the radio about good hot chicken broth for treatment of the common cold being scientifically sound. Have you heard about this? If so, would you please elaborate as I missed most of the particulars.

Mrs. L. Y.

Answer

It's hardly the long-awaited "breakthrough" to end the common cold but it proves that Mother not only knew what was best for us, but had science on her side as well.

Researchers at the Mount Sinai Medical Center, Miami, Florida, have proven that hot chicken soup clears the stuffy nose much better than hot water irrigations or steam inhalations, even when the hot soup was sipped through a straw. No one is quite sure why, but there seems to be some "aromatic substance," as yet unidentified, in the soup that helps to clear the nasal passages.

Interferon, that high-profile antiviral drug of a few years ago, is in the news again. Scientific studies both in Australia and America have shown that interferon nasal spray can reduce significantly the spread of the common cold in a household after one member is stricken with the rhinovirus (the commonest cold-causing virus).

The American research was conducted by Dr. Frederick G. Hayden and co-workers at the University of Virginia Medical School. They treated sixty families with the interferon-laced nasal spray once daily for one week as soon as the first family member reported cold symptoms.

The result was a 60 percent overall prevention in respiratory illness in the sixty families studied. Rhinovirus spread was reduced 80 percent. It should be stressed that this study established the value of interferon, not in curing but in preventing a

cold. The Hayden group is now researching its value in successfully treating a cold once it starts.

The nasal spray (manufactured by Schering-Plough) is
called Alpha Interferon. But don't look for it in your pharmacy
yet. It will probably be a year or so before the FDA (Federal
Drug Administration) gives the nod.

And what should we take in the meantime?

Mother's hot chicken soup, of course.

Addendum (1993): In April 1982, I devoted a column to
interferon nasal spray research conducted by Dr. John Wallace
of Salisbury, England, who found it effective against fifty strains
of cold virus. But since there were at least two hundred strains
currently reported, Dr. Wallace prophetically remarked that "we
have a long way to go yet—five to ten years before interferon
nasal spray is deemed totally effective and generally available
for treatment." It's now 1993 and research continues. Be patient.

Throw in the Towel—You're Beaten!

Dear Dr. MacInnis:

*What should I do about my husband's smoking? When I tell
him all the dire effects of cigarette smoking, he always rejoins,
"I'm 80 now and if I knew I was going to live for so long I would
have taken better care of myself!" Should I give up?*

Mrs. G. Y., Ithaca, New York

Answer

Throw in the towel, you're beaten! And I believe he just
might have a point there. I say this after reading what a research
group from the Department of Geriatric Medicine in a Dunedin
(New Zealand) hospital came up with in studying why some
people seem to age more quickly than others. They also looked
into why certain risk factors produce different effects in older
and younger patients. "Smoking is an important risk factor all
right," they said, "but to a lesser degree than in younger people."

In an ongoing study of risk factors for heart disease, they
showed that in patients over 70, *low blood pressure* was a better

529

predictor of death than *high blood pressure*. This was puzzling but the results suggested that it might be due to older people taking drugs for other conditions.

And the old saw that seniors should not be overweight received a jolt. Said the head researcher, Prof. John Campbell, "obesity should not be regarded as a risk factor after 70. . . . "Rather," he continued, "extreme thinness seems to be also a predictor of death, as this condition is often linked to poor nutrition or underlying disease."

And what about trying to lower cholesterol in old age? "There is no evidence," said Professor Campbell, "that lowering cholesterol in the over 70s will be of any benefit."

Old age does have its compensations!

Chapter 23

Startin' Down the Final Common Path—Last Rights

It seems to me most strange that men should fear,
Seeing that death, a necessary end,
Will come when it will come.
                    —Shakespeare, *Julius Caesar,* Act II, sc. ii

Contrary to popular opinion, the aged are no more preoccupied with notions of death and dying than younger folks, as long as they are in command of their faculties and enjoying a reasonably good quality of life. Indeed, as they in later years "mature," they become, I believe, shielded from "fear of the unknown" and can speak dispassionately, at times wistfully, of the great adventure that beckons down the road. This is particularly true of believers in a hereafter, for to them life is no more than a necessary "stopover" on a journey they implicitly believe will end in heaven for the eternal family reunion. I've known non-believers too, with admittedly nothing to anticipate, who seemed mysteriously sheltered from fear and anxiety, but where sometimes a few "old gamblers," always playing the odds, turned into death-bed believers—just in case!

No business in life, especially in later life, is more important than making a last will and testament which should include a so-called living will that has now the force of law in forty states and, very recently, in two of our Canadian provinces, with indications that it may soon catch on throughout the land. Since the subject is not in my area of expertise, I have invited a lawyer friend well versed in senior legal affairs to contribute what he sees fit to this, my final chapter. My thanks, then, to Don

McCrimmon who will find this an easy assignment, as he currently writes in the Kelowna (British Columbia) *Daily Courier* a column for seniors titled "It's the Law."

The chapter and book end with three of my own columns—two of which attest to the physical futility and, indeed, in my view, the moral obscenity of performing cardio-pulmonary resuscitation (CPR) on the aged, dying patient. The final column addresses the problems surrounding the prolongation of the dying process, ending with the words of Sir Theodore Fox who in his usual elegant prose disposes of this controversial area of medical ethics.

Do I Need a Will?

Your last will and testament is the cornerstone of your estate plan. Upon death, it is the only "say" you have in the distribution of the wealth that took you a lifetime to acquire. It sets out who is to take control of all your affairs (the trustee or executor), who is to be guardian of your dependent children and, of course, it outlines the scheme of distribution of your assets.

Dying without a will (intestate) is an unfortunate situation. If it happens to you, your estate will be distributed according to the intestacy provisions in your state or province. The end result may be quite different than what you would have intended or preferred, especially if there are children involved. Preparing a will allows you to arrange your affairs to suit the needs of your family.

Dying intestate doesn't mean that you have avoided delays, legal fees and court costs. On the contrary, the administration of an intestate's estate is often more expensive and lengthy than the probate of a will. There may be many competing claimants for administration or, more likely, guardianship that necessitates court proceedings. Worse than that, however, is the situation where there are no volunteers to take on the responsibility of administrator or guardian. In the meantime the estate is in limbo while costs mount up.

Unless you die penniless, destitute and alone something has to be done about your estate. The income tax department (the same folks who vexed you during your lifetime) will insist that they be paid in full for income tax or monies you earned in the year of death. They will also want taxes paid on any income earned by the estate after death. Creditors, such as the funeral home, will also want to be paid. Any businesses you had will have to have someone new to run things. None of this can be done without some form of court authority over the estate. As you can see, dying intestate is just additional grief to pile on the ones you leave behind. No one wants to be remembered as "that idiot."

—Don McCrimmon

Making a Will

A will can be anything from a single scrawl on a piece of scrap paper to a video tape to a fifty-page text. It can be prepared by a lawyer, a notary public or the next-door neighbour. In fact, anything that indicates what you want done with your property after your death is a will. The real question, however, is whether or not it is valid and if it will be recognized by the courts.

In most jurisdictions holograph wills (i.e., wills made wholly in the testator's writing and not witnessed) are only recognized as valid under very limited circumstances. If you are not a member of the armed forces or a mariner you can probably forget it. If you make a holograph will in another jurisdiction that does recognize them and happen to die there, the will may only be valid in your home jurisdiction for moveable property (not real estate). In short, a holograph will is usually a complete waste of time. It is, however, cheap.

A videotaped or tape recording of a will has more of a personal touch to it, but it suffers from a serious flaw—because it is not in writing, it is not valid. Video or audio recordings of the testator, while dramatic, are also often a painful reminder to the survivors of the loss they have suffered and, unless there is some special reason for going that route, should probably be

533

avoided. If explanation of the reasons for the testator's choices is required it can just as easily be accomplished by a side memorandum.

Often, a difficult question to decide is at what age beneficiaries should take over their bequests. Some people request wills wherein minor beneficiaries receive their inheritance at age 25 or, for that matter, anytime other than on their majority birthday. This may not be appropriate where the gift or legacy is substantial. For example, many advisors feel it is better to withhold larger sums of money from the beneficiaries until they are old enough and mature enough to handle it wisely. Where a 19 year old might buy a hot car, a big stereo and a boat, the same person at 25 might buy a house, a business and a term deposit. If this situation applies to your family you would probably be well advised to seek legal assistance.

It is possible to prepare a valid will from a stationer's form but you have to be very careful to have it properly witnessed and attested. You also have to be very careful not to allow beneficiaries to act as witnesses. There are, of course, other snags and pitfalls to avoid. The problem with these kinds of wills is that if a question does arise, the preparer of the will is no longer around to answer it. These kinds of wills are greatly appreciated by law firms with large litigation departments as they often result in lucrative law suits. This is seldom the saving sought by the maker of the document.

—Don McCrimmon

Mental Capacity to Make a Will

The classic phrase "being of sound mind" seems simple enough at first glance. The problem, of course, is determining just how sound a mind is needed. As a nineteenth-century English judge said:

Between the extreme case of a raving madman or a drivelling idiot and that of a person of perfectly sound and vigorous understanding there is every shade of intellect, every degree of mental capacity. There is no possibility of mistaking midnight for noon; but at what precise moment twilight becomes darkness is hard to determine.

There are essentially four parts to the test for testamentary capacity, once again provided by a nineteenth-century English jurist. They are as follows:

1. An understanding of the nature of the business in which he is engaged.
2. A recollection of the property he means to dispose of.
3. The persons who are the object of his bounty.
4. The manner in which it is to be distributed between them.

While this sounds somewhat legal and technical it is not necessary for the testator to view his will with the eye of a lawyer. It is sufficient if he has such a mind and memory as will enable him to understand the process, the property and the parties in a simple form.

The first requirement is fairly obvious. You can't have someone making a will if they don't know they're doing it. The second requirement, recalling the property, is a little trickier. It is not necessary that the person instructing the preparation of a will recall every stick of furniture they own or every stock or bond in an extensive portfolio. As one of the once fabulously wealthy Hunt brothers of Texas said, "Anyone who knows how much they're worth ain't worth much."

As for "the persons who are the object of his bounty" the person making the will must not only be aware of the actual beneficiaries but also of those persons who may have a moral claim. In other words, he or she must understand and appreciate not only those who are being favored with a bequest but also those who are being cut out of the will.

Most cases which involve an attack on a will on the grounds of incapacity allege either that the maker of the will suffered from delusions that affected the making of the will or else that the testator suffered from "senile dementia." A delusion, of

535

course, is a belief in the existence of something which no rational person could believe and which cannot be overcome in the testator's mind by reasoned argument. While it is not unusual for people to labour under delusions (such as how good an athlete they once were or how attractive they were/are to the opposite sex) it is relatively rare that such delusions affect testamentary capacity. Far more serious is the presence of senile dementia.

Senile dementia is a legal, more than a medical, term and it presumably includes Alzheimer's disease. Old age, even extreme old age, is not enough. Similarly, the existence of some mental impairment is not fatal. The courts do not "lightly deprive the aged of the right to make a will." What is required is that the testator's mental powers are so reduced by advanced old age that he or she is incapable of understanding the essential elements of will making, that is to say, property, objects, just claims to consideration, revocation, or existing depositions and the like.

Usually the opinion of an attending physician is sought in such cases. Such an opinion is persuasive but not conclusive as laymen of good sense can answer the question just as well as a doctor can. The question of mental capacity is a legal, not a medical one, but if the lawyer taking instruction does a proper job, makes the necessary inquiries, follows the proper procedures and documents his efforts carefully, there is usually no problem.

A simple "mini-mental state" test is easy to perform and generally accepted by the medical profession, as well as the courts, as a fairly reliable indicator of mental capacity. Any reasonably competent legal practitioner should be able to perform such a simple examination. While somewhat time consuming, such a test saves a great deal of argument, time and conflict later on when the testator dies and the will must be admitted to probate, as it considerably reduces the likelihood of an attack on the will's validity.

—Don McCrimmon

536

Living Wills: What Are They?

The term "living will" is commonly understood to mean written instructions which indicate the medical treatment a patient wants or does not want in specified medical circumstances.

The term "living will" is also used to describe a number of similar (but not the same) types of instruments known by such other names as advance directives, patient directives, health-care proxies, advance-care documents, directives to physicians and durable powers of attorney.

Actually, the term "living will" is a somewhat unfortunate choice of words as it is not really a will at all in the normally accepted sense of the word.

A regular will, that is to say a legal will, is of no force and effect while the maker of the document is alive as the maker is always (assuming mental capacity) able to change or amend it.

The living will, on the other hand, only comes into play during the maker's lifetime and then usually when the maker is no longer competent to make changes to it.

The concept of living wills originally came to Canada from the United States. It started in California with the Natural Death Act. Now, in some forty states, there is legislation to regularize the making of such documents and to protect doctors from liability, as they are the ones in the unfortunate position of having to operate under their terms.

In Canada, only Ontario and Manitoba have living will legislation, and it has been been enacted only quite recently. At the moment, there do not appear to be plans in any other jurisdictions to introduce similar laws. This means that in the rest of the country there is no legislation to "breathe life" into such documents.

But that doesn't mean that preparing and executing a form of living will is a waste of time. Any government could introduce enabling legislation in the future that would validate a living will that is now invalid.

The most serious problem with some living wills is that they include some form of statement or declaration that the person does not want any "heroic measures" taken to sustain life in the event that he or she is in a vegetative or permanently comatose state.

They also usually request that death "not be unreasonably prolonged" or that "the dignity of life not be destroyed." While these requests sound very good in theory they are very difficult to put into practice.

Without some definition of what is or is not an "heroic measure" or an "unreasonable prolonging of life" it is left to the best guess of the attending physician or the nearest relative as to what is or is not heroic or unreasonable. Their guess is seldom what was wanted by the original maker of the document.

The unsettled state of the law outside Ontario and Manitoba has left many members of the medical profession understandably confused and concerned. If they abide by terms of a "living will" and do not undertake treatment they may face lawsuits from the patient's family.

If they cease treatment, they may be guilty of negligence of malpractice, or, worse yet, criminal behaviour.

This has led, in many instances, to the doctors opting for their only safe alternative—doing everything possible to extend the lives of the terminally ill, whether the patient wants it done or not.

Like many documents, a living will is usually only as effective as those charged with putting it into practice. To give your living will its best chance of working properly you should discuss it fully with your family and physician.

—Don McCrimmon

The Living Will

To Physicians

I, (Declarant), being of sound mind, willfully and voluntarily make known my desire that my life shall not be artificially prolonged under the circumstances set forth below, and I do hereby declare that:

1. If at any time I should have an incurable injury, disease or illness certified to be a terminal condition by two (2) physicians, one (1) of whom is the attending physician, and where the application of life-sustaining procedures would serve only to artificially prolong the moment of my death, and where my physician(s) determine that my death is imminent whether or not life-sustaining procedures are utilized, I direct that such procedures be withheld or withdrawn and that I be permitted to die naturally.
2. In the absence of my ability to give directions regarding the use of such life-sustaining procedures, it is my intention that this directive shall be honored by my family and physician(s) as the final expression of my legal right to refuse medical or surgical treatment and accept the consequences from such refusal.
3. I have been diagnosed at least fourteen (14) days ago as having a terminal condition by my physician.
4. This directive shall have no force or effect five (5) years from the date filled in below.
5. I understand the full import of this directive, and I am emotionally and mentally competent to make this directive.

Made at Sunshine City, in the Province of Alberta, this _____ day of September, 1993.

_____
(Declarant)

I hereby witness this directive and attest that:

1. I personally know the Declarant and believe the Declarant to be of sound mind.
2. To the best of my knowledge, at the time of the execution of this directive, I:

(a) am not related to the Declarant by blood or marriage;
(b) do not have any claim on the Estate of the Declarant;
(c) am not entitled to any portion of the Declarant's Estate by any Will or by operation of law; and
(d) am not a physician attending the Declarant or a person employed by a physician attending the Declarant.

_____
Witness

Medical Directives

In a previous column I indicated that only Ontario and Manitoba in Canada and forty states in the U.S. had legislation authorizing the use of living wills. In the rest of the country living wills are of very limited force and effect as there is no similar legislation to "put teeth" into such documents. This is not to say, however, that the rest of Canada is without any options for what has been dubbed "death with dignity" because in Canada there *is* a recognized right to the determination of one's own destiny.

There is a common law rule (i.e., judge-made law) to the effect that a competent person should be considered as the absolute master of decisions regarding his or her own body. This has most recently been confirmed by the Ontario Court of Appeal in a civil case which involved a Jehovah's Witness who was taken, unconscious, to an emergency ward after an automobile accident. In her purse she carried a card which identified her as a Jehovah's Witness, explained her strongly held religious convictions and refused any form of blood transfusion. The attending physician, fearing that the woman would die without a transfusion (as, indeed, she would have), ignored the card and ordered the transfusion. In the ensuing civil lawsuit where the patient sued her doctor for giving her a transfusion the court decided against the doctor noting that it was the patient, not the doctor, who had the final decision on whether or not to be treated. The Court upheld the lower court which required the doctor to pay damages for administering treatment against the patient's expressed wishes.

The problem of how to instruct the physician (so that the doctor, too, can place some reliance on the instruction) to withhold unwanted treatment still remains. One solution put forward that holds considerable promise is the medical directive. This document covers preferred treatment goals and specific treatment preferences in several scenarios of incompetence. It also includes the option to designate a proxy decision maker or power of attorney in the event of incompetence, the option to record a personal statement and a place to designate wishes for organ donation. It was designed (by physicians, not lawyers) to be used in consultation with both medical and legal advisors.

The way a medical directive (or advanced medical directive) works is that it considers four different situations in which the patient will be unable to instruct the physician their desired treatment. It requires the maker of the document to consider these situations and decide in advance the treatment they would want tried, what they would not want attempted or the treatment they would want attempted but stopped if not proven effective. Some of the treatment considered, for example, would include such things as cardio-pulmonary resuscitation, major surgery, minor surgery, invasive diagnostic tests, chemotherapy and intravenous feeding.

The four situations include:

1. being in a coma or a vegetative state with no known hope of regaining awareness;
2. being in a coma or vegetative state with a small likelihood of full recovery, a slighter larger likelihood of surviving with permanent brain damage, and a larger likelihood of dying;
3. an irreversible brain disease or brain damage and a terminal illness; and
4. same as 3 but no terminal illness.

The medical directive is a step in the right decision but, as with so many such problems, a simple piece of paper is not the entire answer. The medical directive would be prepared in consultation with the family physician and the other members of the family. They are, after all, the ones who will be turning your instructions into reality and they are also the ones in the best position to scuttle your "best laid plans."

—Don McCrimmon

Cardio-pulmonary Resuscitation in the Aged (Part 1)

Dear Dr. MacInnis:

My aged mother (81), who has Alzheimer's disease, was revived three times in the nursing home by CPR (cardio-pulmonary resuscitation). On the fourth time, all efforts failed and she died from what was called "cardiac arrest." Although her life was prolonged by the first three rescue tactics, I believe inevitable death was just delayed a while at the expense of great psychological distress to the family. I discussed the matter with her doctor but it didn't seem to matter; they went on with CPR just the same.

What could we have done to prevent all of these seemingly useless "rescue attempts" in the first place?

Mrs. A. L., Ontario

Answer

It would appear to me that your nursing home has no code policy in effect. Certainly, it was not operating in your mother's case.

If it was, then her code status would have been discussed with you and your family by your doctor and staff. Normally the patient participates in such discussions, but her loss of awareness (from Alzheimer's disease) would preclude her input. One of the family members would have to be her legal guardian. The result would most likely be a decision for "no heroics" and CPR would never have occurred.

Your letters bring up an important question—one you have pondered, as I'm sure have many other readers: What is the value of CPR in the debilitated elderly?

542

An article in the *Journal of the American Medical Association* (G. E. Taffeta and others, vol. 260 (1988): 2069–72) addresses the subject. They reviewed 399 CPR efforts in 329 veterans at the Houston, Texas, Veterans Administration Hospital.

Results: The elderly did particularly poorly as to outcome. In the 70-year-old group CPR was immediately successful in 31 percent and 92 percent were alive after twenty-four hours. However, none of the patients lived to be discharged from the hospital. A general comment in that, overall, "the long-term outlook is poor at any age. Only 10 to 12 percent ever leave the hospital" (reported by *Internal Medicine Alert*). "Nonetheless," they add, "the decision to code or noncode a patient must be made on an individual basis and not because of a specific diagnosis, e.g., cancer." The authors strongly advise that CPR be administered only to those with the best potential for success.

In our own psychogeriatric department of 212 beds, a situation such as yours would be a rare event indeed. Shortly after admission and initial evaluation, the patient's code status is discussed with the relatives (one who is the legal guardian) and a decision reached as to whether or not aggressive "heroics" should be employed in the case of impending death. (This policy is always subject to periodic review and occasionally the patient's code status may change for the better.)

This policy has resulted in a much better relationship between the relatives and hospital staff. If a "no heroics" policy is instituted in favor of basic terminal care (keeping the patient comfortable), the relatives understand and are grateful, for, in effect, the institution of the code status was theirs.

A code status decision is always mentally traumatic to discuss for the relatives, as well as the medical and nursing staff. But we have found that an early institution of the policy is much less hurtful than a last minute decision, when relatives are never in a position to pass rational judgement in their hour of impending bereavement.

Cardiopulmonary Resuscitation in the Aged (Part 2)

Suppose your spouse or parent (age 70 or over) was suddenly stricken with a cardiac arrest. Would you phone for an ambulance and rush him/her to the nearest hospital? Of course you would. And in the hospital emergency would you expect that everything possible be done in the way of resuscitation? Yes, I believe you would. But if you were told by a competent physician that the situation was hopeless and no amount of heroic intervention would have the slightest effect would you buy that or insist that he "keep on trying"? Even in the face of gigantic odds the answer would again be yes, and only you who have lived the ordeal would understand why. For who of us, in such time of anguish, is capable of dispassionate, rational judgment?

Every year there are over a half-million sudden cardiac deaths in the United States and about 50,000 in Canada. And despite tremendous advances in cardiology, there's been, over the years, little or no improvement in survival.

Cardiopulmonary resuscitation (CPR), involves not only the technique of closed-chest massage (instituted in 1960) but combines with many other life-support measures, which will be described later.

CPR was devised for cardiac arrest mainly in the relatively young adult. But the outcome even in young adult hospitalized patients has been poor, indeed, except perhaps in the treatment of sudden-death threatening disorders of heart rhythm using electrical defibrillation.

Previously published accounts on outcomes of CPR have involved relatively few elderly patients. The large study I will now report appeared in the August 1, 1989, issue of the *Annals of Internal Medicine* on the outcome of CPR on 503 elderly patients age 70 and older. This is by far the largest study of its kind and I commend it not only for the information of the lay public (especially the elderly) but to the medical and nursing professions and administrators in acute- and chronic-care hospitals and nursing homes.

The setting for this study was five Boston, Massachusetts, health care institutions—two acute-care hospitals, two chronic-care hospitals, and one long-term care facility. The 503 elderly patients all received CPR, which included chest massage, oxygen, intubation, intravenous fluids, various cardiac medications, electrical defibrillation, and (in several cases) pacemaker placement. CPR was defined as "successful" when the resuscitated patient could be discharged from hospital.

Patients were divided into out-of-hospital and in-hospital cardiac arrests. The results:

	Out-of-Hospital	In-Hospital
Died immediately	224 (91.8 percent)	167 (64.5 percent)
Died in hospital	18 (7.4 percent)	75 (29.0 percent)
Survived to discharge	2 (0.8 percent)	17 (6.5 percent)

Discussion: Of the 503 elderly patients all of whom received CPR, only nineteen (3.8 percent) survived to discharge.

What happened to these nineteen survivors? Eight were able to return home. The others had physical and mental problems requiring chronic care.

Only 8 of the 503 survived to enjoy a reasonable quality of life.

Who were the best bets for successful CPR? The elderly patient *most likely to survive* was one who, before the arrest, functioned independently with a normal mental status; had an arrest *witnessed* by someone who could detect *one* vital sign (pulse, blood pressure, or breathing); had an initial cardiac rhythm on the ECG of ventricular tachycardia (exceedingly fast ventricular rate) or ventricular fibrillation (fast and chaotically irregular ventricular rate) or who responded *promptly* (within five minutes) to cardiac massage. Of the 209 patients with *no* vital sign or signs, *none* survived.

Conclusion: These grim statistics should be kept in mind by the relatives of elderly people suffering cardiac arrest so they can better understand the exceedingly poor outcome of CPR in most cases.

As an editorial to the article puts it, "For a few elderly patients, CPR may be a blessing. . . . For most it's a curse . . . a misappropriation of previous resources and a growing burden." (My thanks to *Annals of Internal Medicine.*)

Life- (or Death-) Prolonging Decisions

Dear Dr. MacInnis:

My aged mother (83) recently died from a long-standing dementing illness. Mental death occurred about four years ago.

Since that time she never recognized my father or any of the children. Although she became doubly incontinent and had to be diapered and spoon-fed by family members (aided by home care), we finally had to give up and arranged for her admission to a nearby nursing home.

During her four-month stay in the nursing home she suffered from "terminal" pneumonia twice and despite our request to the attending doctor to let her die gently in her sleep, she was vigorously treated with antibiotics, intravenous, etc., and each time she "recovered" to her former physical and mental state. On her third bout of pneumonia a different doctor saw it our way and she mercifully passed away in peace.

I sympathize to some extent with doctors who just never give up. I suppose they were taught to consider death as an enemy to be fought at all times. In some instances this may be laudable, but not, I feel, in my mother's case or others like it.

As sometimes happens, something good and positive came out of it all. Our whole family—including our father—is more determined than ever to leave a living will, prohibiting all heroics, which (as in my mother's case) merely prolong the dying process.

It will also relieve the doctors from making agonizing decisions, don't you think?

Answer

I can never understand why some doctors "agonize" over so-called playing God decisions in situations like yours. Such ethico-moral issues certainly don't bother theologians or church leaders. Speaking on this very issue, Pope Pius XII left no doubt in these words, "In deciding whether to apply life prolonging therapy, we may justifiably desist in order to permit the patient, already virtually dead, to pass on in peace." Others, like a former Archbishop of Canterbury, have declared likewise.

And it has absolutely no relation to euthanasia, which is always an act of commission, that is, a deliberate deed calculated to kill—be it a "mercy" kill or not. This is "active" euthanasia.

Contrast, then, active euthanasia, with the decision to no longer use extraordinary means to prolong life and to make sure the patient is pain free, comfortable, and meets death with dignity. So if pneumonia ("the old man's friend") appears on the scene, the doctor, in all good conscience, can leave it be and not "prolong the dying process" as you have said.

I stress that this is never a doctor's decision alone. It's a sacred understanding shared by the family and everyone involved in the final caring—and, happily, sometimes by the patient.

Said Sir Theodore Fox, one-time editor of Britain's venerable medical journal, the *Lancet,* "The doctor's over-riding duty is to treat his neighbour as himself. And so long as there is any real hope of recovery, the doctor is right to preserve life by any means at his command, even though they cause pain—physical or mental. Here his 'cruelty' is a kindness. But if he persists in prolonging a life that can never again have purpose and meaning, his 'kindness' becomes a cruelty."

And to that I say "AMEN."

Index

hernia, 235–38
  groin, 235–36
  hiatus, 236–38
  umbilical (belly button), 236
herpes zoster (shingles), 444–45
high blood pressure (hypertension)
  drugs for, side effects in very old, 158–59
  false, 155–56, 173–74
  fat arm effect in, 155
  high potassium diet for, 126–27
  non-drug management, 156–58
  risk factors for, 156–58
Hirschsprung's disease, 257–58
hirudin (from leech), 149–50
Huntington's disease, 213–16
hypertension. See high blood pressure

ibuprofen. See NSAIDs, 218–19
implant, lens, 332–33
implant, penile, 273–75
impotence. See Chapter 11: elder sexuality, page 267
  products and devices for, 273–81
incontinence, female stress, 292–97
  collagen injections for, 297–99
  Kegel exercises for, 293
incontinence, males
  Kegel exercises for, 310–11
  collagen treatment for, 310
Indocid, 431–33
infarction, myocardial, 142–43
insomnia. See Chapter 20, page 463
  Halcion for, 471–73
  chloral hydrate for, 471
  non-drug management for, 464–66
ions, positive and negative, 286–88
insulin. See Chapter 16: diabetes in elderly, page 389
itch, perineal, 398–99

jaundice, 38
jogging, 509–11

jogging vs. walking, 511–12
joint (hip) replacement, 227–28

Kegel exercises, 293, 310–11
kidney failure, 153–55

LactAid, 232
lactose intolerance, 232–33
last rights, 531
lecithin, 45
leeches (in medicine), 149–50
legs, restless, 427–29
legs, cramps, 429–30
lens implant, 333
life expectancy, 14–17
life span, 14–17
longevity, 14–17
low vision (services offered), 317
lung cancer, 348–49
L-lysine (cold sores) 451–54

macula, 316
macular degeneration, 316–17
MedicAlert, 263–65
menopause, 382–84
  male, 385–86
methotrexate, 219–21
multiple small strokes. See TIAs
myopia, 336
  excimer laser treatment of, 336–37

nails
  fungus infection of, 433
  ridging of, 458–59
nap, power, 519–20
neuropathy, diabetic, 395–96
nitroglycerine, 141–42
  patch, 162–63
nonagenarians, 7–11
nose, stuffy, 195–96
NSAIDs, 218–19

Osteoarthritis
  NSAIDs for, 218–19, 433

methotrexate for, 219–21
myochrysine for, 222

saltpeter, 499–500
selegilene. *See* deprenyl and Eldepryl
"senility," 57. *See* Alzheimer's disease, Chapter 5
"sex shots," 273
sexuality, elder. Chapter 11, page 267
shingles (herpes zoster), 444–46
shingles, post-herpetic neuralgia, 444–45, 449–50
sick sinus syndrome, 186–87
sight problems. *See* Chapter 13, page 315
Sinemet, 200–207
sinusitis, 193–95
skipped (heart) beats, 151–53
smell, loss of, 345–46
smoking. *See* cigarette smoking
stomach (and bowel) disorders: Chapter 10, page 231
streptokinase, 117, 181
stroke. *See* Chapter 7, page 109
surgery (in the aged), 244–45
swelling (legs and feet) 153–55
Symmetrel (amantadine), 208–9

tacrine, 79–80
Tagamet (cimetidine), 238
tangles (neurofibrilary), 55
tar ointments, 455–56
taste, loss of, 344–46
taxol, 349–50
Tegretol (carbamazipine), 428
THA (tetrahydroaminoacridine), 78–80
TIAs, (little strokes). *See* Chapter 7, page 109
ticlid, 132–33
tinnitus, 341–42
tongue, sore red, 411
TPA (tissue plasminogen activator), 117

tremor: Parkinson's, 200; essential, 202–3
TURP (transurethral resection of prostate), 301–3, 305–6

ulcer, diabetic, 394–95
ulcer (peptic), 247–49
ultrasound, 312–13
urinary problems (in elderly): Chapter 12, page 289
urinary tract infections, 290–92
urushiol, 439, 442

vaccines, flu and pneumonia, 191–92
vaginal dryness, 272
vaginal itchiness, 399
varicose veins, 187–89
vegetarians, 421
vitamins:
  E and C (antioxidants), 406–9
  B-carotene (antioxidant), 354–56
  vitamin C (best food sources), 410
  megavitamins, 411–13
  pros and cons, 413–15
  vitamin B_2 deficiency, 411
  vitamin supplements, 412–13
  vitamin D (from the sun), 445–47
vitiligo, 454–55
Voltaren, 219. *See* NSAIDs

warfarin (Coumadin), 114–15
walking (exercises), 511–12
white coat syndrome, 189–90
will:
  do I need it?, 532
  making a, 533–34
  mental capacity to make, 534–36
  living will, 539
  living wills, what are they?, 537–38
  medical directives, the, 540–42
winter itch, 448
wrinkles, 481

Xanax (alprazolam), 202–3

About the Author

Recently retired after seventeen years as clinical director of geriatric and psychogeriatric medicine at Alberta Hospital, Edmonton, Alberta, Canada, Dr. Frank MacInnis was born in Prince Edward Island, is a graduate of Queen's University Medical School, Kingston, Ontario, and is a specialist in internal medicine, with special interest in the care of the elderly. He is a Fellow of the Royal College of Physicians in Canada and a Fellow of the American College of Physicians in the United States.

Since 1981, Dr. MacInnis has been the author of "Senior Clinic," the internationally syndicated newspaper column that addresses exclusively the medical, surgical, psychiatric, and social issues of middle age and older, and is the only doctor-written feature of its kind in the newspaper field.

The Aging Game is an updated compilation of the best of "Senior Clinic" written over the past twelve years.

Dr. MacInnis now resides in British Columbia.